Quick Reference to

Medical-Surgical Nursing

J. B. Lippincott Company Philadelphia/Toronto

Quick Reference to

Medical-Surgical Nursing

Ellen Baily Raffensperger, R.N., B.A.
Staff Nurse, Progressive Care Unit
Sibley Memorial Hospital
Washington, DC

Mary Lloyd Zusy, R.N., B.A., M.A.
Formerly Medical-Surgical Clinical Instructor
Montgomery College
Takoma Park, Maryland

Lynn Marchesseault, R.N., B.S.N.
Instructor, Pharmacology in Nursing
Montgomery College Community Services
Bethesda, Maryland

Sponsoring Editor: Diana Intenzo
Manuscript Editor: J. Bruce Martin
Indexer: Sue Reilly
Art Director: Tracy Baldwin
Designer: William Boehm
Production Supervisor: N. Carol Kerr
Production Assistant: J. Corey Gray
Compositor: Hampton Graphics
Printer/Binder: R. R. Donnelley & Sons Company

6 5 4 3 2 1

Library of Congress Cataloging in Publication Data

Raffensperger, Ellen.
  Quick reference to medical-surgical nursing.

  (Lippincott's quick references)
  Bibliography
  Includes indexes.
  1. Nursing—Handbooks, manuals, etc.   I. Zusy,
Mary Lloyd.   II. Marchesseault, Lynn.   III. Title.
[DNLM: 1. Nursing—Handbooks.   2. Surgical nursing—
Handbooks.   WY 150 S96L]
RT51.R26   616'.0024613   81-18653
ISBN 0-397-54358-1   AACR2

The authors and publisher have exerted every effort to ensure that drug selection
and dosage set forth in this text are in accord with current recommendations and
practice at the time of publication. However, in view of ongoing research, changes in
government regulations, and the constant flow of information relating to drug
therapy and drug reactions, the reader is urged to check the package insert for each
drug for any change in indications and dosage and for added warnings and
precautions. This is particularly important when the recommended agent is a new or
infrequently employed drug.

To quality patient care, and to the nurses who provide it

Contents

Preface

Our goal in preparing *Quick Reference to Medical–Surgical Nursing* has been to provide the most needed information for medical–surgical nursing practice in a format that provides a quick and easily available reference. We have attempted to provide answers to the most common problems encountered in giving direct nursing care to patients in the general hospital or nursing home. This manual is designed as an on-the-spot source of information to meet immediate needs. It is to be used while you work, providing answers to problems as you meet them.

Because of the limits of size set by our desire to put this much-needed information literally into your pocket, we have continually asked ourselves, "Is this of immediate need?" "Is this a common enough problem or situation to deserve coverage here?" These were criteria for the selection of what to include. We have taken a functional approach, focusing on nursing care in every section. In our section Nursing Responsibilities for Diagnosis and Treatment, we offer tips on how to make procedures work and how to prepare the patient for common diagnostic tests. The procedure book and laboratory manual used in your institution should be your first references in this area. Physician's orders provide the specifics of individualized patient care.

In selecting drugs for the pharmacology section, we have tried to highlight those with special nursing implications, as well as those most frequently used in the medical–surgical setting. Whenever possible drugs are presented in families or prototypes to emphasize their common characteristics. Therefore, it is essential to read the presentation for the family of drugs before going to the specifics of dosages, common side-effects, and nursing implications of individual ones. The separate pharmacology index includes both generic and common trade names for each drug.

The book is divided into several sections. We have attempted to cover each subject only once. Therefore, cross-referencing directs the reader to the place where additional information on related subjects can be found. The code for the different sections is as follows:

LAB	Clinical Laboratory Tests
MNS	Management in Special Nursing Situations
NR	Nursing Responsibilities for Diagnosis and Treatment
PH	Pharmacology
SS	Systems and Specialties

Topics in each section are arranged alphabetically, but because some topics could conceivably be under several names (*e.g.,* urinary calculi, renal calculi, kidney stones), the general index is the ultimate source for quick referral.

We hope that the use of this book will add to the pride and satisfaction to be found in providing quality nursing care for the medical–surgical patient. We have attempted to answer many of the questions that come up in daily practice, especially those which ask "how?" We encourage you, the reader, to delve into references of greater depth—textbooks, journals, and the wealth of nursing literature now available—to answer more fully the questions of "why?"

Ellen Baily Raffensperger, R.N., B.A.
Mary Lloyd Zusy, R.N., B.A., M.A.
Lynn Marchesseault, R.N., B.S.N.

Acknowledgments

Our appreciation goes especially to our husbands, Maurey Raffensperger, Fred Zusy, and Bill Noellert, for their active support and, at Lippincott, to David T. Miller, Vice President, who encouraged the fulfillment of our idea for this book, and to Diana Intenzo, Executive Editor, and Bruce Martin, Manuscript Editor, who helped us along the way.

The content of this book has benefited significantly from reviews and suggestions by the following individuals:

William Battaile, M.D.
Sibley Hospital,
Washington, DC

Charles P.H. Carroll, M.D.
Washington, DC

Dorothy Deters, R.N.
Headnurse, ICU,
Sibley Hospital,
Washington, DC

Gary P. Fischer, M.D., F.A.C.C.
Chevy Chase, Maryland

Mary DiFrancisco, M.D.
Georgetown University
   Hospital,
Washington, DC

Lillian Fink, R.N.
Headnurse, Orthopedic Unit,
Suburban Hospital,
Bethesda, Maryland

Elizabeth Fleming, M.T.,
   A.S.C.P.
Sibley Hospital,
Washington, DC

Mary Ellen Galloway, R.N.
Headnurse, Urology Unit,
Suburban Hospital,
Bethesda, Maryland

Margaret S. Gieger, R.N.
Nurse Epidemiologist,
Sibley Hospital,
Washington, DC

Thomas C. Havell, M.D.
Washington, DC

Alice Irving, R.N., M.S.
Home Care Unit,
Holy Cross Hospital,
Silver Spring, Maryland

Lisa L. Kelber, R.N., B.S.N.
Formerly at Burn Unit,
Washington Hospital Center,
Washington, DC

Bryan Larson, R.R.T.
Chief Respiratory Therapist,
Sibley Hospital,
Washington, DC

Fred R.T. Nelson, M.D.,
F.A.O.S.
Rockville, Maryland

Robert J. Ollins, M.D.
Sibley Hospital,
Washington, DC

Richard Pollen, M.D.,
F.A.C.P.
Kensington, Maryland

Maura A. Raffensperger, R.Ph
Clinical Pharmacist,
Santa Monica Hospital,
Medical Center,
Santa Monica, California

Silvia Hasmelek Reid, R.N.
Montgomery General
Hospital,
Olney, Maryland

Linda Riffle, R.N., B.S.N.
Clinical Coordinator,
Sibley Hospital,
Washington, DC

Mary Spellman, R.N.
I.V. Specialist,
Suburban Hospital,
Bethesda, Maryland

David Shea, M.D., F.A.C.P.
Washington, DC

Joanne McCarron, R.N.
Headnurse, PCU,
Sibley Hospital,
Washington, DC

Frederick Schattenstein,
C.R.T.T.
Washington, DC

Timothy Tehan, M.D.,
F.A.C.P.
Washington, DC

Rachel Thrasher, R.N.
Formerly Headnurse,
Ophthalmology,
National Institutes of Health,
Bethesda, Maryland

Vivian Weatherby, R.N., E.T.
Silver Spring, Maryland

A special word of appreciation is given to Amy Beyers, Patricia A.
Blank, Bernice Johnson, and Susan Zusy for assistance in preparation
of the manuscript, and also to Annie B. Footman, Librarian, Sibley
Hospital.

1

Clinical Laboratory Tests, Their Implications, and Related Nursing Responsibilities (LAB)

Tables: Blood chemistry, hematology, urinalysis, miscellaneous tests
Arterial blood gases (ABGs)
Cultures
Testing for occult blood
Urine specimen collection
   Clean catch method
   Fractional urine method
   Timed urine method
   Testing for glucose and acetone (ketones)
   Testing for specific gravity

TABLES: BLOOD CHEMISTRY, HEMATOLOGY, URINALYSIS, MISCELLANEOUS TESTS

Description

Laboratory examinations of blood and urine are done to obtain a biomedical evaluation of the patient. The following five tables indicate standard tests and normal values. The values vary slightly depending on the equipment and techniques used in individual laboratories.

TABLE 1-1. **Commonly Done Blood Chemistry Tests as Related to Human Physiology and Disease**

Blood Tests			
LDH SGOT	} Necrosis and infarction		
Bilirubin, total			
Bilirubin, direct (If total is elevated)			
SGPT		Hepatic	
Total protein			
Albumin			
Globulin			
A/G Ratio			
Alkaline phosphatase			
Calcium Phosphorus	} Parathyroid disease		} Bone and joint
Uric acid	] Gout		
Urea nitrogen (BUN) Creatinine	} Kidney		
Glucose	] Diabetes		
CO$_2$ Chloride Sodium Potassium	} Electrolytes		
Triglyceride Cholesterol	} Lipid metabolism		

(Courtesy of Central Diagnostic Laboratory, Tarzana, California)

TABLE 1-2. **Blood Chemistry Evaluations and Their Normal Values**

Test	Normal Values
Albumin	3.5–5.0 g/100ml
Alkaline phosphatase	79–258 IU/l
Bilirubin, direct (Done if total is elevated)	0.01–0.50 mg/100 ml
Bilirubin, total	0.01–1.00 mg/100 ml
Calcium	8.6–10.7 mg/100 ml
Chloride	95–109 mEq/l
Cholesterol	147–318mg/100 ml
CO_2	20–33 mEq/l
CPK	5–200 IU/l
Isoenzymes	
MBCPK is elevated in cardiac injury	Female—5–25 U/ml Male—5–35 U/ml
MMCPK is elevated in skeletal muscle damage	Female—55–170 U/l Male—30–135 U/l
BBCPK is elevated in brain tissue damage	Female—5–25 U/ml Male—5–35 U/ml
Creatinine	0.7–1.3 mg/100 ml
Globulin	2.4–3.0 g/100 ml
Glucose, fasting	65–110 mg/100 ml
LDH	56–194 IU/l
Isoenzymes	
Fraction 1 } elevated in cardiac necrosis Fraction 2 }	20–30% 27–37%
Fraction 3 } elevated in pulmonary infarct Fraction 4 } and CHF	16–24% 7–15%
Fraction 5 elevated in liver damage	9–17%
Phosphorus	2.5–4.5 mg/100 ml
Potassium	3.4–5.0 mEq/l
Serum osmolality	280–295 mOsm/l
SGOT	8–36 IU/l
SGPT (Done to confirm whether elevated SGOT and LDH are caused by liver or cardiac injury. Elevation of all three indicates liver damage.)	2–32 IU/l
Sodium	135–145 mEq/l
Total protein	5.9–8.0 g/100 ml
Triglycerides	47–155 mg/100 ml
Urea nitrogen (BUN)	7–21 mg/100 ml
Uric acid	Female—2.0–7.0 mg/100 ml Male—2.5–8.0 mg/100 ml

TABLE 1-3. **Hematology Examinations That Evaluate the Structure and Function of Blood Cells**

Test Description	Value
RBC (red blood cells—erythrocytes)	Male—4.6–6.2 million Female—4.2–5.4 million
Reticulocyte (immature erythrocyte)	0.5–1.5% of erythrocytes
Hematocrit (Hct): volume percentage of erythrocytes in 100ml of blood	Male—42–52% Female—37–47%
Hemoglobin (Hgb): oxygen-carrying pigment of erythrocytes; reported in grams per 100 ml of blood	Male—14–18 g Female—12–16 g
Mean corpuscular volume (MCV): refers to the size of individual erythrocytes; reported in cubic microns	Male—87 ± 5 cuμ Female—85 ± 5 cuμ
Mean corpuscular hemoglobin concentration (MCHC): the concentration of hemoglobin in 100 ml of erythrocytes; reported as a percentage	34 ± 2%
Mean corpuscular hemoglobin (MCH): the hemoglobin content of individual erythrocytes; reported in micromicrograms	29 ± 2 $\mu\mu$g
Platelets: necessary for coagulation of blood	150,000–350,000 cu mm
Sedimentation rate (ESR): rate at which erythrocytes settle in uncoagulated blood (Wintrobetest)	Male—0–9 mm in 1 hour Female—0–15 mm in 1 hour
WBC (white blood cells—leukocytes)	4800–10,800 cu mm
Differential Count—identifies types and numbers of WBC	
Neutrophiles—elevated in most bacterial (Segmented or mature cell) infections, inflammatory diseases, and cancer	40–60%
Bands—elevated in leukemias and acute infections	2–6%
Eosinophiles—elevated in allergic conditions	1–3%
Basophiles—secretes heparin but function is uncertain	0–1%
Monocytes—elevated in most bacterial infections; elevated in monocytic leukemia	2–8%
Lymphocytes—elevated in many viral infections, in lymphocytic leukemia, and in stress reactions, for example, burns and trauma	20–40%

TABLE 1-4. **Urine Examinations**

Test	Comments	Normal Values
Color	Dark urine suggests bile or blood; many drugs result in colored urine.	Yellow
pH	Urine is alkaline with an elevated pH in urinary tract infections or when left standing at room temperature. pH measurement is inaccurate with hematuria, diuresis and contrast media.	4.6–8
Specific gravity (sp.gr.)	Specific gravity is obtained by comparing weight of urine to an equal amount of water. Lowered sp.gr. reflects kidneys' inability to concentrate urine. If kidneys lose ability to function, the excreted urine will become fixed at 1.010.	1.001–1.035
Glucose	Blood sugar is usually greatly increased before glucose appears in the urine.	None
Ketones	Ketones occur in diabetes, starvation.	None
Protein	When more than a trace is present, a 24 hour urine is usually done.	0–Trace
Blood	Blood may occur with cystitis or renal calculi.	0
Microscopic UA		
RBC	⎫	0–1
WBC	⎬ Elevated values indicate kidney disease.	1–3
CASTS		Rare Hyaline
Epitheliel cells	⎭	0
Crystals	Type depends on whether urine is acidic or alkaline.	0

TABLE 1-5. **Miscellaneous Tests of Blood to Determine Toxicity or the Effect of Certain Drugs**

Test	Normal Level	Theraputic Level
Barbiturates	0	
Digoxin level	0	0.6–2.0 ng/ml
Dilantin	0	10–20 µg/ml
Ethanol—Maximum allowable by courts is 0.15%. Intoxication = 0.3–0.4%. Stupor = 0.4–0.5%.	0.0–0.05%	
Gentamycin level	0	4–12 µg/ml
Lithium		0.5–1.5 mEq/l
PT (Prothrombin time)	12–14 seconds	1½–2 times the normal level
PTT (Partial thromboplastin time)	35–45 seconds	1½–2 times the normal level
Quinidine level	0	3–6 µg/ml
Theophylline (aminophyllin) level	0	10–20 µg/ml

ARTERIAL BLOOD GASES (ABGs)

Description

Arterial blood gases (ABGs) are done to determine the ability of the lungs to perform O_2 and CO_2 transfer. ABGs also establish the kidneys' level of function in secreting or absorbing bicarbonate ions, which aids in maintaining the acid–base balance of the body (see Table 1-6).

TABLE 1-6. **Arterial Blood Gases**

Gas	Normal Values	Comments
P_AO_2	80–100 mmHg partial pressure (room air)	Higher altitude = lower O_2 Older ages = lower O_2
P_ACO_2	38–42 mmHg partial pressure	40 is the average
HCO_3^{-1}	24–28 mEq/l	The bicarbonate is regulated by kidneys
pH	7.35–7.45	Above 7.45 = alkalosis Below 7.35 = acidosis

ALKALOSIS

Patients can tolerate a mild alkalosis, which may result from either respiratory or metabolic imbalance.

Respiratory alkalosis results from "blowing off" too much CO_2.

- Treatment consists of building up CO_2 by breathing into a bag or by decreasing the respiratory rate.
- The primary indicator of respiratory alkalosis is a significant decrease in $PACO_2$, with a lesser decrease in HCO_3^{-1} and some increase in pH.
- Typical symptoms are inability to concentrate and dizziness.
- Watch patients with a central nervous system (CNS) disease or injury who may have uncontrolled rapid breathing.

Metabolic alkalosis results from too much base, which may be caused by excessive ingestion of antacids or by the loss of too much acid by way of the GI tract or kidneys (through suction, vomiting, or excessive use of diuretics with resulting low potassium).

- Treatment consists of correcting the cause.
- Be certain that IVs run on time in patients with n.g. suction.
- An adequate potassium level is necessary to correct alkalosis resulting from a loss of HCL.
- The primary indicator of metabolic alkalosis is a significant increase in HCO_3^{-1}, with a lesser increase in $PACO_2$ and pH.
- Typical symptoms are muscle weakness, confusion, or paralytic ileus due to abnormal losses of potassium.

ACIDOSIS

Patients cannot tolerate acidosis, which may result from either respiratory or metabolic imbalance.

- Acidosis requires immediate correction.

Respiratory acidosis results from CO_2 retention, which may be caused by chronic obstructive lung disease or chest trauma.

- The treatment is improved air exchange; intubation or tracheostomy may be necessary.
- The primary indicator of respiratory acidosis is a significant increase in $PACO_2$, with a lesser increase in HCO_3^{-1} and some decrease in pH.
- Typical symptoms are restlessness, confusion, and tachycardia.
- If untreated, respiratory acidosis leads to coma and death.

Metabolic acidosis results from diabetic ketoacidosis, uncontrolled diarrhea, shock, or renal failure.

- The treatment is to correct the specific cause.
- The primary indicator is a significant decrease in HCO_3^{-1}, with some decrease in $PACO_2$ and pH.

- The HCO_3^{-1} bicarbonate may fall so low in its effort to correct acidosis that IV replacement is given.
- Typical symptoms are stupor, deep rapid breathing, and fruity odor to breath.

Nursing Tips

- If the patient is on oxygen, check with the physician to see if ABGs are to be drawn on oxygen or room air. If they are to be taken when the patient is on oxygen the correct liter flow rate must be maintained for 20 minutes before the blood is drawn. Mark on the lab slip the number of liters. If on room air, write "room air."
- A special kit is usually provided for this procedure. The blood is drawn by designated personnel in each hospital (*e.g.,* nurses or respiratory therapists).
- Alert the laboratory when the ABGs are about to be drawn.
- The specimen must be placed immediately in a container of ice, and the specimen should arrive in the laboratory within 5 minutes.
- Pressure should be maintained on the withdrawal site for at least 5 minutes.
- When anticoagulants are in use, prolonged bleeding at the withdrawal site may occur.

CULTURES

Description

Cultures of body fluids or secretions are done to identify bacteria. Sensitivity determinations are usually done concurrently to identify the antimicrobial drugs effective in destroying the bacteria (see Table 1-7).

Nursing Tips

- Use sterile technique in obtaining all cultures except those for stool examination. Specimens contaminated with normal skin flora are misleading and another culture will be required.
- Do not contaminate the outside of the container.
- Send cultures immediately to the laboratory for accurate examination results. Specimens that have been allowed to dry out or stay at an incorrect temperature are useless.
- Label directly on the container as well as on the laboratory slip. Include the time the specimen was obtained.
- If an infectious disease is suspected, write this on the label.
- No antibiotic should be started until after a culture specimen is obtained. If this is not possible, the antibiotic should be noted on the laboratory slip.

TABLE 1-7. **Specimen Collection**

Site	Amount Required	Container	Pathogens	Procedure
Throat	Through swabbing	Swab replaced in sterile container	Group A strep: β-hemolytic	Inspect throat with a flashlight before swabbing to identify both tonsils and posterior pharynx.
Wound (decubitus ulcer)	The applicator should go as deeply as possible into the wound and then be swabbed on tissues surfaces	Swab replaced in sterile container	S. aureus; Group A strep: β-hemolytic	Avoid swabbing pus on the skin surface. Wash off the skin with saline to lessen contamination with normal skin flora. If a large area is involved, take specimens from different sites.
Stool	Size of a pea	Clean container	Salmonella, shigella ova, and parasites	A rectal swab may be sufficient; check with laboratory. Stool must be free of barium for parasite studies. Stool should not be more than 1 hour old.
Urine	5ml	Syringe or sterile container. (See clean catch urine.)	Any organism greater than 50 to 100,000 cu mm	When the tip of an indwelling catheter is sent to culture, cleanse the meatus before withdrawing the catheter. Cut off the catheter top with a sterile scissors. Never collect a specimen from a urinary drainage bag. Specimens may be taken from an indwelling catheter by first cleansing the specimen port in the catheter with alcohol. Specimens should not be more than 1 hour old. (There is an extremely high incidence of urinary tract infection (UTI) after 3 days use of an indwelling catheter.)

Sputum	3–5ml	Sterile container	Any predominant organism	Preferably, early AM sputum (not saliva) obtained after a deep cough. May be obtained by suctioning or a Lukens tube. TBC may not culture out for several weeks.
Cerebrospinal fluid (CSF)	10ml or more	3 sterile containers marked 1–2–3	Any organism	Must be sent to lab IMMEDIATELY.
Blood	Usually done by lab personnel	Check with lab if to be done by other than lab personnel	Any organism	Blood usually taken 3 or 4 times at 30-minute intervals to avoid missing an organism and to confirm the diagnosis. Should be taken between chill and fever spikes.
Body fluids (pleural fluid)	Check with the lab.	Sterile container. Check with the lab; may require special container.	Any organism	Should be processed immediately.

- A tentative identification of organisms takes 24 hours, and final results take 48 hours or more, with the exception of tubercle (TBC) bacilli, which may take several weeks.
- Physicians should be notified immediately of pathogens appearing in cultures.

TESTING FOR OCCULT BLOOD

Description

Testing for occult blood may be done on the unit in emergency situations by using a test tape or slides (*e.g.*, Hemocult). Read the manufacturer's directions carefully.

Nursing Tips

- In preparation for a routine laboratory examination of the stool for occult blood, the patient's diet should be restricted for 2 days. During this time no meat, turnips, horseradish, aspirin, or over 250 mg of vitamin C per day should be consumed.

URINE SPECIMEN COLLECTION
CLEAN CATCH METHOD

The clean catch method is considered a satisfactory means of obtaining an uncontaminated urine specimen.

Nursing Tips

- This should be the first morning specimen after the bladder has been emptied initially upon awakening.
- Instruct the patient to wash the hands and then to cleanse the periurethral meatus thoroughly with two antiseptic towelettes. The patient starts the urine stream, stops, and then voids directly into a sterile container.
- This specimen should go directly to the laboratory.

FRACTIONAL URINE METHOD

A fractional collection of a urine specimen before meals (a.c.) and at bedtime (h.s.) is done with diabetic patients to test for sugar and acetone.

Nursing Tips

- Specimen should be from the *second voiding* at the hour specified. The patient empties his bladder approximately 30 minutes before the time of specimen collection.
- At the time of collection, the patient voids again, and this specimen is tested for sugar and acetone. The test indicates whether sugar

or acetone is being excreted at that time, not whether they have been stored in the bladder.

- If specimen is being collected from an indwelling catheter, one collection is sufficient because the bladder is essentially empty at all times.
- A specimen from an indwelling catheter is aspirated through the collection port, *never* from the drainage bag.
- A report from a patient or nursing assistant that a urine test indicates that more than a trace of sugar is present requires another test by the nurse before insulin is given or the physician is notified.

TIMED URINE METHOD

Timed urine collections are done to determine metabolic function.

Nursing Tips

- Obtain a container which will accommodate the entire specimen.
- Add the preservative in the laboratory if it is necessary for the test. Refer to Table 1-8 for the tests requiring a preservative.
- Instruct the patient to start the collection by voiding and discarding this specimen. Note the time on the container.
- Instruct the patient to save all urine voided during the time period required. Complete the collection by having the patient void for the last specimen at the closing time.
- Caution the patient not to void directly into the container.
- All timed specimens must be kept on ice or refrigerated during their collection.
- Label the container with the patient's name, room number, and hospital number. Include the name of the test, the starting and ending time of collection, and the date.
- Deliver the total specimen to the laboratory as soon as possible. The specimen must be accompanied by the appropriate slip.

TESTING FOR GLUCOSE AND ACETONE (KETONES)
Description

Urine obtained from diabetic patients as stat specimens or fractionals is tested for acetone and glucose. The results help determine daily insulin doses and additional insulin coverage as necessary.

Testing Methods
Acetest

Tablet test for acetone
- Place one tablet on paper towel
- Place one drop of urine on tablet
- Wait 30 seconds

TABLE 1-8. **Preservatives for 24-Hour Urines**

Use No Preservative	No Preservative Necessary; However, 10 ml conc. HCl Will Not Interfere
Amylase	Catecholamines
BUN	Estrogen
Calcium	Follicle-stimulating hormone
Creatinine	17-Hydroxycortico-steroids
Glucose	17-Ketogenic steroids
Heavy metals	17-Hydroxysteroids
Hydroxy proline	17-Ketosteroids
LDH	Pregnanediol
Oxalates	
Phosphorus	
Porphobilinogen	
Potassium	
Pregnanetroil	
Quantitative HCG	
Sodium	
Uric acid	
Urine total protein	

Miscellaneous Preservatives	
VMA (Vanillylmandelic acid)	10 ml conc. hydrochloric acid
Aldosterone	15 ml 30% acetic acid or 4.5 ml glacial acetic acid plus 10.5 ml water
5 HIAA	25 ml glacial acetic acid
Metanephrine	5 ml conc. hydrochloric acid
Porphyrins	5 g Sodium carbonate
Uroporphyrins	5 g Sodium carbonate
Coproporphyrins	5 g Sodium carbonate
Cortisol	2 Boric acid tablets

- Read by acetest color chart. Values are in shades of purple. Results indicate negative, small, moderate, or large amounts of acetone in the urine.

Ketostix

For ketones (acetone)
- Estimate amount of ketones in urine as small, moderate, or large. Test for ketones when urine sugar measures 1% or more. Levodopa, phenylketones (PKU), or Bromsulphalein (BSP) may cause a false-positive result.

Dip-and-Read Reagent Strips

For glucose and acetone
- Throw-away strips of reagent paper are passed through urine stream or dipped into urine, then compared with accompanying color chart to estimate amounts of glucose and acetone in urine.

Diastix

For glucose
- Large quantities of ketone bodies, ascorbic acid, or L-dopa may depress color development.

Clinistix

For glucose
- This 10-second test shows only whether glucose is present or absent, so it is most useful for well-controlled diabetic patients who need only periodic checks of urine for glucose. High doses of aspirin or vitamin C may affect test results.

Keto-Diastix

For acetone and glucose
- Test designed for diabetics whose control is uneven enough to warrant regular ketone (acetone) testing at the same time as glucose testing. (For occasional ketone testing use Ketostix or Acetest.)

Tes-tape

For glucose
- A dip-and-read test for glucose that comes in a tape dispenser. Sometimes difficult to read.

Clinitest

Tablet test for glucose (5-drop and 2-drop methods)
- Except for the difference in the number of drops of urine, the procedure is the same, though one must compare the specimen with the appropriate (*i.e.,* 5-drop or 2-drop) color chart. The 2-drop method is more accurate and is used especially for the patient whose diabetes is difficult to control. It estimates sugar concentration from 0% to 5%. The 5-drop method estimates sugar concentration from 0% to 2%.

- Procedure
  1. Collect urine in clean receptacle. Place 5 (or 2) drops of urine in a clean test tube. Rinse dropper and add 10 drops of water to test tube.
  2. Drop one tablet into test tube. Watch reaction as it takes place. If color should rapidly "pass through" from bright orange to dark brown or greenish brown, it indicates that sugar is over 2%. Record this or try the 2-drop method for more accurate results.
  3. Do not shake test tube during reaction or for 15 seconds after boiling stops.

4. After 15-second waiting period, shake test tube gently and compare with color chart.
5. Record and report results. Check the physician's orders for appropriate insulin coverage.

Nursing Tips

- Clinitest tablets are *poisonous* and may cause chemical burns. Do not touch them with wet fingers. They should be kept in a dry, dark, safe place.
- Clinitest tablets will react with any sugar in the urine (not only glucose). Clinistix or Diastix are specific for testing the presence of glucose, so they could be used as a second test as necessary.
- Large quantities of ascorbic acid, nalidixic acid (NegGram), cephalosporins (Keflin, Keflex, Loridine), and probenecid (Benemid) may cause false-positive results with Clinitest. Use another test method when patients are receiving these drugs.
- Be consistent in the method used to test urine on each patient. Inform the physician of the test being used.
- A report from a patient or nursing assistant that a urine test indicates more than a trace of sugar requires another test by the nurse before insulin is given or the physician is notified.
- Use percentage of glucose present in the urine rather than "plus one, two or three" when reporting results.
- Patients with renal insufficiency may not show glucose in their urine until the blood glucose is elevated highly.

TESTING FOR SPECIFIC GRAVITY
Description

The specific gravity (sp.gr.) of urine is its weight compared with the weight of an equal volume of water. It indicates the kidneys' ability to concentrate and dilute urine. A low sp. gr. occurs with overhydration or renal failure. A high sp. gr. indicates a low fluid intake or excessive fluid loss. The normal range of urine sp. gr. is 1.001 to 1.035.

Nursing Tips

- The equipment to test sp. gr. includes a cylinder to contain the urine (about 10 ml) and a urinometer.
- Use a freshly voided specimen, and fill the cylinder about 3/4 full of urine.
- Place the urinometer into the cylinder; gently spin it; when it comes to rest, read at eye level where the meniscus crosses the scale on the urinometer. This is the sp. gr. reading.
- Record and report results.

BIBLIOGRAPHY
BOOKS

Tilkian S, Conover MB, Tilkian AG: Clinical Implications of Laboratory Tests, 2nd ed. St Louis, CV Mosby, 1979

Wallach J: Interpretation of Diagnostic Tests, 3rd ed. Boston, Little, Brown, 1979

JOURNALS

Carlson M: Demystifying diagnostic procedures. Journal of Practical Nursing 29:16, May, 1979; 29:31, July, 1979

DeHaff J: What you should know about interpreting cardiac enzyme studies. Nursing 76 6(9):69, 1976

McGuckin M: The problems with respiratory tract cultures and what you can do about them. Nursing 76 6(2):76, 1976

McGuckin M: What you should know about collecting stool culture specimens. Nursing 76 6(3):22, 1976

Watson EM, Neufeld AH: Your guide to clinical laboratory procedures. Canadian Nurse 75:25, September, 1979

Worthington L: What those blood gases can tell you. RN Magazine 42(10):22, 1979

2
Management in Special Nursing Situations (MNS)

Alcoholic patient in withdrawal
Decubitus ulcer prevention and treatment
Disoriented patients
Night and evening duty
Pain management

ALCOHOLIC PATIENT IN WITHDRAWAL

Description

Recognizing the symptoms of alcohol withdrawal may be a matter of life or death. Over 15% of patients who experience delirium tremens (DTs) die despite treatment. Patients admitted to the hospital with alcohol on the breath and showing symptoms of intoxication are easy to identify. Suspect those admitted with diagnoses of diseases that are alcohol-related; those with burns, evidence of falls, and bruises; or those who do not respond in the usual way to normal doses of medications, particularly sedatives. Often alcoholics are also heavy smokers.

The goal of treatment is to avoid the toxic crisis of DTs by staying ahead of symptoms with medication. Accurate, continuous assessment is vital.

What to Look for

History of patient's alcohol-use habits should be included in *all* nursing histories. Question the patient in a matter-of-fact way. Be nonjudgmental.

- "When did you have your last drink?" Answer is important because if it was 4 hours ago, you have a little time. If it was 8 hours ago, he may already be in withdrawal and will need to be medicated immediately.
- "What happens when you stop drinking?" "How much alcohol do you drink each day?" Follow by saying that it makes a difference in the dosage of drugs he will be receiving. Assume that an alcoholic does not want to reveal the amount of alcohol he has actually been consuming.

Early symptoms of alcohol withdrawal include

- Headache, slurred speech, poor coordination, staggering gait, nausea and vomiting, diarrhea, insomnia, failure to respond to average doses of tranquilizers or sedatives.

Later symptoms include

- A fluttery feeling, minor anxiety, intention tremor (difficulty lighting a cigarette or holding a cup of coffee), leg jerks, disorientation, agitation, nausea and vomiting, diaphoresis (profuse perspiration), hallucinations (may be visual, auditory, or tactile), seizure.

Symptoms of DTs include the following in addition to all of the above:

- Fever over 100°F or 38°C, pulse over 120, diaphoresis, thrashing, and extreme psychotic behavior.
- One of the keys to the differential diagnosis between a withdrawal reaction to alcohol and to drug overdose is that in alcohol with-

drawal all vital signs are elevated; in drug overdose they are depressed.
- DTs may occur anytime from the 3rd to the 7th day after withdrawal, or sooner if trauma or injury are present. DTs may occur as a result of reduction of alcohol use from heavy to moderate, rather than total cessation of drinking, thereby modifying the time of onset of the delirium.

Treatment

- Sedation in sufficient doses to control the symptoms; the patient is sedated to a point where he can be aroused but still without symptoms. Drugs must be given around the clock (if necessary, patient must be wakened to take medication). Diazepam (Valium), chlordiazepoxide hydrochloride (Librium), or thioridazine hydrochloride (Mellaril) given p.o. or parenterally. *(See PH)*
- Anticonvulsant medications (Valium is one of the best anticonvulsants. Dilantin is also frequently prescribed). *(See PH)*
- Antiemetics
- Maintenance of fluid and electrolyte balance.
- Reestablishment of adequate nutrition.
- Early involvement in an alcohol rehabilitation program.

Nursing Tips

- Provide a calm, safe, nonstressful environment.
- Delirious patients may be very frightened by their hallucinations; they can become very agitated, even suicidal.
- Give quiet reassurance. Help patient stay in touch with reality. Keep room well lit 24 hours a day.
- Stay with the patient, if possible, or have a member of the family come in to stay with him. Keep directions simple.
- Restrain with Posey vest, if needed. Use leather wrist cuffs only if absolutely necessary.
- Have padded tongue blade available. Try to protect patient from head injuries.
- Monitor vital signs for alertness and responsiveness every two hours (q. 2 h). Assess for response to drug therapy q. 4 h. Remember, medications are given around the clock. Communication and follow-up between nursing shifts is essential.

Sources of Information

- National Council on Alcoholism, 1917 Eye St., NW, Washington DC, 20006
- Alcoholics Anonymous Grapevine, Grand Central Station, P.O. Box 1980 New York, NY, 10017 (or your local chapter)

DECUBITUS ULCER PREVENTION AND TREATMENT

Description

A decubitus ulcer (pressure sore, bedsore) is the result of skin breakdown and subsequent necrosis of underlying tissue, fat, and muscle. The usual cause is a sustained pressure (2 or more hours) on the skin surface, resulting in an interruption of the blood supply.

What to Look for

- Reddened area of skin that blanches with pressure.
- Cyanotic area of skin that does not blanche with pressure.
- Blistered area of skin, signifying that necrosis of superficial layers of underlying tissue has occurred.
- Open necrotic area of deep tissue, which is very susceptible to infection.
- Casts or braces which rub and cause skin irritations.
- Common sites are indicated in Figure 2-1.

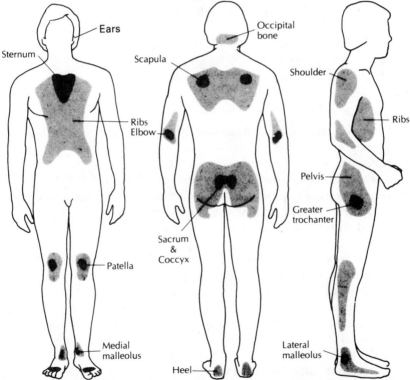

FIG. 2-1. *Sites of potential pressure sores.* (King EM, Wieck L, Dyer M: Illustrated Manual of Nursing Techniques, 2nd ed, Philadelphia, JB Lippincott, 1981)

Treatment

- Prevention is much easier than actual treatment.
- When possible, ensure frequent ambulation (10 minutes every 2 hours), and prevent sitting for more than 2 hours.
- Encourage strict adherance to a 2-hour turning schedule if bed-ridden.

For Reddened or Cyanotic Unbroken Skin

- Wash the area, and pat dry thoroughly; do not use talcum powder.
- Gently massage around the area; do not use alcohol, because it dries the skin, or lanolin, because of a possible allergic reaction. Some caution against massaging directly over the reddened area because injury to subcutaneous fat and muscle has already occurred.
- Use foam-rubber padding, cut to encircle the area. Several pieces of a foam-rubber pad may be stacked together to provide more relief from pressure. The wider the piece of cushioning material used, the more evenly the weight will be distributed.
- It is important to avoid pressure, friction, and moisture on the damaged area. Use a sheepskin to absorb perspiration and to help in lifting the patient.
- Place a flotation or eggcrate mattress on the bed.

For Broken Skin Without Necrosis

- Continue treatment as described above for the surrounding, unbroken skin area.
- Continue to relieve the pressure on the area.
- Use sterile technique in tending broken skin areas.
- Consult with the physician on the advisability of flushing with an antiseptic cleaning agent, *e.g.*, povidone-iodine (Betadine), followed with a saline irrigation to eliminate the possibility of irritation.
- Once every 8 hours, after drying the area, one of the many healing agents may be used. Some of these are antacids, *e.g.*, Maalox paste, thought to neutralize acid conditions of open wounds; Karaya powder, believed to stimulate granulation tissue; heat lamp, used when warm air and heat are prescribed; Granulex, a combination of emollients and the enzyme trypsin, which does light, surface debriding; and Decubitex, containing scarlet red, said to promote granulation tissue (not useful on necrotic tissue). The area must be kept clean and dry between treatments.
- To cover or not to cover is often the question. Antacid pastes must

be thoroughly dry before covering with a light, sterile dressing, taped only on the sides to allow air circulation. An occlusive dressing, using a transparent material (*e.g.*, Op-site) to form a second skin, may be used. This is applied over the decubitus after the area is cleaned and the surrounding area is dry. It serves as a permanent dressing until healing occurs.

For Broken Skin With Necrosis

- Continue treatment as described above for the surrounding, unbroken skin area.
- Use sterile technique in caring for the decubitus.
- Consult with the physician for specific treatment orders.
- A wound culture should be obtained to determine the appropriate topical antibiotic.
- Wash the decubitus with normal saline, hydrogen peroxide, or povidone-iodine (Betadine) to clean and debride necrotic tissue. Whenever these last two agents are used, flush them off with normal saline, and pat the area dry with sterile gauze.
- In some cases, special debridement procedures may be required. Instructions for the use of special medications for cleaning and debridement, such as dextranomer (Debrisan) or collagenase (Santyl), must be carefully read. These medications should not contact normal skin. Discontinue as soon as necrotic area is clean. They are applied once a day.
- Wet-to-dry dressings may be used for debridement and to eliminate infections. Sterile technique is always used. Soak single layers of noncotton sterile gauze with a prescribed sterile solution and squeeze the excess out. Pack this gently into the wound, covering all exposed surfaces. Apply a thin layer of dry sterile gauze, and finish with a 4 × 8 full thickness of sterile gauze (do not use the thick ABD pads). Tape only around the edges so that the gauze will dry. With this treatment the dressing should be dry in 6 to 8 hours. When the dry gauze is removed, necrotic tissue will be caught in the mesh and will be removed. The disadvantage is that newly formed skin may also be pulled away.
- If the area is infected, a topical antibacterial agent (e.g., Neosporin) is commonly applied after debridement.
- Follow with an application of one of various healing agents and dressings as described above for broken skin without necrosis. When a second skin material is used over an infected decubitus, it should be changed daily.
- Surgical debridement, followed by skin grafts, may be necessary for some necrotic decubitus ulcers.

Nursing Tips

- A nursing care plan, with step-by-step directions, is essential for the consistent treatment of a decubitus ulcer. *Consistent* is the key word!
- Any immobilized or edematous patient is at high risk for decubiti. Additionally, patients receiving narcotics for pain are not sensitive to pressure discomfort. Diabetics and those on high doses of steroids should be watched because of an increased susceptibility to skin breakdown.
- Pressure on any skin area for more than 2 hours will cause a loss of blood supply at the center of the pressure area, with increased vulnerability to decubitus ulcers. The use of an alternating pressure or eggcrate mattress does not eliminate the need for turning.
- Turn any immobilized patient every 2 hours. This should follow a sequence of right side—back—left side—abdomen. The patient is often not able to tolerate the abdominal position for as long as 2 hours.
- Post a chart at the patient's bedside with a turning rotation schedule (see Fig. 2-2). Sometimes a total change in position is impossible, but range of motion exercises can be done, and pressure points can be relieved. Note this on the chart.
- RS = Right side; B = Back, LS = Left side; A = Abdomen; ROM = Range of motion
- Under comments, note intolerance to any position.
- Do not schedule position changes at change of shift.
- Lift, do not drag, the patient up in bed.
- Prolonged wheel-chair sitting also causes pressure sores. Be sure a pad (*e.g.,* eggcrate or flotation) is placed on the seat. Patients must also shift their weight every 15 to 20 minutes.
- Alternating pressure mattresses must be inflated before placing the patient on them.
- Do not pull sheets tight over eggcrate mattresses.
- Cotton bath blankets can be used to cover plastic mattress covers and to absorb perspiration.
- Elderly patients do not require a daily bath. Their bath water may have an oil added to prevent dry skin, if they are not allergic to these lubricants. A dry skin is conducive to skin breakdown. Vaseline is an excellent lubricant.
- Give a backrub at least once a day and include all the bony prominences. Use a lotion, and rub it into the skin to avoid leaving a wet surface. Do not use talcum powder; however, cornstarch is acceptable. Remove crumbs and foreign objects, and tighten the bottom sheets.

12^M Position, Comment	Initial
2	
4	
6	
8	
10	
12^N	
2	
4	
6	
8	
10	

FIG. 2-2. *Sample chart for turning rotation schedule to avoid pressure sores.*

- Some patients are allergic to chemical detergents used in washing linens, and this results in skin breakdown.
- Keep the heels from rubbing on the mattress by placing a folded blanket under the ankles, or use heel protectors.
- Never allow the legs to rest on top of one another. Use a pillow or folded blanket to prevent pressure.
- Moisture is a major factor in causing skin breakdown. Be sure that urine and feces are completely washed off the skin of incontinent patients. When the skin is excoriated, avoid using soap, and pat dry or use a hair dryer (set on cool setting) to completely dry the skin. A product such as Peri-wash is very useful in cleaning the skin of incontinent patients.
- When a 2-hour toileting routine is not possible, the only alternative is to keep the skin as clean and dry as possible. The prolonged use of indwelling catheters almost always leads to urinary tract infection.
- High-caloric, high-protein diets are essential for good skin conditions and proper healing. Vitamin C supplement is also used to stimulate wound healing.

- A Stryker frame or Circ-O-lectric bed may be used when it is impossible to otherwise relieve pressure on skin areas.
- Enterostomal therapists are often referred to as "the skin care specialists." Consult with them for skin care problems.
- Physicians will usually follow what the nurse suggests as effective decubital treatment.
- Read the insert on any preparation specifically for decubitus care. Special wound-cleaning procedures may need to be followed.
- Topical applications of ointments containing debriding agents are also used in treating leg ulcers.

DISORIENTED PATIENTS

Description

- A mild degree of disorientation can be expected in any patient, since the hospital environment is quite different from that normally encountered.
- This type of mental confusion is very common in older patients who become perturbed when their established daily routine is disrupted.
- Also, patients with brain damage are vulnerable to psychosis and to an inability to perceive reality.
- Serious disorientation may occur as a result of metabolic changes or imbalances due to an illness.
- Imbalance of electrolytes, BUN, blood sugar, or ABGs, elevated temperature or blood pressure, or withdrawal from alcohol and other drugs are common causes of disorientation.
- Occasionally, change of medication or use of a new medication may result in disorientation.
- Mental confusion may be evident shortly after admission, or as in the case of alcohol withdrawal, it may not occur until 2 or 3 days after admission.

What to Look for

- Early symptoms of confusion may appear gradually. These include increasing restlessness, emotional irritability, apprehension, difficulty in identifying familiar people or objects, and picking at air or bedding.

Treatment

- The common drug of choice in controlling severe agitation and hallucinations is haloperidol (Haldol). It should be regularly scheduled around the clock, *never* just p.r.n. It should be gradually discontinued over a period of several days.

Nursing Tips

- It is important to obtain a nursing history that details medication presently being taken and the amount of alcohol normally consumed daily. The probability of mental confusion occurring increases with the number of medications being taken.
- Explain the hospital routine and attempt to learn the patient's regular routine, especially what he does at night (*e.g.*, frequency of use of the bathroom and usual pattern of sleep). Emphasize that nurses and other hospital personnel will be entering the patient's room at night.
- As much as possible, schedule medications, treatments, and procedures so they do not interrupt sleep.
- A bed near a window, a calendar on the wall, and a clock that the patient can see promote contact with reality. A day-night reversal pattern may develop.
- Oxygen administration often relieves confusion caused by cerebral anoxia. (*See NR, Oxygen administration*)
- Confusion is most severe in twilight or darkness. The addition of flashing lights on an IV pump, suction machines, or unfamiliar noises in a dark room heighten anxiety. Patients with eye patches have an increased tendency to disorientation.
- Keep normal lights on, since partial darkness causes shadows. Keep hearing aids, eyeglasses, and dentures in place on the patient. The head of the bed should be kept elevated; hallucinations increase when a patient is flat in bed. A radio left on day and night is helpful in providing a feeling of companionship.
- The hospital intercom may be left on to monitor activity but do not use it to talk to the patient. A disembodied voice increases confusion.
- A gentle, caring touch may help, because it communicates that "I care."
- In cases of extreme agitation, a family member or friend should be asked to sit with the patient, especially at night. Restraints should be a last resort.

NIGHT AND EVENING DUTY

Description

The successful management of patient care depends more completely upon the individual nurse during the evening and night shifts than during regular daytime hours when support from the hospital staff is generally available.

Nursing Tips

- After day or evening report, the oncoming nurse should make rounds and do patient assessments. Dressings need to be checked, and drainage stains should be outlined with pencil for future reference. Levels of fluid in IV or drainage containers and the IV flow rate should be noted. Be sure that oxygen settings are correct and humidifiers have sufficient water. Call lights should be in place, side rails should be up, and restraints should be applied to those who need them.
- A roll of 1-inch tape, scissors, an alcohol sponge, a Band-Aid, and a small flashlight carried in a pocket can be invaluable.
- Be familiar with the duties of nurse's aides. Make out a work sheet, and discuss it with each aide. Point out the patients that need assistance with eating, including any special orders for increased or limited fluid intake, as well as those patients who need intake and output recorded. Clearly identify to the aide those patients that require specimen collections, fractional urines, or timed collections, elevated temperature procedure, and ambulation or turning or positioning.
- Bedside tables and the areas around patients' beds should be cleared because dim lighting and unfamiliar surroundings increase the possibility of accidents.
- Tell patients early in the evening if they are going to be n.p.o. after midnight.
- Oral temperatures above 99.4°F (37.5°C) or 1° higher for rectal temperatures should be taken about 8 PM. After this time, schedule temperature and routine vital signs assessment with medication administration to minimize frequent interruptions of sleep.
- The day's postoperative patients or any patients who have had an indwelling catheter removed should have orders covering the possibility of their not voiding spontaneously within 8 hours.
- An adequate supply of each patient's medicines should be on hand for the entire night. To avoid late night calls to the physicians, orders for sedation or sleep should be obtained as early as possible in the evening.
- Sleep medications should be withheld until midnight if there are other medications or treatments scheduled for that hour. Repeat sleep medication should generally not be given after 3AM.
- Ideally, noisy or disoriented patients should be in private rooms. When this is not possible, move them for the night into any available room (*e.g.,* treatment room) or to a wheelchair at the nurse's station.
- When there is any doubt about calling a physician at night, first

call the nursing supervisor. When a physician is called, know the patient's current and previous vital signs.

PAIN MANAGEMENT

Description

For the patient experiencing pain, relief is vital, both for the patient's comfort and—for one experiencing chronic pain—his quality of living. Pain control is important to recovery following surgery.

Assessment of pain is difficult. The experience of and response to pain varies widely from person to person. In general, anxiety is usually associated with acute pain, while depression more commonly accompanies chronic pain. It is the person who is experiencing it who is the ultimate judge of the pain's severity.

Frequently, patients (sometimes fearing drug addiction) feel that they must or should "tough it out." They will not ask for medication for pain when it is indicated. But experience has shown that anticipation of pain magnifies it, and if pain is relieved before it becomes intense, lower doses of medication are required.

Following major surgery, patients may require medication around the clock for the first 2 or 3 days. Most often analgesics (*e.g.*, meperidine (Demerol) or morphine sulfate) are ordered by the surgeon to be given every 3 or 4 hours as indicated, with gradually decreasing dosages *(see PH)*. Medication should cover the pain, within safe limits.

Nursing Tips

- Remember that respiratory depression and signs and symptoms of shock may be side-effects of almost all narcotics.
- Maximum respiratory depression will occur within 30 minutes after administration.
- Plan nursing care so that the analgesic can be given a few minutes before any painful treatment. The patient will be better able to move, cough, deep breathe, and ambulate.
- Extend the effect of pain-relieving medication with nursing measures.
  1. Teach the patient to splint a surgical incision when he coughs and deep breathes. *(See NR, Deep breathing techniques)*
  2. Relaxation and breathing techniques used in natural childbirth have been found to be helpful in relieving other types of pain. A back rub may help the patient to relax.
  3. Diversion is believed to decrease pain's intensity. Such activities as watching television, reading, and visiting with friends may help relieve pain.
  4. Provide a calm, restful environment.

BIBLIOGRAPHY

ALCOHOLIC PATIENT IN WITHDRAWAL
JOURNALS

Kurose K, Anderson T, Bull W et al: A standard care plan for alcoholism. Am J Nurs 81(5):1001–1006, 1981

Lewis LW: The hidden alcoholic: A nursing dilemma. Nursing 75 5:20–30, July 1975

Ufer L: How to recognize and care for the alcoholic patient. Nursing 77 7:37–38, Oct., 1977

UNPUBLISHED WORKS

Jeferson L: The alcoholic in the acute care setting. Lecture presented at Seminar for Nurses, sponsored by Hospital Temporaries, Washington DC, June, 1980

DECUBITUS ULCERS

Altman MI, Goldstein L, Horowitz S: Collagenase. An adjunct to healing trophic ulcerations in the diabetic patient. Podiatry Assoc 68(1): 11, January, 1978

Cameron G: Pressure sores: What to do when prevention fails. Nursing 79 9(1):43–47, January, 1979

Cooper-Smith F: Prevention of pressure sores. Nursing Times 75:1294–5, August 2, 1979

Kavchak-Keyes M: Four proven steps for preventing decubitus ulcers. Nursing 77 7(9):58, September, 1977

Kavchak-Keyes M: Treating decubitus ulcers using four proven steps. Nursing 77 7(10):44, October, 1977

Ritchie KB et al: Pressure sores. Journal of Physician Assistants. 8:17–19, Spring, 1978

Snowden D: Decubitus ulcer. Nursing Mirror 148:26–27, Feb 1, 1979

Woodbine A: Pressure sores: A review of the problem. Nursing Times 75:1087–8, June 28, 1979

DISORIENTED PATIENTS
BOOKS

Farrah S: The Nurse—The Patient—The Touch. Current Concepts in Clinical Nursing, Vol III, pp 247–259. St Louis, CV Mosby, 1971

JOURNALS

Coping with agitated patients. Emergency Medicine 11:83, August 15, 1979

Davidhizar R: Recognizing and caring for the delerious patient. J Psychiatr Nurs 16:38, May, 1978

Goodykoontz L: Touch: Attitudes and practice. Nurs Forum 18(1):4, 1979

Kroner K: Dealing with the confused patient. Nursing 79 9(11):71, November, 1979

Trockman G: Caring for the confused or delerious patient. Am J Nurs 78(9):1495, September, 1978

PAIN MANAGEMENT

Cummings D: Stopping chronic pain before it starts. Nursing 81 11(1):60–62, January, 1981

Fagerhaugh SY, Strauss A: How to manage your patient's pain. . . and how not to. Nursing 80 8(2):44–47, February, 1980

Hudson S: Teach breath control to ease your patient's post-op pains. RN Magazine 40(1):36–38, January, 1977

Jacox AK: Assessing pain. Am J Nurs 79(5):895–900, May, 1979

McCaffery M: Understanding your patient's pain. Nursing 80 10(9):26–31, September, 1980

Steele BG: Test your knowledge of post-operative pain management. Nursing 80 6(3):76–78, March, 1980

3

Nursing Responsibilities for Diagnosis and Treatment (NR)

Bone marrow aspiration and biopsy
Cardiopulmonary resuscitation
Cast brace
Cast care
Central venous pressure
Chest tube drainage (thoracic drainage)
Crutch measurement
Deep breathing techniques
Electrocardiogram (ECG/EKG) leads and how to place them
Electroencephalogram (EEG)
Endoscopic procedures
External fixation device
Gastrointestinal intubation (nasogastric and nasoenteric tubes)
Hypothermia blanket
Intravenous therapy
   Hyperalimentation therapy (total parenteral nutrition)
   Intravenous fluids
   Blood and blood component transfusion
   Electrolyte imbalances
Isolation technique
Liver biopsy
Nasopharyngeal or oropharyngeal suctioning
Ostomies, fistulas, and draining wounds
Oxygen administration
Paracentesis (abdominal)
Postural hypotension (orthostatic hypotension)
Range of motion exercises
Renal biopsy
Rotating tourniquets
Scans
   Computerized axial tomography (CAT)
   Nuclear
Sengstaken-Blakemore tube

Thoracentesis
Tracheostomy care
Traction
Ultrasound (sonograms)
Urinary bladder catheterization and drainage
  Catheterization
  Continuous bladder irrigation
  Intermittent bladder irrigation
  Suprapubic catheters
X-ray preparations

BONE MARROW ASPIRATION AND BIOPSY

Description

The bone marrow has as its principal function the manufacture of erythrocytes, leukocytes, and platelets. Bone marrow aspiration and biopsy are done to determine the effectiveness of this function.

Nursing Tips

- These two procedures may be done at the bedside or in a treatment room.
- Contact the laboratory for proper container and preservative.
- A bone marrow aspiration may be done on the sternum or iliac crest. When a biopsy is done, the iliac crest is used.
- This procedure causes momentary but sharp pain when the marrow is aspirated.
- Apply pressure to the site for 3 to 5 minutes to prevent bleeding. Check back in 15 minutes for any bleeding.

CARDIOPULMONARY RESUSCITATION (CPR)

Procedure

1. Place victim flat on his back on a hard surface. If unconscious, open airway (see Fig. 3-1). Lift neck to tilt back, or lift chin to tilt head back.
2. If person is not breathing, begin artificial breathing with four quick breaths mouth to mouth with the nose pinched closed. A manual resuscitation bag may be used. If a tracheostomy is present, the artificial breathing is applied to the stoma.
3. Check carotid pulse.
4. If pulse is absent, begin artificial circulation. Depress sternum 1½ to 2 inches. With one rescuer: 15 compressions alternating with two quick breaths. With two rescuers: 5 compressions alternating with one quick breath. Continue uninterrupted until advanced life support is available.

CAST BRACE

Description

Following a period of traction providing acceptable alignment, a *cast brace* may be used to reduce rehabilitation time for fractures of the femoral shaft or tibia by allowing for early ambulation and weight bearing. In long-leg cast bracing or standard bracing, a quadrilateral socket form (frequently called a *quadsocket brace*) is now most often used (see Fig. 3-2).

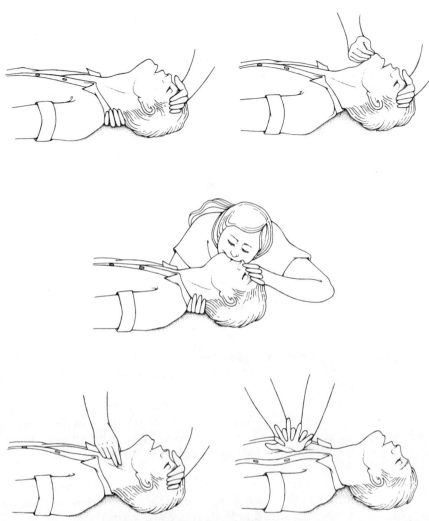

FIG. 3-1. *Cardiopulmonary resuscitation.*

Skeletal traction is maintained until the fracture site is stable (usually about 4 to 6 weeks) before these devices are fitted *(see NR, Traction)*. The cast brace includes a thigh cuff of plastic or plaster and a short-leg walking cast that are joined at the knee with metal hinges.

Nursing Tips
- Vigorous quadriceps and hamstring exercises started during the period of traction are continued throughout treatment.

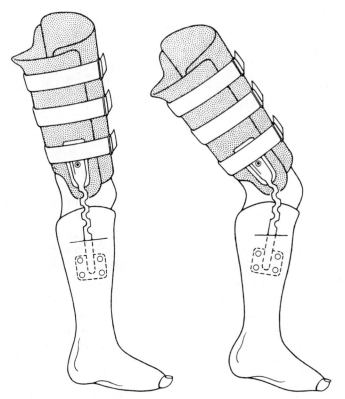

FIG. 3-2. *Example of a cast brace with adjustable quad socket.* (Pope brace, orthopedic division of Parke, Davis).

- Once the brace is applied, watch for swelling of the knee. If apparent, elevate the extremity. Apply ice packs, if ordered.
- Watch for signs of circulatory or neurological impairment caused by the cast. They are pallor, pulselessness, pain, paralysis, or paresthesia (tingling or numbness).
- Inspect knee hinges for firm attachment.
- If ordered, teach the patient how to inspect and tighten screws with the special instruments provided by the manufacturer. Some physicians prefer to make all such adjustments themselves.
- Unless specifically ordered, neither nurse nor patient should attempt to adjust the brace. It's function is that of a cast.
- Provide assistance with exercises and ambulation.

CAST CARE

Description

Casts are used to immobilize a bone or joint in alignment, to reduce fractures, and to correct and prevent deformities. They may be made of layers of plaster-of-paris bandages or of plastic material.

What to Look for

- Unrelieved pain, pallor, pulselessness, paralysis, or paresthesia (tingling or numbness) are all signs of possible neurovascular impairment caused by edema under the unyielding cast. After application of a fresh cast, observe the patient frequently during first 48 hours, at the beginning of each shift, and p.r.n. thereafter. Report the presence of any of the above symptoms immediately. The cast may need to be altered, bivalved (split in half), or removed. *Pain must always be investigated.* Do not mask it with medication until the cause is determined.
- All toes and fingers should be warm and pink, should have feeling, and should be capable of flexion and extension.
- Decreased capillary filling in nail beds: test by applying pressure to finger or toe nail. Normally, when pressure is released the nail becomes pink almost immediately. A delay in return of normal color indicates impaired circulation. *Report immediately.*
- *Caution:* Compartment syndrome (Volkmann's contracture) is a dreaded complication of compromised blood supply (ischemia) to a muscle group (usually in the arm or hand) that, if unrelieved, can cause permanent disability within 6 hours. The cast must be released. The cast can be changed, the contracture cannot.
- Bleeding: circle outer border of area of apparent bleeding and mark the time. Check underside of cast; blood tends to pool at the bottom of a cast.
- "Hot spots" felt on a dry cast or a musty odor coming from it could be signs of skin breakdown underneath it.
- Signs of pressure on the heel or Achilles tendon (burning sensation over heel area) in patients in leg casts.
- Signs and symptoms of complications of immobility (*e.g.,* pneumonia, constipation, renal calculi, or neurovascular problems).

Nursing Tips

Preparation for the Cast

- Skin under the cast should be clean, dry, and in good condition.
- Patient should be told that as cast dries it will give off heat and grow lighter.

- Casting may be postponed to allow for reduction of swelling. Provide pain medication and gentle handling in the interim.

Care of New Casts

- Plaster may require 24 to 48 hours to dry depending upon variables such as humidity and the thickness of the cast.
- To promote drying:
  1. Expose all sides of the cast to the air. Cast dryers are dangerous; if ordered, use on cool setting only. Lamps and lights are discouraged; if used they should be 15 to 18 inches away from the cast.
  2. Keep cast uncovered.
  3. For a large body cast (*e.g.,* a hip spica), turn the patient every three hours.
     a. Turn carefully as a unit with three or four people supporting the areas of greatest strain.
     b. Usually, turn with the affected limb up (*i.e.,* turn toward the unaffected side).
     c. Handle only with the palms of your hands.
     d. Never place wet cast on flat, hard surface or where there are sharp edges that will alter the shape of the cast.
     e. Ice bags, if ordered to reduce edema, should be filled only 1/3 full and placed against the sides of the cast with care so as not to dent it.
     f. Do not use the abduction bar on a hip-spica cast for turning. When patient is prone, toes should hang over end of bed.
- If practical, elevate the affected part of a little above the level of the heart to reduce edema. The head of the bed should be lower than the casted extremity.
- Pillows not covered with plastic (plastic retards drying) should support the curves of the cast, so that it will not become flattened over boney prominences (*e.g.,* sacrum or heel).
- A firm mattress with a bed board and trapeze is useful when the patient has a hip spica or a large body cast.

Protection of the Cast

- "Petal" the edges of the cast with short strips of adhesive with rounded corners on one end. Tuck rounded end under; secure it; pull other end over the edge of the cast and secure it. The next petal will overlap slightly.
- Dry clean small areas of the cast with a damp cloth and scouring powder. Be careful not to dampen the cast.
- To decrease odor, a 1:750 solution of benzalkonium chloride (Zephiran) may be sponged lightly on soiled areas.

- Put plastic up under the buttocks and around the perineal area of the hip-spica cast. Use fracture bed pan with the head of the bed slightly higher than the foot of the bed. Place a small pillow under the patient's back to prevent cracking the cast.

Itching Under the Cast

- A gauze strip placed next to the skin and under the cast may be moved back and forth, up and down.
- Air may be blown under the cast with a large syringe or a hair dryer with a "cool" setting.

Cast Removal

- Equipment required:
  1. Cast cutter (a saw with dull teeth), cast knives, spreaders.
  2. Solution of 1 part vinegar and 4 parts water may be used to soften cutting line on cast.
- Advise patient that procedure is noisey and may feel warm, but will not hurt.
- Elevate and support the affected body part after cast removal. There is always some swelling.
- Gently clean the skin with lanolin or lotion, followed with mild soap and water.
- Never force movement in a joint.
- Physiotherapy or hydrotherapy, or both, should be ordered to help the patient regain motion and learn crutch walking, if required.

CENTRAL VENOUS PRESSURE

Description

Central Venous Pressure (CVP) describes the pressure in the right atrium of the heart, which receives the venous blood returning from all parts of the body. This pressure is determined by the volume of blood, the condition of the heart muscle, and vascular tone. The CVP is useful for monitoring the administration of fluid into the vascular system.

Starting and Maintaining the CVP Measurement

- The physician inserts an IV catheter through the basilic, subclavian, or internal jugular vein into the superior vena cava or right atrium. This is then connected to IV tubing that has a manometer connected to it through a three-way stopcock. This IV tubing must be filled (primed) with fluid, usually D_5W (5% dextrose in water), prior to being connected to the catheter.
- The manometer must be taped on a pole in an upright position

with the zero point on the manometer at the level of the right atrium. Mark this atrium location on the patient with a permanent ink mark at the midaxilary line. Check for proper alignment at every reading.

- A three-way stopcock at the base of the manometer allows IV fluid to flow to the patient, usually at a slow KVO (keep vein open) rate (20 to 30 ml per hour), when readings are not being taken. This keeps the tubing patent (open).
- To obtain a reading, place the patient flat in bed. When this cannot be done, be certain that all readings are taken at the same head-of-bed elevation. These readings will not be as accurate as when the patient is flat in bed.
- Adjust the stopcock so the IV fluid fills the manometer to about the 20-cm level. Then open the stopcock to the patient. The fluid level will fluctuate with respirations. A lack of fluctuation indicates a kink or a clot in the tubing. Read the fluid level in the manometer where the meniscus stabilizes. This is the CVP reading.
- Return the stopcock to resume KVO IV to the patient.
- A normal CVP reading ranges between 5 to 12 cm of water, as long as right heart valvular disease and pulmonary hypertension are not present. Changes in the reading are more important than values. To establish values for a patient, begin taking CVP readings every 15 minutes for an hour, and then as often as ordered.
- A significant decrease in pressure may indicate hypovolemia; an increased pressure to above 12 cm may indicate right ventricular failure or hypervolemia.

Nursing Tips

- False CVP readings may be due to a misplaced venous catheter, the use of intermittent positive pressure breathing (IPPB) or respirators (these must be momentarily disconnected while the CVP is read), or a kink in the tubing.
- Hourly urine outputs are needed when a CVP is being monitored.
- Sepsis is always a risk with IV catheters; therefore, IV tubing and dressing must be changed with strict aseptic technique every 48 hours.
- Establish with the physician the CVP reading changes that should be brought to his attention.

CHEST TUBE DRAINAGE (THORACIC DRAINAGE)

Description

Drainage of air and fluid from the pleural cavity is accomplished by gravity flow or aided with suction. A water-seal bottle system or disposable plastic unit (*e.g.*, Pleur-evac), is used to collect air and fluid. Either system must be kept 2 to 3 feet below the patient's chest. The mattress may be kept at the elevated position to ensure that the 2 to 3 foot difference between the patient and the collection unit is maintained. Bottles should be in a rack or should be taped to the floor. The plastic unit, Pleur-evac, hangs from the bedframe at the patient's feet. All connections within any system should be taped to avoid air leakage. These drainage systems rely on a seal that acts as a one-way valve to prevent the evacuated air and fluid from flowing back into the pleural space. Commonly used systems have a water seal, and the fluid in the water-seal tube will normally fluctuate approximately 6 cm between inspiration and expiration, but continous bubbling in the water seal indicates a leak in the system. An obstructed chest tube may stop the fluctuation. These water-seal systems have an opening to the atmosphere to either vent evacuated air or to allow automatic control of the amount of suction. *Do not obstruct this opening.*

ONE-BOTTLE WATER-SEAL GRAVITY DRAINAGE

Drainage is collected and air is expelled using just the one container. See Figure 3-3*A*. Evacuated air is released to the atmosphere through an air vent. The end of the glass tube connected to the patient must always be submerged 1 to 2 inches in sterile water or saline to produce a water seal. This allows air and fluid to leave pleural space but makes it impossible for outside air and fluid to reenter. Mark the level of sterile fluid before drainage enters for accurate intake and output. As the fluid level rises due to the accumulating drainage, the glass tube needs to be raised so that it continues to be submerged 1 to 2 inches, thereby maintaining a low pressure that the drainage must overcome. This is the principal disadvantage of a one bottle system. Remember, the end of the glass tube must always be 1 to 2 inches below the fluid level.

TWO-BOTTLE WATER-SEAL GRAVITY DRAINAGE

In a 2-bottle water-seal system, drainage collection and water seal are in two separate bottles. They are connected as shown in Figure 3-3*B*. The water seal is independent from the drainage collection, which provides an advantage over a one-bottle system.

SUCTION WITH WATER-SEAL DRAINAGE

See Figure 3-3*C* and *D*. Suction creates negative pressure within the closed system. This negative pressure sucks air and fluid from the pleural space faster than the gravity drainage system. In addition to a 1- or 2-bottle drainage and water-seal system as described earlier, this method includes another bottle for suction control. The former

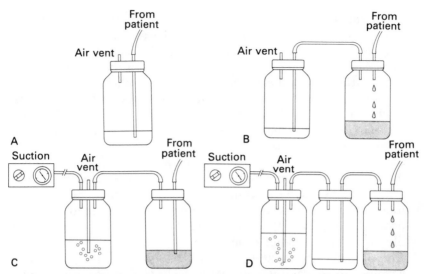

FIG. 3-3. *Types of water seal drainage. (A) 1-bottle water seal gravity drainage; (B) 2-bottle water seal gravity drainage without suction; (C) suction with water seal drainage, 2 bottles; (D) suction with water seal drainage, 3 bottles.*

air vent opening on the gravity system water-seal bottle is attached to the suction bottle as shown in the figures. The long glass tube in the suction bottle is the suction-control tube. The upper end must always be kept open to atmospheric air. The depth to which the tube is submerged beneath the fluid level establishes the suction pressure; this is always ordered by the physician as 10 cm or 15 cm or 20 cm of water. It is prudent to mark the fluid level at the beginning of suction and then to check hourly that the tube remains submerged the proper number of centimeters. There will be continuous bubbling in a suction control bottle because this is what maintains the desired amount of suction. The other bottles function the same as described earlier for the gravity system.

Nursing Tips

- Remember, continuous, as contrasted to intermittent, bubbling in the water-seal bottle in either gravity or suction sets probably indicates an air leak. Check all connections, starting at the chest catheter site. This air leak must be stopped because air is entering the system and the pleural cavity. Notify the physician if the air leak cannot be stopped.
- When you receive a report on a patient with a chest tube, find out how much bubbling is going on and where.
- Two large clamps should be kept taped to the head of the bed of any patient with chest tubes. They are to be used only in an emer-

gency situation to prevent outside air from entering the pleural space. They are clamped as close to the chest as possible, are *never* covered up, and are clamped for as short a period of time as possible. The danger of clamped chest tubes is that trapped air in the pleural space will cause a tension pneumothorax.

- Vertical loops of chest tubing hanging from the mattress or kinks in chest tubing defeat gravity drainage. Coil any loops of tubing horizontally on the mattress, but *never pin*. A kink in or pressure on suction tubing lessens the suction.
- Chest tubes with draining fluid may develop clots. These tubes must be "milked" every hour for the first 24 hours and then every 4 hours. This may be uncomfortable for the patient. Stabilize the tube at the chest insertion site with one hand and gently squeeze down the tube with the other hand. Move hands as necessary all the way to the drainage collection unit.
- The drainage from chest tubes will be bloody at first, gradually changing to serosanguineous. Mark the level of drainage each hour for the first 24 hours and then every 4 hours. If there is more than 200 ml per hour the surgeon must be notified.
- Following a pneumonectomy there may be a chest tube, but it is never on suction because scar tissue formation in the cavity is desired.
- A plastic disposable unit (*e.g.,* Pleur-evac) duplicates in one unit a three-bottle system. The same principle applies regarding keeping the Pleur-evac 2 to 3 feet below the patient's chest. Read the manufacturer's directions carefully.
- When starting suction, increase it until steady bubbling appears in the suction bottle or chamber. Do not increase suction beyond this point, since proper operation is established when steady bubbling occurs.
- Always keep a spare bottle set or Pleur-evac ready for replacement usage when either is in use.

CRUTCH MEASUREMENT

Nursing Tips

- When measuring for crutches, make sure the rubber tips are on the crutches.
- With the patient standing, measure 2 inches from the axillary fold to a position on the floor 4 inches in front of the patient and 6 inches to the side of his toes. (There should be 2 finger widths between the axillary fold and the arm piece.)
- With the patient lying down, measure from the anterior fold of the axilla to the sole of the foot, and add 2 inches.

- The location of the handgrip should allow 20° to 30° flexion of the elbow.

DEEP BREATHING TECHNIQUES

Abdominal breathing may be taught by having the patient place one hand on his chest and one on the abdomen to determine proper abdominal movement. When breathing is done correctly, the abdomen moves, while the chest remains immobile. The most complete lung expansion occurs when arms are placed above the head. This technique is especially useful for the patient with chronic obstructive pulmonary disease (COPD). *(See SS, Chronic obstructive pulmonary disease)*

Incentive spirometers are especially useful in promoting deep breathing because they enable the patient to actually see and measure the effectiveness of his deep breathing efforts. Directions for the use of incentive spirometers usually come with the product and vary slightly according to make.

Intermittent positive pressure breathing (IPPB) is administered by the respiratory therapy department. (The usefulness of IPPB is currently being questioned; some evidence links the treatment with spread of infection through the equipment.)

Sustained maximal inspiration (SMI) is essentially a yawn technique. The patient is instructed to draw in one or more slow deep breaths in succession before exhaling.

Forced expiration (coughing) should only be done when the incision is splinted either with a pillow or with both hands. Increasingly it is being encouraged only if secretions are auscultated in the chest.

Cooperation in deep breathing effort postoperatively is improved if nursing care can be planned so that the patient will have been medicated for pain a few minutes before deep breathing is attempted.

ELECTROCARDIOGRAM (ECG/EKG) LEADS AND HOW TO PLACE THEM

Description

A standard twelve-lead EKG (ECG) includes six limb leads and six chest leads. The six limb leads are obtained from only four limb electrode placements. The electrodes are applied to the right and left arm and right and left leg.

Nursing Tips

- Tell the patient that you are preparing for an EKG (ECG). Also, tell him that the attached wires do not conduct electricity to the body. If possible, have the bed flat.

- Emphasize the importance of not moving during this procedure, since movement interferes with the electrical signals being measured.
- The limb electrodes are metal and are attached by means of wide rubber bands to the patient's extremities. A saline pad or an electrode gel should be placed between the skin and the electrode.
- Place the electrodes on the insides of the forearms and ankles. If these areas are unavailable, any area on an extremity may be used. The cables which connect the electrodes to the machine are color-coded on the plug ends which insert into the electrodes. They are marked as follows:

  RA (right arm) with white letters
  LA (left arm) with black letters
  RL (right leg) with green letters
  LL (left leg) with red letters

- The cable-electrode connection should be tight. Twisting or bending of the cable should be avoided.
- To obtain chest leads, an electrode is placed at six different positions around the chest (see Fig. 3-4). The electrodes are attached by suction cups which adhere to the skin with the aid of electrode paste.
- Mark chest lead positions with electrode gel.
- Use sufficient gel to produce good suction between the cup and the skin surface.
- Depending on the machine, either one chest-lead suction cup with a cable will be moved through each of the 6 positions at the direction of the person operating the EKG (ECG) machine, or 6 chest-lead suction cups with cables will be attached to the patient at the same time.

ELECTROENCEPHALOGRAM (EEG)

Description

An electroencephalogram (EEG) is a recording on paper of electrical activity within the brain. It is used to diagnose epilepsy and brain death, and may also indicate changes related to other brain abnormalities.

Nursing Tips

- No anticonvulsants, tranquilizers, or alcohol for 24 hours preceding the test. The diet should contain no caffeine during this period.
- It is important for the patient to know there will be no electric shock used. The electrodes attached to the head are for recording electrical activity within the brain.

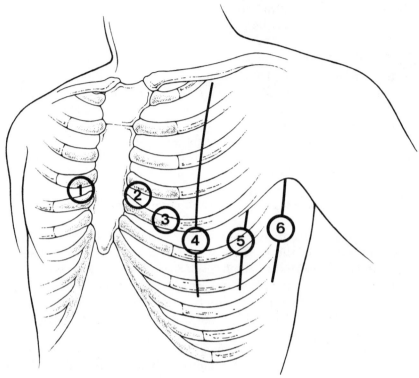

FIG. 3-4. *Standard positions for "C" (also called "V") chest leads.* 1, *4th intercostal space to right of sternum;* 2, *4th intercostal space to left of sternum;* 3, *midway between V_2 and V_4;* 4, *5th intercostal space midclavicular line;* 5, *5th intercostal space between V_4 and V_6;* 6, *5th intercostal space midaxillary line.*

- The conduction paste used on the head should be either shampooed or washed away with alcohol as soon as possible after the EEG.

ENDOSCOPIC PROCEDURES

Description

Endoscopic procedures refer to the viewing of hollow organs or body cavities through the use of a tubular metal instrument with a light source. Flexible fiberoptic endoscopy (FFE) describes special plastic-coated scopes which are very maneuverable and have excellent optics. They contain bundles of light fibers which conduct light to an area, and other bundles which send magnified images back to the viewer, a camera, or a TV screen. There are channels in the scope for insertion of a variety of instruments, such as grasping devices, biopsy forceps and electrocautery tools. There are also air, water, and suction channels. Malfunction and disease may be seen clearly, and special procedures may be performed.

Diagnostic Tests

- Bronchoscopy provides a visual examination of the lung and permits a biopsy. FFE allows a more complete viewing of the respiratory tree, compared with the inflexible metal bronchoscope.
- Proctoscopy or sigmoidoscopy provide a visual examination of the sigmoid or lower colon and permit a biopsy.
- Colonoscopy, using FFE, may be used to view as far as the sigmoid or all the way to the cecum. This is used frequently in the removal of polyps.
- Cystoscopy provides a visual examination of the bladder and permits a biopsy.
- Mediastinoscopy provides a visual examination of organs and lymph nodes in the mediastinum, and permits a biopsy. The instrument is inserted through a small suprasternal incision.
- Peritoneoscopy/laparoscopy provides a view of the contents of the peritoneum. It is especially useful for viewing the liver and obtaining a biopsy. The instrument is inserted through a small incision in the abdomen.
- Panendoscopy (or EGD), using FFE, permits the viewing of the esophagus, stomach, and duodenum, where ulcers, tumors, hiatal hernia, esophageal varices, and origins of bleeding may be seen. Biopsies are often done.
- Endoscopic retrograde cholangiopancreatography (ERCP) is performed with a special side-viewing FFE instrument. This is passed down into the duodenum, and a small catheter is inserted through the papilla of Vater and into the common bile duct. A contrast material is then ejected through the catheter to enable fluoroscopic or x-ray visualization of the pancreatic duct and biliary tree beyond the scope. Endoscopic electrosurgery may also be done to open the papilla of Vater and allow stones to be released into the duodenum.
- Athroscopy is used to view the interior surface of a joint; most commonly it is used to look at the knee. Through the use of this procedure, diagnostic and surgical procedures (e.g., biopsy or the removal of loose bodies) can be performed.

Nursing Tips

- The procedure must be fully discussed with the patient by the physician, and a signed permit must be obtained. Informed consent should include the explanation of the possibility of complications. Perforation, bleeding after biopsies, or mucosal irritations are rare but may occur. If there is a possibility of a polypectomy or stone removal, this should be written on the permit.

- Always find out if the patient is on aspirin or an anticoagulant. Frequently a PT, PTT, and type and crossmatch are done beforehand. *(See LAB)*
- In lieu of special orders the evening before, keep the patient n.p.o. after midnight for the day of the examination.
- An intravenous is often started beforehand to allow immediate vein access in case medication is needed after the procedure is started.
- Laxatives and enemas are given in preparation for bowel examination. It is usually a 2-day preparation.
- When a scope is introduced through the mouth, the throat is anesthetized. Nothing p.o. is allowed afterwards until the gag reflex has returned, usually in about 2 hours. A sore throat lasts a day or two.
- Wheezing may indicate laryngospasm or tracheal edema necessitating immediate medical treatment.
- In order to permit better viewing, carbon dioxide or air is insufflated into the bowel during a colonoscopy, causing spasmlike pains. This is also done in the abdomen when a peritoneoscopy/ laparoscopy is performed, and abdominal distention and cramping may result.
- The incisions for a mediastinoscopy or peritoneoscopy/laparoscopy are usually covered with only a Band-Aid.
- It is imperative that the nurse know when the patient returns to the floor whether an operative procedure such as liver biopsy or polypectomy was done in order to be alert to possible internal hemorrhage *(see NR, Liver biopsy)*. The patient needs to know of any limitations to activity following any procedure.

EXTERNAL FIXATION DEVICE

Description

An external fixation device provides for reduction and stabilization of complicated fractures, especially ones where skin is broken or there is evidence of infection (see Fig. 3-5). The device (Hoffman is one commonly used type) consists of wires or pins that are inserted through the fractured bone and attached to an external metal frame. It may be used for upper or lower extremities or the pelvis.

Nursing Tips

- At first, inspect and cleanse each pin site, removing crusts, twice daily. Later, cleansing once a day may be sufficient.

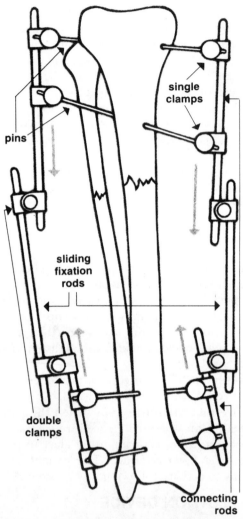

single
clamps

pins

sliding
fixation
rods

double
clamps

connecting
rods

FIG. 3-5. *External fixation site. Pins inserted through the bone proximal and distal to the fracture site are connected in pairs with metal rods and clamps. Adjustable sliding fixation rods join the pairs of pins and, as they tighten, pull the pins toward each other (see arrows). The resulting pressure holds the pieces of bone in proper alignment.* (RN, December, 1979; courtesy Lou Bory Assoc.)

1. Cleanse with hydrogen peroxide applicator.
2. Rinse with sterile normal saline.
3. Apply nonocclusive antibacterial agent (*e.g.,* Neosporin ointment or Helafoam) with sterile applicator. (Use of povidone-iodine is discouraged because it tends to corrode the metal.)

- Cleanse fixator with alcohol wipes daily.
- Encourage self-care of pin sites and fixator.
- Elevate affected body part, postoperatively. Support foot to prevent foot drop.
- Until patient is able to move the extremity himself, move it by grasping frame of fixator, not limb itself.
- Active motion of adjacent joints is usually begun, after initial swelling has gone down, in an exercise program developed by a physiotherapist. Early weight bearing is usually not allowed.
- Treatment of soft tissue wounds, if present. *(See SS, Open fracture)*

GASTROINTESTINAL INTUBATION

Description
Intubation of the stomach or intestine is done
- To empty or decompress, by removing gas and stomach or intestinal contents by suction (done especially in cases of bowel obstruction).
- To diagnose certain conditions by analysis of aspirated material.
- To wash out the stomach (lavage) following ingestion of poisonous substances, of to constrict blood vessels in the stomach lining in cases of gastrointestinal bleeding (iced lavage).
- To provide nutrition by gavage (enteral feeding) for the patient who is unable to take food by mouth.

The tube is usually passed through the nose, though it may be introduced by mouth. *Nasogastric* or *n.g.* (from nose to stomach) and *nasointestinal* or *nasoenteric* (from nose to intestine) are terms commonly used to describe these tubes. A *gastrostomy* tube is inserted directly into the stomach from an opening made in the abdominal wall; an *enterostomy* tube is inserted into the intestine; and an *esophagostomy* tube is inserted into the esophagus.

Equipment
- Short tubes are for placement in the stomach, and are usually about 127 cm (approximately 4 ft) long.
  1. *Levin tube:* a single-lumen tube which comes in several sizes; 16 French is used most commonly for adults. Low intermittent suction is used when suction is required.
     a. Rubber Levin tubes: Chill to stiffen before insertion by putting in the refrigerator or by placing in a pan of chipped ice.
     b. Plastic Levin tube does not require chilling.
  2. *Gastric sump tube (e.g., Salem, Ventrol):* a double-lumen tube (tube within a tube) with two ports, one for suction, and the other a "pigtail" port to allow for the flow of air.

    a. Continuous low suction (30 mm Hg) is preferred. If unavailable, intermittent suction should be set at "high."

    b. The vent tube (pigtail) should give off a hissing sound. If it does not, or if fluid comes out of the vent, reposition the patient to reposition the port of the tube. Then—only with a physician's order—gently irrigate the vent tube with 10 ml of normal saline followed by 10 to 20 cc of air.

    c. Vent lumen must be kept above patient's midline, (*i.e.,*pinned to gown on upper chest). Collection trap must be kept below midline.

3. Newer, smaller, softer, more pliable tubes for n.g. feedings.

    a. *Keofeed:* a silicone rubber tube weighted at the end. Sizes 7.3 to 9.6 French are most commonly used. Most formulas will drip by gravity. Patient cooperation is required for insertion. Keofeed Tube Guide (made of gelatin) may aid in passing tube.

    b. *Dobbhoff tube:* polyurethane, weighted at the end.

    c. *Med Pro:* a silicone rubber tube enclosed in a stiff, outer polyvinyl chloride tube, which is withdrawn after tube is passed. This tube is easier to pass in the patient who is unable to cooperate. It usually requires a pump for continuous infusion.

    d. *Small Levin tube:* 6 to 8 French.

- Long tubes: used to decompress the bowel (usually 6 to 10 ft long).

    1. *Miller–Abbott:* double-lumen tube is passed; then balloon is inflated with air, or partially filled with mercury, to facilitate passage of tube through the pylorus into the small intestine. Suction lumen should be marked, so that it can be differentiated.

    2. *Cantor:* a single-lumen tube with a small rubber bag at the distal end that is filled with mercury before insertion.

- *Gastrostomy tube:* a large rubber catheter (20 to 22 French or Malecot) may be sewn into place in the stomach at first (enterostomy tube goes directly into intestine). After wound has healed, tube may be withdrawn and reinserted p.r.n.

- *Sengstaken-Blakemore tube:* used for compression of bleeding esophageal varicies. *(See NR, Sengstaken-Blakemore tube)*

- Suction: for decompression. It should also be available for the unconscious patient or one in danger of aspirating regurgitated enteral feeding.

    1. Wall suction: a suction device built into the wall at the patient's bedside.

    2. Portable suction machines, (*e.g.,* Gompco) in most cases provide intermittent suction at "high" and "low" settings.

- Pump for volumetric or drop administration, required for some enteral formulas.
- For enteral feedings:
  1. An administration set (manufactured or improvised), with an IV pole for continuous feeding.
  2. 50-ml syringe and a cup of water for intermittent feeding.
  3. Formula containing balanced nutritional elements and electrolytes appropriate to patient's needs (*e.g.*, Isocal, Ensure Plus, Vivonex).

Nursing Tips

- Check your agency procedure book for step-by-step instructions regarding these procedures. The following are tips on how to make them work.
- Check level of fluid drainage in bottle at beginning of each shift.

Inserting the Tube

- Place patient in high Fowler's position, unless contraindicated.
- Measure distance between bridge of nose and earlobe plus distance from earlobe to tip of xiphoid process, and mark tube with tape. This represents the approximate distance the tube should be inserted for placement in the stomach.
- Choose the nostril with greatest air flow, unless you are changing tubing (when you will use the other naris). When tube is passed through the mouth (the last choice), patient's dentures must be removed.
- Curve the end of the tube by curling it around your finger. With patient's head back against the pillow, insert the tube, trying to point the end downward towards the ear. Once past the back of the nasopharynx (where there may be slight resistance), pause; have patient bring his head forward; rotate tube 180° and advance it down the esophagus as the patient swallows sips of water or sucks in air through a straw.
- Check with flashlight that tube is advancing correctly. Unusual discomfort or unusual resistance during insertion may indicate that tube is curled up in the back of the throat.
- Excessive coughing, cyanosis, or the patient's inability to talk during the insertion of the tube are signs that the tube has gone through the vocal cords and is in the trachea. Withdraw it.

Checking the Placement of the Tube in the Stomach

- Check immediately upon insertion of tube, before each intermittent gavage feeding, and at least every 4 hours when patient is on continuous enteral feeding.

1. Inject 10 cc of air while auscultating over the stomach. If placement is correct, you will hear a "swoosh" sound.
2. Aspirate stomach contents. If nothing is aspirated and there are no other signs suggesting that tube is in respiratory tree, advance the tube a little and attempt to aspirate again.

Taping the Tube
- Never tape tube to the forehead. Pressure on the naris can cause tissue necrosis. Use hypoallergenic tape to secure tube as shown in Figure 3-6. Attach end of tube (if it is free), to patient's gown with rubber band and safety pin.
- Long tubes used for intestinal decompression are *never* taped while they are being advanced.

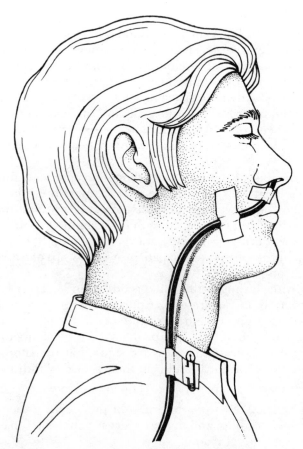

FIG. 3-6. *Method for taping nasogastric tube.*

Gastric Analysis

- Specimens are taken of stomach contents. Procedure is prescribed by the physician, depending upon diagnostic needs.

Lavage

- To wash out the stomach, fluid (usually water or normal saline) is repeatedly introduced and aspirated.
- Iced lavage: to remove clots and to reduce and stop gastric bleeding by constricting blood vessels of the stomach by chilling.
  1. The physician will order the specifics.
  2. Gastric tube will be passed into the stomach.
     a. Large size (36 to 40 F) may be passed orally.
     b. A double-lumen gastric tube provides for more rapid continuous lavage. Iced solution is fed through smaller tube; suction is attached to larger port. Bag within a bag (one for ice and one for solution) may be used for delivery of iced solution.
  3. If single-lumen gastric tube is used, instill at least 200 ml of cold solution (iced saline or water), and allow it to remain in the stomach for 1 to 2 minutes. Then aspirate.
  4. Manual irrigation will remove clots more effectively than intermittent suction. Note and record the amount, color, and consistency of aspirated fluid.
  5. Monitor patient's vital signs.
  6. Keep patient warm during the procedure.

The Long Tube: Intestinal Intubation for Decompression of the Intestines

(See SS, Obstruction of the GI tract)

- Position patient on his right side to facilitate tube's passage through the pylorus, with specific changes of position ordered after x-ray confirms that tube has passed into the small intestine. Ambulation may then be encouraged.
- Advance tube 2 to 4 inches at a time according to physician's order. Slow advance decreases possibility of kinks.
- *Never* tape tubing until it has reached its destination.
- Attachment of tubing to suction as it advances or after it reaches the obstruction may be ordered.
- If irrigation of tube is ordered, irrigating fluid may be difficult to aspirate. Irrigating fluid which goes in is counted as intake. All drainage, including what is aspirated, is counted as output. Observe and record character and color of drainage, as well as amount.
- Mouth care is essential. An antibiotic mouthwash may be ordered.

Removal of Gastrointestinal Tubes

- Clamp tube to prevent aspiration of drainage.
- Nasogastric tube is pulled out in one continuous, moderately rapid motion with patient exhaling slowly and deep breathing.
- Intestinal tube is withdrawn slowly. Patient may feel nauseated. Deep breathing may be helpful.
  1. Weighted tip may be brought out through patient's mouth for removal. The rest will be pulled out through the nose.
  2. Tube may have a fecal odor. Give mouth care immediately.
  3. If tube has passed through the ileocecal valve, tube may be allowed to pass out through the rectum.

Keeping the Tube Open

- Vomiting around the n.g. tube, unrelieved gastric distention, and no drainage are signs that suction is not functioning properly.
  1. Repositioning the patient may help by moving tube's sucking ports away from stomach or intestinal wall.
  2. Check suction mechanism by disconnecting the tube and testing to see whether water can be sucked up. If it cannot, replace suction machine.
  3. Milk n.g. tube toward the machine, then check its patency by gentle aspiration. Irrigation with 30m of normal saline, if ordered, may open the tube. What goes in is counted as intake, what is aspirated, as output.

Relieving Discomforts of Intubation

- Dry lips and mouth, sore throat, hoarseness, earaché, and dry nose are common complaints. Relieve them with lip pomade, Vaseline applied to lips and nose, gargles, throat sprays, lozenges, and antibiotic mouthwashes, p.r.n. and as ordered. Try to prevent parotitis (surgical mumps) by giving excellent regular mouth care.

Gavage (Enteral Feeding)

- Elevate the head of the bed at least 30° during and for an hour following gavage feeding, if not contraindicated for other reasons.
- Check placement of the tube before every intermittent feeding and every 4 hours with continuous feeding.
- Check for residual during continuous feedings by aspirating every 2 to 4 hours. Residual over 150 ml is considered evidence of delayed gastric emptying; the rate should be slowed, and the physician should be notified. Aspirated residual should be slowly refed.
- Never attempt to catch up on volume. Retape bottle with new times when necessary.

- Restrain the hands of the restless or disoriented patient to prevent his removing the n.g. tube.
- Intermittent enteral feeding:
  1. Administer slowly by gravity, taking 15 to 20 minutes for 250 ml of formula, followed by 50 ml of water. Feeding should be at room temperature.
  2. Too-rapid administration may cause diarrhea and other gastrointestinal symptoms.
- Continuous enteral feeding:
  1. Infusion rate should be consistent. Check q. 30 min if being administered by gravity, every hour if by pump.
  2. Delivery sets vary in terms of delivery of gtt/ml. Check tubing package. Label tubing with gtt/ml delivered by this set.
  3. Calculate gtt/min as with intravenous sets.

$$\frac{\text{gtt/ml}}{60 \text{ min/hr}} \times \text{ml/hr} = \text{gtt/min}$$

Example problem:
> Physician's order: Continuous gavage feeding at 75 ml/hr. Delivery set delivers approximately 20 gtt/ml.

$$\frac{20}{60} \times 75 = 25 \text{ gtt/min}$$

  2. Do not hang more than a 4-hour supply at one time.

Recognize and Attempt to Prevent Complications

- Metabolic disturbances because of the high glucose content of many formulas may cause
  1. Diarrhea, nausea, dehydration
  2. Glucosuria with diuresis
  3. Hyperosmolar, hyperglycemic, nonketotic coma preceded by symptoms of lethargy, thirst, glucosuria, and polyuria.
- Slowed infusion rates may help, but antidiarrheal agents (*e.g.,* Lomotil, paregoric) may be ordered. *(See PH)*
- Diabetic patients and those on steroid therapy require special observation for glucose intolerance.
- Urine should be checked for sugar q 4 to 6 hours in patients with symptoms of glucose intolerance. *(See LAB)*
- Blood glucose should be checked periodically for patients with glucosuria. Insulin may be ordered. *(See LAB and PH)*
- Aspiration pneumonia:
  1. To avoid aspiration of regurgitated formula, have suction equipment at the bedside of unconscious or semiconscious patients. Suction p.r.n.

2. Interrupt continuous feedings while patient is receiving other treatments (*e.g.*, respiratory therapy). Resume feeding 30 minutes later.
3. Gastrostomy and enterostomy feeding are being used in some cases both for patient comfort and in the attempt to avoid this common complication of gavage feeding.

- Monitor for electrolyte imbalances. *(See LAB)*
- Watch for gastric distention; prevent it by periodically aspirating for residual (see above).

Administration of Medications Through the Nasogastric Tube

- Liquid medications or non–enteric-coated tablets (crushed) mixed with a small amount of water may be given by n.g. tube, using the same precautions as with enteral feedings. Always follow by injecting 30 ml of water.
- Discontinue suction, if it is being used, for 30 minutes after administration of medication, so that it can be absorbed.

HYPOTHERMIA BLANKET

Description

A hypothermia blanket is made from rubber or plastic. A cooled solution of alcohol and water circulates in coils within the blanket. The blanket is attached to a refrigeration machine which is set, by physician's order, at the body temperature to be maintained. A rectal probe connects to the machine and indicates on a control panel a continuous body temperature reading. Hypothermia blankets are used to reduce prolonged, highly elevated body temperatures. The blanket is usually placed under the patient; however, two blankets may be used, with one covering the patient.

Starting and Maintaining the Hypothermia Blanket Procedure

- Bathe and oil the patient's skin before using the blanket. During hypothermia blanket use, baths are not given; however, the skin should be kept well-oiled during the procedure.
- Prior to using the blanket, an IV or n.g. tube should be in place. These patients will be n.p.o. Also, an indwelling urinary catheter should be inserted and a cleansing enema given prior to the hypothermia procedure.
- Wrap or pad areas of pressure (*e.g.*, heels, elbows, and sacrum) to prevent tissue breakdown.
- Secure rectal probe with paper tape.
- Take baseline vital signs prior to starting the procedure.
- Read the manufacturer's directions for proper use of the machine.

- Set the machine at the temperature to be maintained. Check for correct placement of the rectal probe every hour. Take a rectal temperature with another thermometer every 2 hours to verify the rectal probe's accuracy.
- Shivering must be avoided because it increases metabolism and prolongs the time necessary to decrease temperature. Chlorpromazine hydrochloride (Thorazine) *(see PH, Psychotrophics, major tranquilizers)* is often given to prevent shivering.
- Turn the patient every hour and check the skin for areas of irritation.
- BP, pulse, and respirations must be taken every 2 hours. Heart rate, respirations, and urinary output decrease during hypothermia. Cardiac irregularities and respiratory depression may develop at low body temperatures.
- Hypothermia blankets may be in use for several days. When they are removed, continue to check the temperature every 2 hours until it stabilizes.

INTRAVENOUS THERAPY

Description

Intravenous administration is necessary when taking fluids by mouth is impractical or contraindicated, or when direct access to the blood stream is required. The type, amount, and flow rate of IV fluid and electrolyte replacement is determined in accordance with the physical needs of the patient. It is very important to maintain the prescribed flow rates to prevent fluid and electrolyte imbalances. An IV may also be used to provide quick vein access for emergency medication administration. The solution commonly used for the KVO (keep vein open) IV is D_5W (5% dextrose in water). The KVO delivery rate is 50 ml or less per hour, depending on the cardiac or renal status of the patient.

Starting and Maintaining the IV

- Thorough handwashing before this procedure is required to prevent infection. The use of an antiseptic hand cleaner is recommended.
- Preoperative IVs should always be started with a #19 needle or catheter in case a blood transfusion in necessary.
- Use a microdrip or pediatric drip set for KVO IVs (60 gtt = 1 ml).
- Solutions are ordered by the physician in ml per hour, but the nurse regulates the flow rates in drops (gtt) per minute. The formula needed to convert from ml/hr to gtt/min is

$$\text{gtt/min (flow rate)} = \text{gtt/ml (from calibration of set)} \times \frac{\text{ml/hr}}{60}$$

- Size of drop varies according to the calibration of the set. Standard or macrodrip sets are calibrated so that 10 gtt = 1 ml, 15 gtt = 1 ml, or 20 gtt = 1 ml. Microdrip or pediatric drip sets are calibrated at 60 gtt = 1 ml. This information is found on the package of the IV tubing.
- Fill the drip chamber half full before opening and priming the tubing. This will elminate air bubbles.
- Always maintain a primary IV line into which an additive line (*e.g.,* piggyback tubing) may be connected.
- Infusion pumps should be used when the IV flow rates are extremely critical (*e.g.,* in hyperalimentation or with heparin or theophylline). Check the pumps every 30 minutes.
- If the present container of IV solution contains less than 50 ml at the change of shift, replace with a full container prior to shift change.
- Every 24 hours the IV site dressing must be changed and ointment applied to the insertion site. The IV tubing should be changed every 48 hours. Both dressing and tubing must be marked with date and initials.
- Intravenous tubing often becomes permanently compressed by the mechanism in infusion pumps, and the flow stops. To prevent this, change the tubing every 12 hours.
- The smallest possible container of IV fluid should be used to maintain a KVO IV. It must be discarded and a new container must be hung every 24 hours.

The IV Site

- It is standard practice to use arm veins; IVs in the lower extremities have a high risk of thromboembolism. When possible, start IVs in hand veins that are satisfactory for KVO IVs. Use the larger veins above the hand for rapid infusions, blood, or medications that are going to be regularly added by piggyback. The antecubital vein should be saved for routine blood work.
- Wrapping the arm with warm towels for 15 to 20 minutes is helpful in raising veins. Holding the arm below the heart level also helps identify veins.
- Seventy-two hours is considered the maximum time a needle may be in a vein without an increased incidence of infection and phlebitis. Metal needles should be changed every 48 hours, and plastic over-the-needle catheters should be changed every 72 hours, or as recommended by hospital policy.
- After withdrawing an IV needle or catheter, apply pressure with a sterile pad to stop the bleeding. If the patient has been on anticoagulants, the bleeding may not stop immediately.

Factors Disturbing the Flow Rate

- The IV container should be at least 3 feet above insertion.
- When a clot occurs in a needle or catheter, *gently* irrigate with normal saline. If resistance is met, discontinue and start a new IV
- If the needle or catheter position has changed, remove the dressing, gently realign it into the vein, and retape.
- Check for infiltration by applying a tourniquet above the insertion site. If the needle is in the vein, the IV will stop.
- Ambulatory patients should be instructed to keep the IV arm at waist level to prevent blood from backing up in the tubing. If blood does appear, increase the flow rate for a minute to flush it through.
- Blood appearing in the tubing, a wet IV dressing (infiltration or detached needle), pain at or above the insertion site, and coldness, swelling, or redness in the arm are indicators of a disturbed flow rate. Instruct patients to alert a nurse if these symptoms occur.
- Patients may cause the IV to malfunction by handling the tubing. This is especially true of disoriented patients.

Precautions When Medications Are Used in IVs

- Check patient's allergies before giving or starting any IV medication. Watch carefully for reaction during the first 15 minutes of any infusion.
- Always check with a pharmacist before adding anything to an IV solution if there is a question about it's compatibility with the solution. For instance, diazepam (Valium) *(see PH, Psychotrophics, minor tranquilizers)* and phenytoin sodium (Dilantin) *(see PH, central nervous system, anticonvulsants)* are *never* given in an IV solution, only as an IV bolus.
- Know the rate of infusion for medications by piggyback. In most cases a delivery rate of 100 ml per hour is well tolerated for piggyback medications in a volume of 50 to 100 ml. However, some antibiotics are particularly irritating, *e.g.,* penicillin, erythromycin, and the tetracyclines *(see PH, antimicrobials)*. They must be more dilute to be comfortably administered.
- When medications need to be added to an IV container, be sure to rotate the container to thoroughly mix the solution. Attach a label with the name and amount of additives. Avoid adding medications to hanging IV containers: use a new container.

Complications of IV Therapy

- Infections may result from skin bacteria entering at the insertion site because of poor aseptic technique. When a patient develops signs and symptoms of sudden systemic infection (*e.g.,* chills, fever, nausea) while receiving an IV, discontinue the IV and send tubing, needle, and container to the lab for examination. This also applies when an infection appears at the IV site (*e.g.*, purulent drainage).

- Speed shock may occur as a result of too-rapid administration of drugs.
- Circulatory overload occurs with too-rapid infusion. This may result in congestive heart failure or pulmonary edema. Be alert for shortness of breath (SOB), coughing, rales, dilation of neck veins, and decreased urine output in comparison to fluid intake.

HYPERALIMENTATION THERAPY
Description

- Hyperalimentation therapy, also called total parenteral nutrition (TPN), provides necessary calories, amino acids, and electrolytes in small volume. The solutions, designed to meet the patient's requirements, are prepared by pharmacists according to a physician's prescription. They must be kept refrigerated until used. These solutions are highly concentrated, requiring the use of a large-size catheter or needle inserted into a large vein. The subclavian or internal jugular is generally used. A chest x-ray is necessary to ascertain proper catheter placement before TPN solution is administered.

Nursing Tips

- The risk of sepsis is high, and nothing other than the TPN solution should be run into the IV line.
- An IV pump must be used for delivery of TPN. Microdrop or pediatric sets are often not suitable for these viscous solutions. Check the pump every 30 minutes.
- The TPN tubing and dressing must be changed every 48 hours using strict sterile technique. Refer to individual institution's procedure book concerning technique for and frequency of filter and tubing change.
- TPN can provide about 1000 calories per container. Metabolic and electrolyte abnormalities may occur. Hypoglycemia can result from the abrupt cessation of hyperalimentation.
- Patients receiving TPN must have their temperature taken and their fractional urines tested for glucose, acetone, and specific gravity every 6 hours. Insulin coverage is usually ordered for 1% or 2% urine glucose (*see LAB, Urine specimens*). Daily weights done at the same time each day and intake and output (I and O) are extremely important.
- Check infusion site once each shift for signs of leaking, swelling of the neck, hand, or face, and distention of neck or arm veins. Report any of the above to the physician.

- Hyperglycemia may be present as the body adjusts to the high glucose content of the TPN solution even though insulin is included in the solution.
- TPN solutions are prepared to be given in sequence. Never speed up or slow down the delivery rate or change the sequence without an order.
- A complication of long-term TPN is a decrease in fatty acids. Thus fat emulsions (*e.g.,* Intralipid) may be required 1 to 2 times weekly. There are 550 calories in 500 ml. These may be given in peripheral veins. Again, this line must not be used for any other solution. Use the tubing that comes with the solution. Do not use a filter.
- The initial flow rate for administering fat emulsions is 1 ml/min for 30 minutes, then proceed as ordered. Observe closely in the first 30 minutes for allergic reactions.

INTRAVENOUS FLUIDS

The various kinds of IV fluids, their actions, and important considerations in their administration are listed in Table 3-1.

Nursing Tips

- Isotonic (iso-osmotic) IV solutions do not cause fluid to be drawn out of or into blood cells. A common isotonic solution is normal saline (0.9% sodium chloride).
- Hypotonic (hypo-osmotic) IV solutions cause blood cells to draw fluid inward and may cause them to burst (lyse). Hypotonic IV solutions can also cause fluid to move from the plasma to interstitial space. One-half normal saline (0.45% sodium chloride) is a common hypotonic solution.
- Hypertonic (hyperosmotic) IV solutions draw fluid out of blood cells. They can also cause fluid to move into the plasma from interstitial space. Dextrose 10% in Water ($D_{10}W$) is an example of a hypertonic solution.

TABLE 3–1. **Intravenous Fluids**

Fluid	Action	Comments
Dextrose in water		
5%	Replaces fluid Provides calories	170 calories per liter
10%	Replaces fluid Provides calories	Irritating to peripheral veins. Dextrose concentrations higher than 10% should not, in general, be given in peripheral veins

(Continued)

TABLE 3–1. **Intravenous Fluids** *(Continued)*

Fluid	Action	Comments
50% as a 50ml bolus	Corrects hypoglycemia Osmotic diuretic	Given over a period of 5 minutes
Sodium chloride 0.9% (normal saline)	Isotonic fluid replacement Corrects mild sodium depletion (used to precede a blood transfusion)	Use with caution in patients with CHF, or poor renal function
0.45% sodium chloride (½ normal saline)	Replaces fluid without large amount of sodium	Used most often in diabetic ketoacidosis
3% or 5% sodium chloride (hypertonic)	Used to correct severe hyponatremia	May cause death if too much is administered. Always be sure of order before administering
Dextrose/Saline combinations, *e.g.*, $D_5\frac{1}{2}NS$, D_5NS, $D_5\frac{1}{4}NS$, $D_5\frac{1}{3}NS$	Replaces fluid Dextrose provides calories	
Lactated ringers (Hartman's solution) Contains sodium, chloride, potassium, calcium, lactate, and water	Balanced electrolyte solution, roughly equivalent to electrolyte concentration of potassium, calcium, sodium, and chloride in the plasma. Lactate is a bicarbonate precursor in persons with normal blood perfusion and normal liver function	Can cause lactic acidosis in patients with poor perfusion (*i.e.*, shock) or liver disease
Ringers solution	Higher concentrations of sodium and chloride than Lactated Ringers	Useful for patients with poor perfusion (*i.e.*, shock) or during surgery
Balanced electrolyte solutions (*e.g.*, Ionosol, Isolyte-M)	Replaces fluids with approximately the normal serum electrolyte concentrations	These solutions have a fixed electrolyte concentration, which does not allow for individual variations.
Amino acids (*e.g.*, Amigen, Aminosol)	Provides amino acids and calories for patients unable to eat or drink	May be given peripherally.
Hyperalimentation solution	Depending upon the formulation, can provide approximately 1000 calories per liter for patients who are unable to eat or drink or who have an absorption deficiency	May cause severe metabolic and electrolyte imbalances. Solutions must be given in proper sequence as provided by pharmacy. Urine test for sugar, acetone, and specific gravity every 6 hours because of high glucose content of fluid.

(Continued)

TABLE 3–1. **Intravenous Fluids** (Continued)

Fluid	Action	Comments
Hyperalimentation solution (Continued)		*Do not add anything to bottle or piggyback into the same line without checking hospital policy.*
Fat emulsion	Concentrated amount of calories in small volume, 500ml = 550 calories. Often given as adjunct to hyperalimentation because these solutions are deficient in fatty acids	Don't use a filter. Run at 1 ml per minute for the first 30 minutes to check for reaction (*e.g.*, nausea or headache). May deliver 500ml in 4 to 6 hours. A peripheral vein may be used. Do not add anything to the solution or piggyback into the IV line
Human serum albumin 5% iso-osmotic to plasma 25% hyperosmotic to plasma	Both solutions are used as plasma expanders. The osmotic pressure of the 25% solution will rapidly pull fluid into the bloodstream from surrounding interstitial space at a rate 3% times the amount infused in 15 min, causing hemodilution and diuresis in a hydrated patient with normal renal function The 25% solution is useful in patients whose fluid and sodium intake must be kept low.	The 5% solution is administered at a rate of 2 to 4ml/min, the 25% solution at 1ml/min. They may however be administered very rapidly in cases of hypovolemic shock. Monitor blood pressure. Watch for signs of circulatory overload (*e.g.*, SOB, chest pain.) *Note:* Salt-Poor Albumin is a misnomer used for 25% Human Serum Albumin: the sodium content is approximately equivalent to that of blood.
Plasmanate 5% iso-osmotic to plasma	Same actions as 5% albumin	Rapid infusion (greater than 10 ml/min) may cause hypotention and also vascular overload. Watch for chest pain and shortness of breath
Dextran	Synthetic plasma expander (crossmatching of blood must be done prior to administration of dextran)	Watch for allergic reactions. Start at 1 ml per minute
Hetastarch (Volex, Hespan)	Synthetic volume expander	Does not interfere with blood typing. Causes fewer allergic reactions than dextran
Mannitol	Osmotic diuretic	Do not give if crystals are present in the solution. Use a filter

BLOOD AND BLOOD COMPONENT TRANSFUSION

Description

Blood transfusions are commonly used to replace blood losses or to correct an anemic condition. Blood is typed (A, B, AB, or O) and is further classified as Rh positive or negative. Blood is ordinarily obtainable as whole stored blood, as fresh whole blood, or as packed red blood cells (PBCs), which is whole blood that has 80% of the liquid plasma removed. Whole blood (stored or fresh) is given in cases of sudden and excessive blood loss because it restores volume. Whole blood may be stored in blood banks for up to 35 days, but stored blood has diminished clotting ability. Fresh whole blood is particularly useful in cases of massive hemorrhage because fresh blood contains necessary clotting factors. Fresh blood must be used immediately. PBCs are commonly given to correct anemia. PBCs may be frozen and stored for up to 3 years.

Starting and Maintaining the Transfusion

- Blood transfusions require meticulous attention to detail. Death may result if the infused blood does not match the patient's blood. Therefore, two nurses together must verify the patient's name by checking his wristband and asking his name. Also, they must double check the number on the lab slip, which must match the number on the container. The Rh and blood type on the lab slip must also match that on the blood container. If there is any question, return the blood to the lab for investigation.
- Vital signs including temperature must be taken before, during, and after a transfusion.
- Start the IV with a #19 needle or catheter and with normal saline infusing through blood administration tubing before the blood is obtained from the blood bank.
- The blood must be hung (transfusion started) immediately.
- Blood and blood-product transfusions should be started at 2 ml/min (20 qtt/min) for the first 15 minutes. This is the period when the most serious reactions are most likely to occur.
- Stop the blood immediately with *any* reaction. Reactions to blood transfusions produce a variety of systemic reactions: fever, chills, back pain, pruritus (itching), or urticaria. Notify the physician and change the tubing, keeping the vein open with normal saline. Follow individual hospital procedure with any blood reaction.
- For those patients who are susceptible to congestive heart failure, infusion time is lengthened up to four hours. Check those patients frequently for signs of fluid overload, *e.g.*, coughing, SOB, rales, or jugular vein distention (JVD). *(See SS, Cardiovascular, congestive heart failure, pulmonary edema)*

- Slow rates of infusion may cause the blood to stop running. If this happens, clamp the blood tubing, and run saline through it for a minute before restarting the blood. Do not repeat this more than twice because it increases the sodium intake.
- The infusion of blood should always be completed within 4 hours because of the possibility of bacterial proliferation and RBC hemolysis occurring at room temperature.
- Whole blood infusion rate is adjusted to the patient's need for blood replacement. PBCs are commonly packaged in 250 ml containers, and this may be infused in 1½ to 2 hours.
- Never add any medications to the infusing blood or the IV line.
- The IV tubing used to transfuse blood should be changed after two units are infused.
- A blood warmer is occasionally used for some patients who have antibodies that react to red blood cells at low temperatures.
- Blood pumping devices are occasionally used when blood needs to be transfused rapidly. Watch these patients extremely carefully for signs of congestive heart failure or infiltration from vein blowout at the needle site.
- Plasma, albumin and dextran are volume expanders and may be given in emergencies until blood is available. They do not need typing and crossmatching.
- Plasma in 250 ml units is infused as rapidly as desired. A "Y" blood transfusion set is used, and normal saline may be run between units of plasma. Albumin comes with special tubing for its infusion, due to the high viscosity. The rate of infusion is 1 ml/min unless otherwise ordered.
- Dextran may cause a reaction, so infusion rate should be 1 ml/min for the first 15 minutes.
- Platelets must be given as soon as they become available because of their short life span. A special platelet transfusion set is used. Depending on the patient, they can be administered as rapidly as 1 to 2 minutes per unit (50 ml to 75 ml).

ELECTROLYTE IMBALANCES

Description

Electrolyte imbalance may result from insufficient or inappropriate fluid intake or from excessive loss of body fluids through perspiration, vomiting, diarrhea, gastrointestinal suctioning, and too-frequent enemas. Diuretic and steroid therapy, as well as severe trauma, chronic blood loss, and long-term immobilization cause losses and abnormal redistribution of electrolytes (see Table 3-2).

TABLE 3-2. **Electrolyte Imbalance**

Electrolyte	Causes	Symptom
Sodium hypernatremia (high sodium, above 145 mEq/L)	Renal impairment Diarrhea Decreased water intake Excessive sweating Fever	Increased temperature Flushed skin Oliguria Thirst Delirium
Sodium hyponatremia (low sodium, below 135 mEq/L)	Water intoxication Repeated use of tap water enemas Pancreatic fistulas Gastric suctioning Vomiting	Confusion Anorexia Diarrhea Seizures
Potassium hyperkalemia (high potassium, above 5 mEq/L)	Renal failure High intake of potassium Massive tissue injury, *e.g.*, burns, trauma Rapid transfusion of stored blood	Intestinal colic Muscle weakness Cardiac arrythmias
Potassium hypokalemia (low potassium, below 3.4 mEq/L)	Loss with diuretics IV replacement fluids without potassium Vomiting and diarrhea and prolonged gastric suctioning Excessive dieting	Muscle weakness Cardiac arrythmias Anorexia
Calcium hypercalcemia (high calcium, above 10.7 mg/100 ml)	Prolonged bedrest or confinement to a wheelchair Hyperparathyroidism Excessive milk intake and vitamin D	Bone pain Calcium deposit in kidney forming stones Decreased tendon reflexes Cardiac arrythmias Hypercalcemic crisis Intractable nausea and vomiting Coma
Calcium hypocalcemia (low calcium, below 8.6 mg/100 ml)	Intestinal malabsorption Hypoparathyroidism Burns Inadequate dietary intake	Abdominal and muscle cramps Osteoporosis Tetany
Magnesium hypermagnesemia (high magnesium, above 2.1 mEq/l)	Epsom salt overdose Severe renal disease	Slowed heart conduction Hypotension Lethargy
Magnesium hypomagnesemia (low magnesium, below 1.3 mEq/l)	Malabsorption syndrome Chronic alcoholism Enterostomy drainage Vomiting and diarrhea Prolonged gastric suctioning	Disorientation Tremors Cardiac arrythmias Hyperactive reflexes

(Continued)

TABLE 3-2. **Electrolyte Imbalance** (Continued)

Electrolyte	Causes	Symptom
Chloride hyperchloremia (high chloride, above 109 mEq/l)	Excessive intake of ammonium chloride	Metabolic acidosis
Chloride hypochloremia (low chloride, below 95 mEq/l)	Loss from prolonged n.g. suctioning without chloride replacement	Metabolic alkalosis, *e.g.,* weakness, tetany, and decreased respirations. Hypokalemia accompanies metabolic alkalosis
High bicarbonate (above 33 mEq/l)	Loss of acid by vomiting n.g. suction, draining fistula Too much bicarbonate of soda or other antacids	Metabolic alkalosis with accompanying hypokalemia, tetany, depressed respirations
Low bicarbonate (below 20 mEq/l)	Diabetic acidosis Chronic kidney failure Starvation	Metabolic acidosis, *e.g.,* deep rapid breathing, weakness, stupor

Nursing Tips

- Check recent electrolyte levels on any patient who has behavioral or physical changes.
- The unit to describe electrolyte chemical activity is called a milliequivalent (mEq), expressed per liter. Be extremely careful in transcribing "mEq" so it does not appear as "mgm."
- Potassium levels below 3.5 or above 5.6 mEq/liter can be life threatening, and the physician must be notified immediately.
- Preoperative requirements for electrolyte levels, especially potassium, vary with institutions. Know what they are so corrective measures may be ordered as necessary.

ISOLATION TECHNIQUE

Description

Isolation technique prevents the spread of communicable disease among patients, hospital personnel, and visitors. The Joint Commission on Accreditation of Hospitals requires all accredited acute care institutions to have an infection control program, implemented by an infection control committee. Information on establishing and maintaining isolation technique must be available on each patient care unit. The card system of isolation is commonly used. Five categories of isolation—strict, respiratory, protective, enteric, and wound and skin—are individually printed on a card. The front of the card lists the type and essential requirements pertaining to a private room, gown, mask, hand care, gloves, and care of articles. The back of the card lists diseases or conditions requiring that particular type of isolation. The card specific to the isolation needed is placed on the patient's bed or door. It may also be put on the front of the patient's chart.

Nursing Tips

- Remember, isolation is for the disease. These patients are often very sensitive about being considered contaminated.
- When conditions appear to warrant isolation, the physician should be contacted. In the event this is not possible, notify the infection control nurse. It is better to "over isolate" than to "under isolate."
- Handwashing is the most important method of preventing nosocomial (hospital acquired) infections. Handwashing should be done before significant contact with any patient, and after contact with any excretions or secretions. Vigorous scrubbing with soap and water for at least 15 seconds followed by thorough rinsing constitutes proper handwashing. The faucet should be turned off with a clean paper towel. The use of an antiseptic hand cleaner is recommended before inserting an IV or urinary catheter.
- Common sources of nosocomial infections are urinary and IV catheters and inhalation therapy equipment.
- Gowns, masks, and gloves must be used only once. Gloves must be changed after contact with secretions and excretions even if patient care is not completed.
- All wounds with excessive purulent drainage should be dressed using one pair of gloves to remove soiled dressings and another pair to apply the new dressing.
- Specimens sent to the laboratory must be clearly labeled "isolation."
- When culture reports are used as a criteria for discontinuing isolation, the negative cultures must be specimens obtained after antibiotic therapy has been terminated.

LIVER BIOPSY

Description

Under local anesthesia, aspiration of liver tissue is usually done at the patient's bedside by closed-needle biopsy. Liver biopsy is also done frequently during peritonoscopy (see NR, Endoscopic procedures). With either method, the chief danger is hemorrhage.

Nursing Tips

- Written permission (informed consent) is usually required.

- Typing and crossmatching is frequently done.
- "n.p.o. after midnight" is frequently ordered preceding biopsy.
- In closed-needle biopsy, position patient on his left side with right arm elevated, or in the supine position (lying on this back), according to the physician's preference. Patient holds his breath during insertion of needle and until it is removed.
- Vital signs are taken preceding the procedure and q.15 min until stable, q.4 hr for first 12 hours.
- Reposition patient on his right side with pillow under the costal margin, a position to be maintained for several hours. Bed rest for 24 hours.
- Observe for signs of complications: hemorrhage, shock, peritonitis, pneumothorax.
  (See SS, Postoperative care, hemorrhage, shock, peritonitis)
  (See SS, Respiratory, pneumothorax)

NASOPHARYNGEAL OR OROPHARYNGEAL SUCTIONING

Description

Suctioning of the nose, mouth, and throat is done to clear and maintain an open airway. Ideally, the objective is to stimulate coughing so the patient may naturally clear the airway.

Nursing Tips

- When there is suspected cerebrospinal fluid discharge from the nose or when there is a bleeding disorder, do *not* do nasopharyngeal suctioning.
- Suction as needed, never routinely, because suctioning is traumatic and tends to stimulate the production of secretions.
- Position the patient at a 45° angle.
- Before suctioning, hyperinflate the patient with a self-inflating bag (*e.g.*, Ambubag), which may be connected to an oxygen source. This aids in stimulating coughing. Hyperventilate the patient after each suctioning.
- Suctioning is always a sterile procedure. Separate sterile suction catheters must be used for the nose and mouth and then are discarded. Catheters may be rinsed during the procedure with sterile water. Dispose of remaining water after each suctioning.
- If the patient is conscious, explain the necessity of the procedure. Lubricate the catheter, a size 14 or 16, with sterile water, and insert it 3 to 5 inches into a nostril. Ask the patient to take deep breaths and cough. This aids in allowing the catheter insertion into the pharynx.

- If the patient is unconscious, grasp the tongue and hold it out of the mouth for ease in passing catheter from nose to throat.
- *Never* apply suction while inserting the catheter. Suction while withdrawing and gently rotating the catheter.
- Suctioning should never exceed 8 to 10 seconds. The setting on wall suction should not exceed 60 to 80 mmHg.
- Prolonged suctioning may result in a slow and irregular heart rate.
- Oropharyngeal suctioning may be impossible if patient bites the tube.
- Suction bottles should be emptied and cleaned every 12 hours.

OSTOMIES, FISTULAS, AND DRAINING WOUNDS

Description

Ostomies, fistulas (abnormal passageways from a normal cavity to another or to the skin), and draining wounds present the patient and the nurse with an unnatural situation in which material from internal organs discharges directly onto the skin. Drainage from the upper gastrointestinal tract is especially irritating to the skin because of its high enzyme content. Ostomies are created in an attempt to improve upon a pathological condition; they may be temporary or permanent. The goal of treatment is the closure of fistulas and draining wounds. These conditions are being considered together because of the commonalities of their nursing care: protection of the skin around the opening, collection of drainage, prevention of odors, and emotional support for the patient. Nursing tips for the care of stomas are adaptable to that of fistulas and draining wounds.

Equipment

Many products are on the market. Select equipment with individual patient's needs in mind. Read accompanying printed material for specifics about each product. The following will provide general guidelines (see Fig. 3-7).

- *Pouches or appliances*
  1. Disposable or temporary: pouch with faceplate with adhesive backing; used in the hospital; cheap and clean.
  2. Reusable (or permanent): may be one unit (pouch and faceplate), or 2-piece with separate faceplate or disc and pouch; may be used at home after stoma has shrunk to permanent size; pouch may last several months with good care. If patient brings one to the hospital, suggest that he send it home. It is expensive and could be lost. Use of a disposable one during hospitalization also saves the nurses 30 to 40 minutes clean-up time.

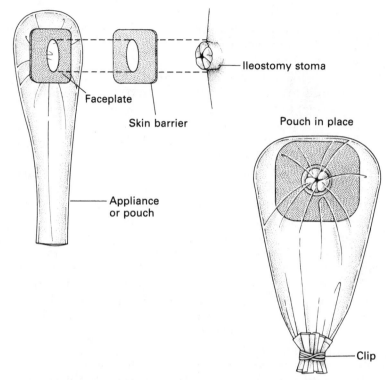

Ileostomy stoma

Faceplate

Skin barrier

Pouch in place

Appliance
or pouch

Clip

FIG. 3-7. *Components of ostomy appliance. The outlet of the punch should be cuffed and doubled back twice. It either should be sealed with a clip or fanfolded and secured with a rubber band.*

3. Pouch adapted to need: may be open-ended drainable; may be closed; may have valve at end to facilitate emptying (for the urinary stoma). Loop colostomies require an extra large pouch at first, selected to fit the gasket. Karaya gasket, cut to fit around the stoma, is applied over a bridge support. The gasket will fit under other types of supports.

4. Adhesive backing of pouch: may have pre-cut opening, or may be cut to fit with $\frac{1}{16}$ of an inch to $\frac{1}{8}$ of an inch clearance around the stoma. Measuring guides are helpful to ensure proper fit, but a pattern may have to be drawn to fit an irregularly shaped stoma. To avoid reversal, place faceplate (or skin barrier) over the pattern as it is fitted around the stoma. Remove both at one time; draw pattern on faceplate (or skin barrier); mark paper with "top" and "right" or "left" side for future use as a pattern; remove paper and apply properly fitted faceplate.

- *Protective skin barriers*
  1. Skin Prep: (a commercial product) coats and protects the skin; apply with spray, brush-on, or Skin Prep wipes.
  2. Karaya: powder, rings, or paste.
     a. Karaya paste comes in prepared form, but when large amounts are needed it can be mixed (karaya powder with glycerine) to the consistency of stiff peanut butter (almost to the point where it can be worked with the hands).
     b. Karaya rings protect skin and have healing qualities; they don't do well with urinary ostomies because urine melts them.
  3. Stomahesive wafers (Squibb): can also be used with urinary ostomy.
  4. ReliaSeal (Davol): can also be used with urinary ostomy.
  5. Tincture of benzoin (plain): wiped on; protects skin.
- *Products for securing appliances*
  1. Adhesive-backed pouches may be attached directly to the skin in some instances.
  2. Skin bond or cement: used for good adherence with some reusable appliances; usually provided by pouch manufacturer. Skin must be dry before application. Cement must be dry before applying pouch to body surface.
  3. Solvents: used to remove cement; must be washed off.
  4. Belts: to support weight of pouch (not hold it).
  5. Hypoallergenic tape: used to "picture frame" the faceplate to the skin for extra security.
  6. Double-faced adhesive discs: may be used instead of cement; usually used with reusable appliance; should be applied over skin barrier.

Nursing Tips

- Patient teaching for the ostomate should begin preoperatively, and should resume as soon after surgery as possible. Mastery of the physical care of the ostomy comes first, and can be introduced in steps appropriate to the patient's condition, readiness, and capability. The goal is acceptance on the part of the patient of the change in his body, and independence in management of the ostomy.
- Gloves are never worn by the nurse in caring for an ostomy.
- Sterile technique is used in dressing draining wounds.
- Montgomery straps facilitate ease of dressing changes in any situation where a wound with copious drainage requires a large dressing. *(See SS, Introduction, Postoperative care, Fig. 5-3)*

Prevention of Leaks Around Appliance

1. Proper fit of appliance is essential. (See above.)
2. Faceplate or skin barrier must be molded smoothly to the skin. Skin should be smooth and taut; this is best accomplished when patient is either standing or reclining. (Concave defects in the skin around the stoma may be filled with karaya paste to provide an even surface for application of the appliance.)
3. When cutting the skin barrier, use the tips of sharp scissors to make the hole in the center, so that it is not bent because that would make a seal more difficult and leakage more likely.
4. A piece can be cut out of karaya rings, and ends brought together for a better fit.
5. *Skin around stoma must be dry* before application of faceplate or skin barrier. A tampon or a 4 × 4 gauze square covered with a medicine cup may be held over stoma to absorb drainage. Fistulas or draining wounds can be packed with sterile gauze. Remove wick or packing when pouch is in place and secure.
6. Have patient lie quietly for 30 minutes after application of pouch so that seal can set.
7. Empty pouch often enough to prevent unnecessary strain on seal by weight of drainage. (Rinse the bag before closing it again). Change pouch often enough to prevent leaks, usually every 2 or 3 days. Leaks cause skin irritation; they may be recognized by the patient by a sensation of burning or itching under the appliance, or by odor coming from it.

For Skin Irritation

● Always wash the skin with soap and water; rinse and dry thoroughly. Depending upon the degree of irritation, one or more of the following approaches will be helpful.
1. A shower, tub bath, and exposure to the air at the time the appliance is changed may be comforting to irritated skin.
2. Weeping skin may be washed with Amphojel or another aluminum hydroxide antacid. It is soothing. Pour off the thin liquid at the top of the bottle, and use the thick, pasty liquid at the bottom. Let dry. Dust with karaya. Spray lightly with Skin Prep (or similar product). Dry and spray again.
3. Karaya powder is an effective skin healer, but the patient should be warned that it will burn. Brush off excess, and add a little extra to oozing areas. Cover with Skin Prep, Tincture of benzoin (plain), or a similar product.
4. Large excoriated areas may be covered by a $\frac{1}{4}$-inch thick appli-

cation of karaya paste (see above), applied with a tongue blade either at one time, or in several layers for quicker drying. "Picture frame" the faceplate of the pouch over the karaya. Any exposed karaya should be covered with paper tape, so that it does not stick to clothing or bedding.

5. Use skin barrier (see above) as second skin. Faceplate is attached to it.

To Control Odors

1. Disposable appliances:
   a. Open-ended: rinse well after emptying; insert deodorant.
   b. Closed-ended: discard after each use.
2. Permanent reusable appliances:
   a. Keep the pouch clean by emptying it as needed and by rinsing with soap and water.
   b. Rotate two or three appliances. Clean with Wisk (household detergent) or specially prepared product. Rinse well and air between uses. Discard if odor lingers.
3. Place Banish, mouthwash, or other deodorizing preparation in pouch.
4. Bismuth subgallate (Devrom) or bismuth subcarbonate p.o. may be ordered to prevent gas formation and odor when gas-forming foods have been eaten. *Caution:* Reversible central nervous system side-effects may occur with prolonged use, so use should be reserved for specific occasions.
5. Release gas by opening pouch in the bath room.
6. Room deodorizers may be helpful. Plan time for colostomy irrigations and similar procedures with consideration for second patient in room.
7. Odors from a necrotic wound may be reduced by cleaning the purulent material with irrigations of sterile solution of $\frac{1}{2}$ normal saline and $\frac{1}{2}$ hydrogen peroxide, and by packing the wound with iodoform gauze, as ordered by the physician.

Colostomy Irrigation

- See hospital procedure book. Cones, the most popular irrigating tip, are easy to use and help avoid accidental perforation of the intestine.

Urinary Ostomies

- Any urinary diversion to the skin, *e.g.,* ileal conduit.
  1. Karaya rings are dissolved by urine. Use instead ReliaSeal or Stomahesive skin barriers, or apply pouch directly to skin. If skin becomes excoriated, karaya powder may be used.

2. Disposable pouches are recommended. If they are not suitable, the build-up of odor and uric acid crystals in a reusable pouch can be controlled by soaking it in a solution of $\frac{1}{4}$ white vinegar to $\frac{3}{4}$ water or a commercial product such as BIZ regularly. Rinse well with cool or cold water. Every other day, while wearing pouch, patient should rinse the pouch and stoma with the vinegar solution for 20 minutes—best done before bedtime—so that solution can be allowed to drain down tubing into night drainage bag.

3. Threads of mucus in the urine of a patient with an ileal conduit are normal, but be alert for signs of urinary tract infection (*e.g.*, foul-smelling urine or pain in the back in the kidney region). Mucus may be dissolved by using a product such as Mucosperse in the pouch.

4. Urostomy bags should be attached with tubing to a drainage bag at the bedside at night.

Sources of Information

- If your hospital has an enterostomal therapist, she is your nearest and most expert source of assistance in your care of patients with ostomies, fistulas, and draining wounds.
- United Ostomy Association, 1111 Wilshire Blvd., Los Angeles, CA, 90017. Telephone: (213) 481–2811. Local branches of the association.
- American Cancer Society, 777 Third Ave. New York, NY, 10017. Local branches of the society.
- Companies that are suppliers of ostomy equipment will do in-service education programs on the use of their products; they offer good written material on their products and on ostomy care.

OXYGEN ADMINISTRATION

Description

Oxygen is a significant component of the air we breathe, and it is essential for sustaining life. When administered artificially it must be handled and considered as a drug, and therefore capable of harm if misused. Oxygen must be administered at the prescribed flow rate, which should be governed by arterial blood gas analysis. Oxygen should be humidified to prevent dryness of the respiratory tract. This humidification substitutes for the natural humidity in normal air. Oxygen is highly combustible, especially when concentrated. Specific precautions need to be taken to avoid open flame or electrical sparks within any area where oxygen is being administered. Oxygen may be administered either by a face mask which covers the nose and mouth or by a nasal tube. In the case of tracheostomy, a "T" tube or special tracheostomy mask is used to introduce the oxygen into the trachea.

Starting and Maintaining Oxygen Therapy
Nasal Prong Method

- The nasal prongs are two small projections that hook onto the nose and direct oxygen into the nostrils.
- Turn the oxygen on at a low flow rate (one liter).
- Insert the prongs in the nose and the tubing over the ears, or secure an elastic strap.
- Turn the oxygen to the prescribed flow rate.
- Sinus pain and sore nostrils often occur due to the direct oxygen flow into the nostrils.

Nasal Catheter Method

- The nasal catheter is a tube that is inserted through one nostril into the throat.
- Measure from the tip of the nose to the earlobe for proper insertion length.
- Turn the oxygen on at a low flow rate (one liter).
- Insert the lubricated catheter into a nasal passage.
- The tip of the catheter should extend to slightly above the uvula.
- Turn the oxygen to the prescribed flow rate.
- Tape the catheter to the nose. Alternate nostrils every 8 hours.
- Check for possible abdominal distention due to oxygen flow to the stomach, which happens if the catheter is advanced too far.

Simple Face Mask

- This mask connects directly to the oxygen-supply tubing.
- Turn the oxygen on at a low flow rate (one liter).
- Explain to the patient that to provide necessary oxygen the mask must be snugly fitted. Exhaled air is expelled through vents in the sides of the mask.
- Turn the oxygen to the prescribed flow rate after the mask is in place.

Partial Rebreathing Mask

- There is a reservoir bag between this mask and the oxygen-supply tubing.
- Turn the oxygen on at a low flow rate (one liter).
- Fill the reservoir bag with oxygen by momentarily closing the opening between the bag and the mask.
- Explain to the patient that the mask must be snugly fitted to provide the necessary oxygen. The reservoir bag should deflate slightly with inspiration.

- Turn the oxygen to the prescribed flow rate after the mask is in place.
- The patient rebreathes approximately 33% of expired air as a result of the reservoir bag. This air still contains a high amount of oxygen.

Nonrebreathing Mask

- This mask is similar to the partial rebreathing mask except that two one-way valves ensure that only the source oxygen is delivered from the bag to the patient. This allows delivery of more concentrated oxygen than with other masks.
- Turn the oxygen on at a low flow rate (one liter).
- Fill the reservoir bag by momentarily closing the one-way valve between the mask and the bag.
- Explain to the patient that the mask must fit well.
- The one-way valves prevent the rebreathing of exhaled air. Be sure the oxygen-delivery tubing is not obstructed. This is the only effective way the patient can receive any oxygen because outside air is shut off by the valve system. Never allow the bag to deflate completely.
- Set the oxygen at the prescribed flow rate.
- Empty any water that may accumulate in the bag.

Venturi Mask

- This mask functions according to the physics of the Bernoulli effect to maintain a constant mixture of air and source oxygen. No reservoir bag is required.
- Venturi masks are used to administer a carefully regulated flow of oxygen to patients who are extremely sensitive to oxygen concentrations.
- Turn the oxygen on at the prescribed flow rate, which is marked on the mask.
- Explain to the patient that room air is mixed with source oxygen to deliver an accurate oxygen concentration.
- The mask must fit well.
- Be sure the air entry openings on the mask are always clear and unobstructed.
- Separate humidification is not required because enough room air is mixed with the oxygen to provide humidification.

"T" Tube Method

- The base opening of a T tube is attached to an endotracheal or tracheostomy tube to conduct warm, humidified oxygen. One arm is connected to the source oxygen nebulizer and the other arm is open to the atmosphere.

- A nebulizer is used to provide the high humidity necessary for patients with a tracheostomy. A continuous mist should exhaust from the T-tube opening that goes to the atmospheric air. This shows that room air is not diluting the source oxygen.
- Water collects in the tubing; the tubing must be disconnected to empty the water out of the system.

Tracheostomy Mask

- This is similar to a simple face mask except that it is shaped to cover the tracheostomy opening.
- See comments under "T" tube.

Nursing Tips

- Inspired oxygen should have minimal bacterial contamination. The oxygen-delivery equipment must *never* be shared among other patients. Humidifiers and nebulizers must be kept scrupulously clean and filled with sterile water. Nebulizers are more apt to cause infection than humidifiers.
- Continuous oxygen therapy, using a mask, should never be interrupted except for short intervals, such as to wash and dry the face in order to prevent necrosis of facial tissues.
- Nasal prongs can be substituted for masks when eating or drinking.
- Portable oxygen tanks should be used by patients on continuous oxygen therapy when they leave their beds.
- Never place oxygen-delivery equipment on a patient before turning on the oxygen. This will avoid a sudden oxygen surge or aspiration of water in the tubing.
- Aspirations can be a problem with masks if the patient vomits.
- No electric razors should be used for patients receiving oxygen.
- ABGs should be done at least daily on patients receiving continuous oxygen.

PARACENTESIS (ABDOMINAL)

Description

Using sterile technique and local anesthesia, aspiration of peritoneal fluid from the abdomen is now done mostly for diagnostic purposes. Fluid (50 to 100 ml) may be removed for examination (*e.g.*, for protein, cytology, and cellular and bacterial content). When ascites cannot be reduced by other methods, and accumulation of peritoneal fluid is causing respiratory embarrassment, therapeutic paracentesis may be done to remove excess fluid (*see SS, Liver disorders*). It is avoided when possible because of the dangers of reducing circulating blood volume and of depleting body protein.

Nursing Tips

Diagnostic Paracentesis

- Informed consent must be signed.
- Patient voids immediately before procedure.
- Position the patient sitting upright, with back supported and feet on the floor.
- Describe appearance and amount of fluid aspirated and how well procedure was tolerated. Label specimens and send to appropriate laboratories for examination, as ordered by physician.

Therapeutic Paracentesis

In addition to those above, these tips apply:

- Slow release of fluid and limit amount released at one time to prevent hypovolemia caused by sudden pressure change.
- Vital signs should be taken during the procedure and frequently thereafter until it is certain that patient's condition is stable.
- Salt-poor albumin may be infused over a 24-hour period following the procedure to counteract removal of protein in ascitic fluid.
- Observe for signs of vascular collapse (increased pulse rate, decreased blood pressure, pallor), oliguria, hyponatremia, infection, and bleeding.

POSTURAL HYPOTENSION (ORTHOSTATIC HYPOTENSION)

Description

Postural hypotension is an early sign of sharply reduced blood volume or hemorrhage. It is indicated by a sharp drop in the patient's blood pressure when the patient assumes an upright position.

How to Check for Postural Hypotension

- Take the patient's blood pressure (BP) and apical pulse (AP).
- Have patient either sit up or stand beside the bed.
- Again take BP and AP.
- If BP has dropped markedly (more than 10 mm Hg) and the AP has increased 20 to 30 beats per minute, it indicates hypovolemia (reduced circulating blood volume).
- Watch for pallor or feelings of faintness. If patient exhibits them, help him back to bed, and assume that he is hypovolemic.

RANGE OF MOTION EXERCISES

Description

Range of motion (ROM) exercises are done to maintain or restore full use of a joint or joints. Moving a joint through its normal range

of motion may be done actively or passively. In passive ROM, someone assists the patient. A physician's order is required if a pathological
condition is present (*e.g.*, arthritis, fracture, or an acute cardiac condition).

Nursing Tips

- Never move a joint to the point of pain. Stop before pain or fatigue
  is felt.
- With the joint supported, move it slowly and rhythmically through
  its ROM about five times.
- When full ROM exercises are ordered, every joint should be
  moved: starting with the head and neck; then the shoulder, elbow,
  wrist, and fingers; then hip to toes. Exercises are usually done
  three times a day.
- Progress from passive to active ROM as soon as possible by teaching patient to do it himself. In case of paralysis, the affected extremity can be assisted by the good one.

RENAL BIOPSY

Description

A percutaneous needle biopsy of the kidney may make possible a
definitive diagnosis by providing information about the glomeruli
and tubules. Hemorrhage—causing hematuria, hematoma, or flank
pain—is a serious risk with this procedure.

Open renal biopsy (with specimen for electron microscopy) is also
done.

Nursing Tips
Percutaneous Needle Biopsy

- An informed consent is required.
- Pressure is applied to the area for 20 minutes following the pro-
  cedure. A pressure dressing should remain on the site for 24
  hours.
- Bed rest for 24 hours.
- Vital signs, color of urine, hemoglobin, and hematocrit must be
  checked frequently.
- Fluids should be forced.

Open Renal Biopsy
- Same nursing care as for kidney surgery.

ROTATING TOURNIQUETS

Description

Rotating tourniquets assist in the treatment of left ventricular heart failure by decreasing the work of the heart. These tourniquets are applied in a rotating sequence to the four extremities to decrease the amount of blood returning to the heart. This is an emergency treatment for pulmonary edema.

Establishing and Maintaining Rotating Tourniquets

- Take the blood pressure before inflating the tourniquets and then every 15 minutes.
- Tourniquets are applied as high as possible on all four extremities.
- Inflate three of the tourniquets to slightly more than the diastolic blood pressure. Distal pulses must always remain palpable. Arterial constriction from overly tight tourniquets must be avoided.
- Rotate inflation of tourniquets so that each extremity has a 15-minute noninflated period out of every 60 minutes.
- No extremity is compressed for more than 45 minutes. In elderly patients, tourniquets may be rotated every 5 minutes.
- The tourniquets are released in a clockwise pattern, and *never* all at the same time. Keep the 15-minute spacing between each release.
- Urine output is checked and recorded hourly.

SCANS
COMPUTERIZED AXIAL TOMOGRAPHY (CAT)
Description

The x-ray CAT scanner was initially developed in 1973 for noninvasive examination of the brain. It was so successful that present-day scanners are designed to examine any portion of the body. Because these scanners are rather complex and very expensive, they are located mostly at major medical centers. Thus this examination may be done only after others have failed to be definitive.

CAT scans require that the patient remain completely immobile while x-ray pictures are taken sequentially by the x-ray mechanism from different angles around the body. As many as 180 x-ray pictures, each at a different angle, may be used. A mathematical technique, using a computer program, compares and combines the density of small parts (called pixels) of each x-ray film. The resulting composite pictures, produced by mathematically analyzing some 30,000 pixels, reveal the internal organs and structures in cross sections, or tomographs. These tomographs have sufficient detail to show abnormalities that would not be apparent from the individual x-rays.

Nursing Tips

- In some cases a contrast material is injected that selectively increases the x-ray density of body structures or organs so as to obtain even more detail in the tomograph.
- Because of the x-ray technique used in CAT scans, the body receives no more radiation than when exposed to the more traditional x-ray studies. They must precede barium examinations.
- In some medical centers CAT scans already have been able to replace most of the more dangerous pneumoencephalography studies and half of the cerebral angiograms and nuclear brain scans.
- Also, a CAT scan is now the preferred procedure in traumatic head injuries because of the speed and definitiveness of the resulting tomography.
- Tomographs of other parts of the body are becoming more common and are now capable of supplanting much of the previously done exploratory surgery.

NUCLEAR SCANS

Radioactive isotopes are used for diagnosis in nuclear medicine. They are given by mouth or IV injection and emit a minute amount of radiation, which is detected by a machine that measures or converts it into an image.

- It is preferable that scans be done before barium studies or x-rays requiring dye injections, and that no other tests be scheduled the day of the scan.

The following is the preferred sequence when a series of scans is to be done:

Thyroid scan—for size, location, and shape of thyroid.

- The patient should be well-hydrated.
- An IV injection or oral dose will be given and a scan done after 20 minutes.

Thyroid Uptake—to test the function of the thyroid.

- It must be established before this scan whether the patient is presently on thyroid or iodine medication or has had an x-ray requiring IV contrast media in the past 5 years (*e.g.*, pyelogram).
- The patient must be able to take a 131I capsule p.o. and must go to the Nuclear Medicine Department the next day for the 10-minute scan.

Xenon Ventilation Lung Scan—to evaluate the air supply to pulmonary tissues.
- There is no injection.
- It is done by inhalation and takes about 20 minutes.

Lung—to identify possible pulmonary emboli, emphysema, or carcinoma.
- The patient should be well-hydrated.
- An IV injection is given, and the scan takes about 20 minutes.

Gallbladder—to analyze the function of the gall bladder, obstructions in it, or acute and chronic gallbladder disease.
- The patient must be n.p.o. after midnight.
- An IV injection is given, and the scan takes about 60 minutes.

Liver–Spleen Scan—to identify the size and shape of the liver or spleen, space-occupying lesions, or a ruptured spleen.
- This scan should be done before a barium enema of upper GI series or after the patient is completely rid of the barium.
- There should be a one-day interval after a bone scan.
- The patient must be well-hydrated.
- An IV injection is given, and the scan takes about 45 minutes.

Renal Flow and Scan—to demonstrate renal blood flow and to identify size, location, and function of the kidneys and ureters.
- The patient should be well-hydrated and sent with a full bladder.
- An IV injection is given, and the scan takes about 30 minutes.
- The patient should force fluids for the rest of the day.
- If the patient has an indwelling urinary catheter, the collection bag should be emptied before the scan on the day of the scan, and then every 2 to 4 hours for the rest of the day.
- Pregnant nursing staff should not care for these patients.

Pancreas—to identify tumor or pseudocyst and the size and shape of the pancreas.
- The patient is kept n.p.o. after midnight until a special pancreatic meal, ordered from the diet kitchen, is given when the Nuclear Medicine Department calls in the morning.
- If ordered by the physician, 1 oz of whiskey is mixed with the meal to enhance pancreatic activity.
- The patient goes immediately to Nuclear Medicine.
- An IV injection is given, and the scan takes about 45 minutes.

Brain—to identify brain tumors, hemorrhage, hematomas, and abscess.
- The patient should force fluids before and during the scan.
- An IV injection is given, and a flow study is done.
- The patient returns to the floor and at least an hour later returns for the second part of the scan, which takes about 30 minutes.

- If the patient has an indwelling catheter, the collection bag should be emptied every 2 to 4 hours.
- Pregnant nursing staff should not care for these patients.

Bone—to identify areas of increased bone metabloism associated with tumors and changes in bone metabolism.

- An IV injection is given; the patient should then drink at least three 8-oz glasses of liquid in the next 2 hours.
- Before the patient goes for the scan, 2 hours after the injection, the bladder should be empty.
- The scan takes 1 hour, and fluids should be forced for the remainder of the day.
- If the patient has an indwelling catheter, the collection bag should be emptied before the scan, and then every 2 to 4 hours for the rest of the day.
- Pregnant nursing staff should not care for these patients.

Gallium—to detect tumors or abscesses in soft tissue.

- An IV injection is given, and scans are done at 24-, 28-, and occasionally 72-hour intervals.
- Each scan takes 1 hour.
- The physician must order a laxative the evening before each scan, then two tap water enemas the morning of each scan.

SENGSTAKEN-BLAKEMORE TUBE

Description

Used to apply direct pressure to bleeding esophageal varices, the Sengstaken-Blakemore is a triple-lumen tube that has an esophageal balloon, a gastric balloon, and a gastric tube with sucking ports (see Fig. 3-8). After insertion, the round gastric balloon will be inflated with about 150 to 250 cc of air, pulled back, and fitted snugly against the esophageal orifice of the stomach. After traction has been applied, the long, narrow esophageal balloon will be inflated to the desired pressure (usually about 25 to 30 mm Hg), which will continue to be measured by a manometer.

Equipment

- Two Sengstaken-Blakemore tubes, which have been tested by inflating them with air. Lumens should be marked appropriately with tape and water-proof marking pen.
- Scissors should be at the bedside. (If the tube displaces upwards and obstructs respiration, you would cut the tube and remove it).
- Some hospitals provide a football helmet on which to secure the tube to apply traction, thus relieving trauma resulting from taping a taut tube to the patient's nose or face.

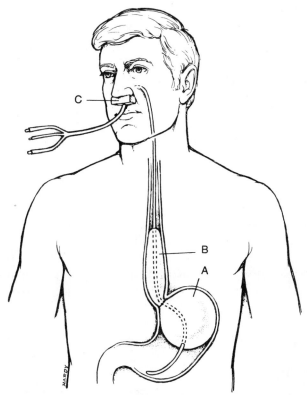

FIG. 3-8. *Sengstaken-Blakemore tube in place. The gastric balloon* (A) *and the esoph-ageal balloon* (B) *are inflated. Traction is maintained by a foam sponge placed about the tube at the external nares and held by tape* (C). *The foam sponge also prevents ulceration of the nasal skin and cartilage. The 3 open tube ends are then connected: The one marked gastric balloon is closed with a screw clamp. The esophageal balloon is connected to a mercury or ancroid sphygmomanometer, and pressure is maintained at 30 mm Hg. The third tube is connected to an intermittent nasogastric suction machine.* (Cosgriff JH, Anderson DL: The Practice of Emergency Nursing, p 327. Philadelphia, JB Lippincott, 1975)

- Manometer to be attached to the lumen of the esophageal balloon.
- Foam-rubber padding to go around the tube and under the nares.
- Suction equipment.
- A tube may be inserted for aspiration of the upper esophagus.

Nursing Tips

- Irrigate gastric suction tube as ordered. Check character, color, and amount of aspirate.
- Keep nostrils clean and lubricated, and keep padding adjusted to prevent pressure.

Preventing Complications

- Aspiration of vomitus as the tube is being inserted is the most dangerous part of this procedure. Have suction equipment available.
- Erosion of the gastric or esophageal mucosae can be prevented by intermittent release of pressure, as ordered. Authorities' opinions vary, but this may involve releasing pressure every 15 to 20 minutes, or deflating the balloon for 5 minutes every 8 to 12 hours. The tube may be left in place 48 hours. Keep pressure in esophagogastric tube at level ordered.
- Complete pharyngeal obstruction may occur if the gastric balloon ruptures and the tube displaces upwards. Watch for signs of acute respiratory distress. If necessary, cut the tube and remove it.
- Esophageal perforation is indicated by sudden back pain, shock, pains in the upper abdomen, and fluid in the chest.
- Aspiration pneumonia is a continued threat, since patient cannot swallow because of obstructed esophagus. Keep patient n.p.o. Encourage frequent expectoration. Suction p.r.n. Give frequent mouth care.

THORACENTESIS

Description

Needle aspiration of either pleural fluid or air from the pleural space may be done for either therapeutic or diagnostic purposes. In some cases, medications may be injected into the pleural space. The procedure is done with local anesthesia, using sterile technique. See your agency procedure book.

Nursing Tips

- Informed consent must be signed.
- Patient's position will be designated by physician. An upright position facilitates removal of fluid.
- Caution patient against sudden movements or coughing during the procedure.
- Monitor pulse and respirations. Observe for untoward symptoms during and after the procedure (*e.g.,* respiratory difficulties including dyspnea, uncontrolled coughing, and blood-tinged or frothy sputum; also, shock, pallor, cyanosis, weakness, diaphoresis, and pain).
- Possible complications include shock, pneumothorax (with possible mediastinal shift), infection, and electrolyte imbalances. (*See SS, Postoperative complications; SS, Respiratory system, pneumothorax*)

- Fluid is removed slowly, the amount limited to 1000 ml at one time.
- After the procedure:
  1. Small, sterile pressure dressing is applied to site.
  2. Position patient so that he is lying with puncture site up to minimize leakage from it.
  3. Vital signs are taken every hour for 4 hours following procedure, longer if indicated.
  4. Record amount and character of withdrawn fluid. Care for specimens appropriately.

TRACHEOSTOMY CARE

Description
A tracheostomy is a surgically provided direct connection using a tube from a neck stoma to the trachea. When it is necessary to artificially maintain an open airway for longer than 72 hours, a tracheotomy is usually performed. An emergency temporary open airway can be obtained without surgery by using an endotracheal intubation tube.

Maintenance and Care of a Tracheostomy
- An extra tracheostomy set should be kept at the bedside with the same size tube. In case of accidental expulsion, keep the stoma open with a hemostat.
- Tracheostomy tubes are made of metal or plastic. The most commonly used in cases of respiratory failure are plastic. These may or may not have removable inner cannulas. Metal tubes have removable cannulas.
- Tracheostomy care must be done with sterile technique. Pulmonary infection is a serious complication of tracheostomies. Dust and lint enter directly into the lungs. Never use cotton-filled gauze for tracheostomy dressings.
- If there is a removable inner cannula, take it out at least every 4 hours, and clean it with hydrogen peroxide, sterile water, and sterile pipe cleaners. Suction the outer cannula before replacing the inner cannula; replace and lock.
- Wash the skin around the stoma with hydrogen peroxide, rinsing with sterile water, and apply an antimicrobial ointment at least every 8 hours. Replace a soiled dressing, and keep the area as dry as possible. Observe for wound infections. Be gentle, the skin is very tender.
- These patients must have a nebulizer to warm and humidify the air *(see NR, Oxygen administration)*. Often a tube from a nebulizer

is attached with a T tube or tracheostomy mask to the opening of the tracheostomy tube. Disconnect the tubing at the tracheostomy tube connection to empty the condensed water that accumulates in the tubing. Check the nebulizer at the beginning of every shift for an adequate water level. All water and medications to be nebulized must be sterile. Equipment and medication must *never* be shared with other patients.

- Plastic tracheostomy tubes have a built-in inflatable cuff which produces a tight seal in the trachea. These cuffs are deflated or inflated according to the physician's orders. It is common practice to inflate the cuff prior to an oral or tube feeding and for 30 minutes afterwards to prevent aspiration.
- To prevent pressure necrosis on the tracheal wall, the cuff must never be over-inflated. It can be kept safely at up to 25 cm of water or 18 mm of mercury. There must be a method available to verify the pressure.
- Always suction the pharynx before deflating a tracheal cuff to prevent aspiration of mucus. Discard this suction catheter and use a new sterile catheter for removing tracheobronchial secretions.
- Leakage of food particles from a tracheostomy indicates a fistula between the esophagus and the trachea. Notify the physician immediately.
- It is important to teach the patient to cough to help prevent pulmonary infection. Often, taking a deep breath and momentarily covering the tracheostomy opening will produce a cough.
- Teach the patient to stabilize the tube with his fingers during a cough. Also, have the patient hold a covering in front of the tracheostomy when coughing.
- When the tracheostomy ties are changed, one nurse should stabilize the tube to prevent accidental expulsion, while the other nurse changes the ties.
- The ties should be tight enough to allow only two fingers beneath them.
- The ties must be knotted at the side of the neck. The gown should have snap closures or should be tied in front to prevent accidental untieing of the knot.
- Unless a laryngectomy has been done, speaking a few words can be accomplished by taking a breath and momentarily covering the tracheostomy opening.
- In the immediate postoperative period (first 24 hours) tracheal suctioning may be required as often as every 15 to 30 minutes. A size 14 catheter is used or one not exceeding $\frac{1}{3}$ the diameter of the lumen of the tube.
- Suction when the patient needs it, never on a routine basis. It is traumatic and tends to stimulate the production of secretions.

- Tracheal suctioning, also called deep suctioning, should never exceed 8 to 10 seconds because of the danger of hypoxia leading to cardiac arrest. Gentle suctioning is necessary to prevent trauma to the trachea. Suction pressure should not exceed 60 to 80 mm Hg.
- The color, amount, odor, and consistency of secretions should be noted as well as the frequency of suctioning. It is important to note any increase in the need for suctioning.
- When no secretions can be aspirated and the patient is congested, it probably means that there is inadequate humidification.
- Hyperventilate (bag) the patient before beginning suctioning with a self-inflating bag (*e.g.*, Ambubag) attached to an oxygen source. This oxygenates and helps loosen secretions.
- Know the patient's ABGs so hypoxic patients can be watched carefully for signs of oxygen deprivation (*e.g.*, cyanosis and tachycardia).
- The suction catheter is inserted 6 to 8 inches toward the bronchus to be suctioned.
- Suction is not applied until the catheter is being withdrawn, using a pill-rolling movement of the fingers to prevent it from adhering to the side walls.
- Hyperventilate after suctioning. If it is necessary to suction again, wait at least 3 minutes.
- Any equipment disconnected from a tracheostomy during suctioning (*e.g.*, a T tube) must be placed on a sterile field.

TRACTION

Description

Traction is a pulling force applied to a part of the body. It provides alignment and stability to a fracture site by reducing the fracture and maintaining correct position. It may prevent flexion contractures, reduce deformity (in scoliosis), and lessen muscle spasm (*e.g.*, back pain). If the part is elevated above the heart, it may reduce edema.

Countertraction is a pull in the opposite direction of the pull of the traction.

Most traction is continuously applied, though cervical and pelvic traction may be intermittent.

- In *straight or running traction* the pull is in one plane, and the body supplies the countertraction (*e.g.*, Buck's; see Fig. 3-9).
- In *suspension or balanced suspension,* there is a lifting force to the extremity as a whole (suspension), which allows the patient movement while the line of traction is still being maintained (*e.g.*, skeletal traction with Thomas splint and Pearson attachment; see Fig. 3-11).

Manual traction would be applied during cast application.

- *Skin traction* (Buck's, Russell's) is applied with tapes adhered to the skin and circumferential bandages or Buck's boot attached to a footplate or spreader with a hook on the bottom, which attaches to a rope, pulley, and weights.
- In *skeletal traction* the traction is applied directly to the bone by inserting into the bones devices such as Steinmann pins, Kirschner wire, or Crutchfield tongs. It is used with balanced suspension.

Equipment

- Bed with a firm mattress, possibly a hinged headboard; in most cases an overbed frame with a trapeze.
- Pulleys, ropes or cords, weights (with specific amount ordered by physician), and bars for attachment of the pulleys.
- In addition to the above, special types of traction may require additional equipment.
  1. Traction for the lower extremity may include
     a. A footplate to maintain normal position of the foot.
     b. A prepadded boot ("Buck's boot") for Buck's traction
     c. A splint to support the part
        (1) Thomas splint (supports thigh), with Pearson attachment (supports calf); used with skeletal traction.
        (2) Böhler–Braun inclined plane splint. Frame rests on the bed; may be used for skin or skeletal traction of lower extremity.
  2. Pelvic traction
     a. A belt, measured to fit. *(See Nursing tips under Pelvic traction)*
     b. Straps that extend from belt to spreader, which is attached to traction rope.
  3. Cervical traction may be provided with one of the following:
     a. Head halter
     b. Crutchfield, Barton, or Vinke tongs for skull traction, with bed frame which provides for turning, *e.g.* Foster or Stryker frame or Circ-O-lectric bed.
     c. Halo-skeletal traction

General Nursing Tips

- Patient's body should be in good alignment; it should provide at least some countertraction. The patient's position in bed and his limitations of movement will be specified by the physician.
- The pull of the traction on extremities should be in alignment with the long axis of the bone.
- Keep patient pulled up in bed. Footplate or knots should not touch pulley or foot of bed. Traction should be continuous (unless otherwise ordered).

- Teach patient to use trapeze to lift back, buttocks, and shoulders off bed in a straight line.
- Eliminate possibilities of friction along the line from the patient to the weights.
  1. Weights must hang free. *Never* remove weights without a physician's order. Keep them off the floor and off the bed.
  2. Keep cords free of obstruction, free of linens.
- Be sure that ropes are not frayed, that knots are well tied (square knots) and taped, and that ropes are on center tract of pulley.
- A sketch of the traction in the Kardex is extremely helpful.
- Bed making is usually easiest from top to bottom.
- Always investigate patient's complaints. Check for signs of neurovascular impairment: pain, pallor, pulselessness, paralysis, or paresthesia (tingling or numbness).
- Prevent complications of immobility
  1. Pulmonary *(See NR, Deep breathing techniques)*
  2. Circulatory *(See SS, Post operative care, preventing vascular complication)*
  3. Constipation and fecal impaction
  4. Decubiti *(See MNS)*
  5. Renal calculi *(See SS, Urinary tract and the prostate)*
  6. Muscular atrophy/contracture
  7. Emotional problems: boredom, depression, and, sometimes, adjustment to changed body image.

BUCK'S EXTENSION

Description

A running skin traction is now most commonly applied with the use of a prepadded "Buck's" boot. It may also be applied with tapes that are adhered to the skin (secured by circumferential bandages, usually elastic) and attached to a foot plate or spreader with a hook on the bottom (see Fig. 3-9). Either setup attaches to a rope, pulley, and weights, with the specific amount of weight prescribed by the physician. Usually ordered for temporary immobilization of hip fractures (particularly subcapital fractures) before surgical fixation, it may also be used to immobilize the leg in abduction following total hip replacement.

Nursing Tips

(See general nursing tips for traction)
- Buck's boot must be the proper size. With physician's order, it may be removed once a day for bathing and inspection of skin.
- Traction tapes can only be applied to skin in good condition. Cir-

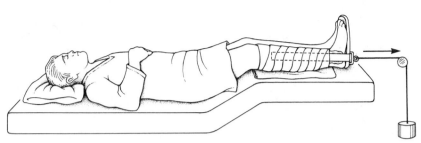

FIG. 3-9. *Buck's traction.*

cumferential bandage should be wrinkle free and not too tight. Spreader must be wide enough to prevent tapes from rubbing ankle. Observe for, document, and report any of the following:

1. Numbness, tingling, swelling and change in color, pain, decreased sensitivity to heat, cold, or touch, disturbance in the mobility of the foot—all are signs of neurovascular impairment. Avoid pressure on the peroneal nerve (3 inches below knee on outer aspect).
2. Complaints of burning or irritation under the bandage, slipping of the tapes, a feeling of sponginess under the bandage (indicating possible skin breakdown).
3. Tightness of elastic bandage caused by swelling.

- With either skin traction or Buck's boot, avoid pressure on the Achilles tendon and the heel by placing a folded bath blanket under the calf or by using heel protectors. Cotton may be used to protect the maleolus.
- Keep patient pulled up in bed, with the body in alignment.
- The patient's position in bed and his limitations of movement will be specified by the physician.
- Usually, patient may be turned to a 45° angle with a pillow between his legs for back care.
- Head of bed may usually be elevated, but it should be lowered several times a day to relieve pressure on sacrum, and to prevent hip contractures.
- Back care is very important. Massage with one hand while pushing mattress down with other. Eggcrate mattress is frequently ordered.

RUSSELL'S TRACTION

Description

A skin traction similar to Buck's, in which balanced suspension is provided by a sling under the knee (see Fig. 3-10). Russell's traction is used in treatment of some femoral fractures (preferred in intertrochanteric and subtrochanteric types), and for some knee injuries.

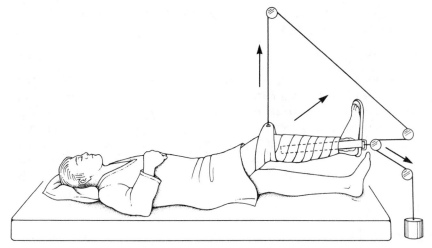

FIG. 3-10. *Russell's traction.*

Nursing Tips

(See general nursing tips for traction)

The physician will leave specific orders for the positioning of the patient and for the limits of his movement. The following are general guidelines that will usually apply.

- The knee sling should elevate the calf enough to produce a 20° angle between the patient's hip and the bed, with the calf parallel to the bed. This relationship should be maintained in all positions. Heel should clear the bed.
- Movement
    1. Patient can lift with trapeze, pushing downward with unaffected leg while keeping waist straight.
    2. External or internal rotation of upper leg is prohibited.
    3. Lower body may be tilted, and movement of the whole body toward the foot or the head of the bed may be permitted for short periods of time only.
- Check popliteal space for evidence of pressure or skin irritation. The area may be padded with a piece of felt or sheepskin.
- Whether or not to have a pillow supporting the calf is part of the physician's traction plan. Find out what it is, and maintain as originally set up. Be sure it is noted on nursing-care plan.
- Check for color, warmth, sensation, and movement of the foot (ability to plantarflex and dorsiflex). Provide a footplate.
- Nursing tips under Buck's extension traction apply here.

THOMAS SPLINT WITH PEARSON ATTACHMENT AND SKELETAL TRACTION

Description

To reduce a fracture of the femur, hip, or lower leg, skeletal traction is applied by inserting a metal pin or wire (Steinmann pin, Kirschner wire) into or through a bone distal to the fracture and then applying traction directly to it. Balanced suspension is supplied by the Thomas splint, which supports the thigh, and its Pearson attachment, which supports the lower leg in a position parallel to the bed (see Fig. 3-11). The knee is flexed about 45°. The advantage of this setup is that the patient can lift his leg and move his body, furthering better circulation.

Nursing Tips

(See general nursing tips for traction)

The physician will leave specific orders for the patient's position in bed and his limitations of movement. The following are general guidelines that will usually apply.

- Movement:
  1. Most movements can be done within limits of patient's tolerance.
  2. External or internal rotation of the leg is prohibited.

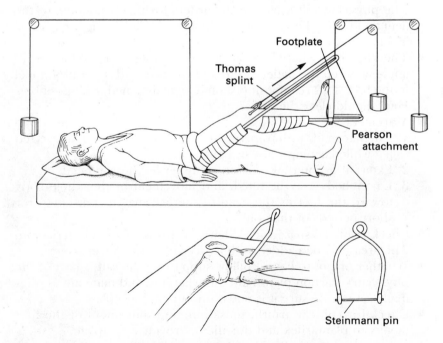

FIG. 3-11. *Skeletal traction with Thomas splint and Pearson attachment.*

3. When raising the body, patient should push downward on unaffected leg and keep waist unbent.

- Check the color, pulse, temperature, ability to plantarflex and dorsiflex both feet at least once each shift. Position footplate appropriately.
- Pressure points that require attention are the popliteal space, the
  Achilles tendon, the heel, and the peroneal nerve (3 inches below
  knee on outer aspect) especially if the splint has tipped with movement. Tendency to invert the foot and difficulty in extending the
  toes are signs of peroneal nerve impairment.
- Material under splint should be smooth; no extra padding between
  leather ring and skin.
- Keep ring of Thomas splint dry and clean, with half-ring positioned over the anterior aspect of the thigh. Check groin and areas
  where ring might rub for signs of pressure or irritation.
- Inspect pin sites every shift for redness or other signs of infection.
  Give pin care, as ordered. Pin care varies, but one method consists
  of cleansing around the site with hydrogen peroxide solution using
  sterile applicators at least every shift during the first postoperative
  days. After 4 or 5 days use alcohol sponges to clean around the
  pin. The area is allowed to remain exposed to the air.
- Cleanse affected leg with either alcohol or lotion.
- Provide back care to prevent skin breakdown. Eggcrate mattress
  or alternating pressure mattress may be helpful.

PELVIC TRACTION

Description

For possible herniated disc or back strain, traction is applied to the
pelvis by means of a girdle or belt worn by the patient. The traction
is frequently intermittent.

Nursing Tips

- Proper fit of the girdle is essential. Measure pelvic circumference
  to ascertain size. Top edge of belt should be at the iliac crest, lower
  part slightly below the greater trochanter.
- Watch for signs of skin irritation over iliac crests.
- Movement and position
  1. Back must be kept straight, level, and in proper alignment.
  2. A pillow may be allowed under the head, and the bed may be
     gatched at the knees with the angle of hips to knees from 45°
     to 60° and with feet level with knees (William's position, see Fig.
     3-12) to provide countertraction.
  3. Patient should not bend or twist his back.
  4. Signal bell must be within easy reach.

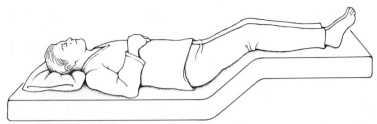

FIG. 3-12. *Williams' position. Degree of flexion at the hips may vary depending upon purpose of positioning.*

- Spreader bar used to maintain equal pulling force on straps must be kept parallel to foot of bed.
- Constipation can aggravate back discomfort. Plan an individualized bowel program to prevent it.
- Lack of sensation in legs should be reported to physician immediately.
- For reapplication of pelvic traction, apply belt carefully, and suspend weights slowly and smoothly.
- Keep patient's feet as well as belt straps free of bed linens.
- Use fracture bedpan if bathroom privileges are not granted.

CERVICAL TRACTION
CERVICAL SKIN TRACTION
Description

Skin traction applied with a head halter is frequently intermittent and is usually used for cervical myositis, dislocations, and minor fractures.

Nursing Tips

(See general nursing tips for traction)
- Spreader must be wide enough to prevent pressure on the side of the head.
- Protect patient's chin, ears, and back of head with padding. Give gentle massage, if permitted.
- Give frequent shampoos for cleanliness and stimulation of the scalp, if ordered by physician.
- Soft foods may be indicated to minimize chewing.

CRUTCHFIELD, BARTON, OR VINKE TONGS
Description

Crutchfield, Barton, or Vinke tongs placed in the top of the skull make possible continuous skeletal traction in cases of severe cervical fractures or dislocation.

Nursing Tips

(See general nursing tips for traction)

- A bed frame that provides for turning (*e.g.*, Foster or Stryker frame, or Circ-O-lectric bed) is required.
- Motor sensory changes should be reported immediately (*e.g.*,loss of muscle strength, projectile vomiting, and respiratory distress).
- Check for bleeding around the tongs and for skin breakdown on the back of the head. (Protect the occipital area from pressure. Massage and shampoo p.r.n. if ordered).
- Turn on frame every 2 hours. See hospital procedure for how to use Stryker frame or Circ-O-lectric bed.
- Because of the difficulty in eating and drinking in the supine position and the danger of aspiration, suction equipment should be at the bedside.
- Make the foundation of the bed with two drawsheets instead of one full-length sheet.
- Prism glasses for reading and for watching television will be helpful for the patient who must remain flat.

HALO-SKELETAL TRACTION

Description

The Halo-skeletal traction device provides another way to immobilize the cervical spine. A stainless steel ring fits around the head and is secured in place with four skull pins. The ring is then attached to a body vest of plaster or plastic to give it stability.

Nursing Tips

- Provide pin care as ordered to keep areas of pin insertion into the skull free from infection.
- Inspect the device to be sure all screws are tight.

ULTRASOUND (SONOGRAM)

Description

Ultrasound uses sound waves with frequencies far above those that the human ear can detect to produce images of internal body organs and structure and also to detect and measure internal movements, such as those produced by a beating heart.

- Ultrasound functions the same as radar and sonar, but produces no radio or x-ray radiation, and it does not require injection of a contrast medium into the blood. It is safe and painless, and does not require invasive techniques.
- The scanner probe must be in good contact with the body.

- In some cases the patient is immersed in water that also contains the probe; in others, a flexible membrane that contains the water and the probe is placed over the organ of interest, in order to effectively couple the probe closer to the body.

Ultrasound has a wide and growing range of application in medical diagnosis. It has already virtually replaced other imaging methods in obstetrics, and the ultrasound noninvasive examinations of the heart have been able to reduce the need for hazardous cardiac catheterization.

- Ultrasound doppler-type scans can detect and locate deep venous thrombosis and, also, stenosis (constriction) in arteries.
- The more sophisticated machines can even discover if there is a plaque buildup on the inner wall of an artery.

Current research is now identifying and cataloging how different tissues absorb, scatter, and otherwise modify the ultrasound waves so that body tissue of all types may be identified. There are preparations for some types of sonograms.

Nursing Tips

- Patients scheduled for abdominal sonograms are n.p.o. after midnight preceding the scan.
- A pelvic scan requires a full bladder.
- Gallbladder scans necessitate a fat-free diet the day before and then n.p.o. after midnight.

URINARY BLADDER CATHETERIZATION AND DRAINAGE

CATHETERIZATION

Description

Recognition of the high incidence of bladder infection associated with catheterization has made this a procedure that is ordered only if absolutely necessary. Nursing measures should be used to promote normal emptying of the bladder (*e.g.*, a warm bed pan, a comfortable position, privacy, and the sound of running water). When all else fails, catheterization is still ordered in some cases to relieve urinary retention, to measure for retention, occasionally to collect a sterile urine specimen, and to insert an indwelling or retention catheter for continuous urinary drainage or irrigation. Maintaining sterile technique during the procedure is essential. Avoiding contamination of the closed urinary drainage system and providing appropriate catheter care for the indwelling catheter, including hand washing before handling catheter or drainage equipment, are other musts.

Equipment

- Prepackaged catheterization kits with sterile contents available in most hospitals contain catheter, cotton balls, lubricant, disposable forceps, cleansing solution, specimen cup, gloves, and drapes. Kits with urinary drainage bag and tubing included may be requested. Instructions on how to do the catheterization procedure are usually included in the kit.
- Take a second catheter and pair of sterile gloves with you to the patient's bedside for use if needed. They can be returned, if not contaminated.
- Have tape on hand if a retention catheter is being inserted.
  1. Commonly used types of catheters:
     a. French or Robinson: usually used in "in and out" catheterization.
     b. Foley—two lumen (one for balloon) or three lumen (third lumen for irrigant): the most commonly used retention catheter.
     c. Coude: a stiffer catheter with a curved tip, especially useful for relieving retention caused by an enlarged prostate because tip rides over it.
  2. Size in the French, Robinson, or Foley catheters:
     a. The larger the number, the larger the catheter.
     b. Adult females: usually 14 to 16.
     c. Adult males: usually 16 to 18, though some urologists recommend sizes 18 to 20 because the larger, blunter tip causes less damage to an enlarged prostate.
  3. Material: rubber, latex, and 100% silicone
     a. 100% silicone should be used if the catheter is to be retained more than a week.

Nursing Tips

Catheterization Procedure

- See hospital procedure book or directions included in kit.
- Sterile technique is essential.
- Cut tape, if it will be needed, before starting procedure.
- For the female patient:
  1. Side lying, or lateral position, makes procedure technically simpler for nurse and more comfortable for the patient.
  2. Before opening the sterile kit, put on unsterile gloves and find the landmarks: the urinary meatus, the clitoris, and the vagina (see Fig. 3-13). Be sure you can see the urinary meatus clearly.
  3. If the first catheter goes into the vagina, leave it there as a landmark. Insert the second catheter into the meatus.

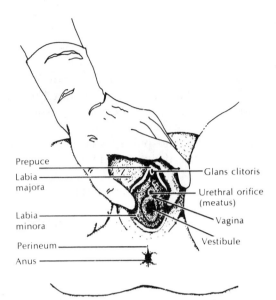

Prepuce

Labia majora

Labia minora

Perineum

Anus

Glans clitoris

Urethral orifice (meatus)

Vagina

Vestibule

FIG. 3-13. *Female structures in the perineal area.* (Wolff L, Weitzel MH, Fuerst EV: Fundamentals of Nursing, 6th ed, p 472. Philadelphia, JB Lippincott, 1980)

- For the male patient:
  1. Grasp the penis firmly (grasping it too lightly may stimulate an erection). With the patient's legs drawn up slightly, hold the penis at a 60° to 90° angle slightly towards the legs.
  2. Insert the well-lubricated catheter into the urinary meatus using scrupulous sterile technique. Slight resistance may be felt as the catheter passes the internal urethral sphincter. Use gentle constant pressure. *Never* force the catheter.
- Decompression of the bladder should be done slowly. The maximum amount of urine to be withdrawn at one time is 300 ml. Allow another 300 ml to escape 15 minutes later. Continue in this fashion until bladder is empty.

Indwelling or Retention Catheter

- Try to reduce incidence of infection.
  1. Wash hands before touching catheter or any part of the urinary drainage system.
  2. Force fluids, unless otherwise contraindicated. Monitor intake and output carefully.
  3. Never place a patient with a closed urinary drainage system in a room with another patient with any kind of infection. Try to avoid placing two patients with closed urinary drainage systems in the same room.

4. Catheter care (the value of which is now under study)
   a. The entire shaft of the catheter and the area around the meatus must be kept scrupulously clean, dry, and free from mucus and crusts.
   b. Wash with soap and water or cleanse with povidone-iodine at least twice a day. Be systematic. Agency procedures vary, so check yours.
5. In an attempt to decrease bacterial growth in cases where long-term catheter use is expected, some physicians order 1 g of ascorbic acid q.d. to acidify the urine. Cranberry juice will acidify urine, but the amount needed to be effective (six to eight glasses per day) makes it impractical.
6. Recent studies indicate that periodic instillation of hydrogen peroxide into the urinary drainage bag significantly decreases incidence of catheter-related urinary tract infections. If ordered, 30 ml of 3% hydrogen peroxide is introduced into the bag after each time it has been emptied, either through the outlet tube or through closed additive sites found in some new bags.
7. Signs of urinary tract infection (UTI) include burning around the catheter, fever, chills, and cloudy, foul-smelling urine. If a UTI is suspected, the physician will usually order a specimen sent for culture and sensitivity before beginning treatment.

- Taping the retention catheter:
  1. Catheter should be taped so that it has some give, so that it will not pull, and so that it will not be directly against the skin. Physicians' preferences vary somewhat on how or whether to tape. Inquire. General guidelines include the following:
     a. Female patient: catheter is taped against inner aspect of the thigh.
     b. Male patient (see Fig. 3-14): catheter is taped so that penis rests on the abdomen or laterally, preventing fistula development or abcess formation at the penal-scrotal angle.
- Leaking around the catheter:
  1. Leakage around the catheter is caused by the use of a catheter that is too small, by inadequate inflation of the balloon, or by bladder spasms, usually following surgery of the prostate. *(See SS, Prostate)*
     a. Balloon sizes vary; they usually hold between 5 to 30 ml of water. Most standard Foley kits contain catheters with 10-ml balloons. Larger balloon sizes may be ordered by the physician.
  2. Check the balloon by withdrawing water from it through its port with a syringe. Refill with sterile water to its ordered capacity.

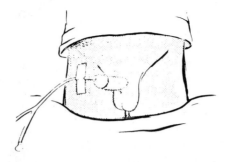

FIG. 3-14. *Method of taping catheter in a male patient.* (Lewis LW: Fundamental Skills in Patient Care, 2nd ed, p 176. Philadelphia, JB Lippincott, 1981)

3. If leakage continues, the physician may order a balloon with increased capacity.
4. Any problem with a retention catheter inserted during genitourinary (GU) surgery should be reported to the physician.
- Urinary drainage bags: receive urine in a closed system; usually attach to bedside or chair. Smaller "leg" bags may attach to ambulating patient's leg.
  1. Wash hands before touching catheter or urinary drainage system.
  2. Never lift the bag above the level of the bladder. Avoid reflux (the backward flow of urine from the system into the bladder).
  3. Keep bag on side to which patient is turned. Avoid occluding the tubing by preventing kinks in it and by positioning patient so he is not lying on tubing.
  4. A urine meter, as part of the drainage system, makes possible accurate hourly measurement of urinary output.
  5. Empty the bag at least every 8 hours, and record output. Keep the emptying tube clean and away from the side of the graduate into which urine is being emptied. Use a separate disposable graduate for each patient. Wipe the tip with alcohol before reinserting it into its holder.
  6. Check and follow agency procedure as to when bags are to be changed. If there is white sediment in the bag or if the tubing when rubbed between fingers feels sandy, it is time to ask. Always use new bag and tubing when catheter is changed.
- Collection of specimens from closed urinary drainage systems (see Fig. 3-15):
  1. Never violate the integrity of a closed system by disconnecting the catheter from the tubing to collect a specimen.
  2. Avoid clamping tubing for specimen collection. Let urine collect in tube as it lays on the bed.

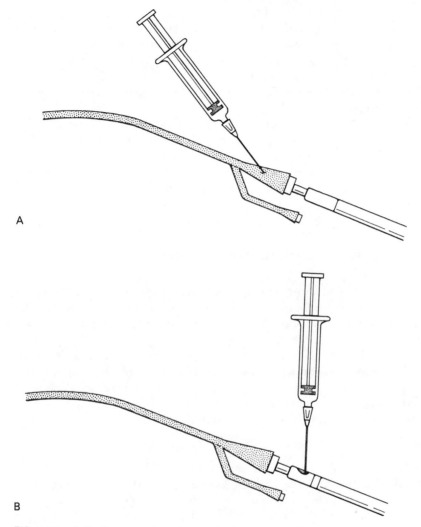

FIG. 3-15. *Collecting a specimen from a closed urinary drainage system.* **A.** *Aspiration from catheter.* **B.** *Aspiration from drainage port.*

3. Sponge the trap or the area between balloon arm and connecting tube on a rubber catheter with an alcohol wipe. (Silicone and plastic catheters are not self-sealing, so the trap is the only place from which urine can be withdrawn).

4. Withdraw amount of urine needed with sterile needle and syringe. In many hospitals, if the specimen is for culture, it is sent to the laboratory in the syringe in which it is collected, with needle covered. Chance of contaminating it by putting it in another container is thus avoided.

- Removal of the indwelling catheter:
  1. Remove water from the balloon through its port with a syringe (do not cut the end), and gently withdraw catheter.
  2. Encourage fluid intake, if not otherwise contraindicated.
  3. Measure and record intake and output accurately.
  4. Encourage ambulation (if allowed) to reinstate normal voiding patterns.
  5. Record amount of urine in patient's first voiding after catheter removal. Note position of the bladder. Some patients void but incompletely empty the bladder (retention). If patient has not voided or shows evidence of a distended bladder 6 hours (or at a time specified by the physician) after the catheter's removal, notify the physician.

CONTINUOUS BLADDER IRRIGATION
Description

Continuous bladder irrigation may be ordered following surgery of the prostate or bladder to reduce clot formation; or it may be ordered in an attempt to reduce multiplication of bacteria in a closed urinary drainage system. A three-way catheter (one lumen for drainage, one for inflation of the balloon, and one for the irrigating solution) is used. Antimicrobial solution (usually 1 ml of Neosporin GU irrigant added to 1000 ml sterile, normal saline, intravenous solution) is delivered by intravenous tubing or special GU irrigant tubing at approximately 125 ml/hr, or at a rate specified by the physician.

Nursing Tips

- Irrigating solution should be at room temperature.
- Care of the catheter and the system is like that of any retention catheter and closed urinary drainage system. *(See Catheterization)*
- Calculate the urinary output by subtracting the amount of irrigating solution that has gone in from the total amount in the drainage bag. Bags should be emptied, and output should be recorded at least every 8 hours.

INTERMITTENT BLADDER IRRIGATION
Description

Intermittent bladder irrigation may be ordered to flush a retention catheter, or to flush clots and to keep the catheter patent following GU surgery.

Nursing Tips

- Aseptic technique is essential.
  1. Cleanse junction of catheter and tubing before disconnecting.
  2. Use new sterile syringe for each irrigation.
  3. Use small bottles (200 ml to 500 ml) of irrigant so that it can be used in 24 hours. Refrigerate leftover solution between uses to reduce bacterial growth. Warm before using by placing bottle in warm water in basin or sink.
- Insert 30 to 50 ml of irrigant into catheter at one time. Allow to drain, or use gentle suction to aspirate. This procedure is usually done two or three times. If there is no return from the catheter, notify the physician immediately. Never use force to aspirate a catheter unless specifically ordered.
- Note character and color of aspirated bladder contents. Chart.

SUPRAPUBIC CATHETERS
Description

Suprapubic catheters are inserted directly into the bladder through the abdomen about 2 inches above the symphysis, under strict aseptic technique. Several types of catheters may be used, for example, the dePezzer (mushroom), the Bonanno, and the Cystocath. Sutured into place, these catheters are started by siphonage and drain directly into closed systems. They are being used in a variety of gynecological, bladder, and prostate surgeries because they are relatively infection and pain free, and seem to promote earlier spontaneous voiding.

Nursing Tips

- Distinguish between obstruction and bladder spasms the first postoperative day by checking hourly.
  1. Obstruction—indicated by decreased urinary output, distention, and tenderness—is dangerous and must be corrected immediately. Catheter must remain patent.
  2. Bladder spasms usually subside in 48 hours. They are painful, but do not affect urinary output, and may be relieved with sitz bath or an antispasmodic. *(See PH)*
- Continue to monitor amount of urine flow and its character.
- Prevent undue tension on the catheter or tubing. Avoid kinks or other occlusion of the tubing.
- Protect skin around the catheter; apply antimicrobial ointment; maintain sterile dry dressing.
- The physician may order intermittant clamping of the tubing to restore bladder tone and function as he prepares for removal of the catheter.

X-RAY PREPARATIONS

TABLE 3-3. **X-Ray Preparations**

Study	Preparation
Gallbladder series (Oral cholecystogram)	1. 6:00 PM, fat-free supper 2. 10:00 PM, six (6) Oragrafin capsules 3. n.p.o. after midnight 4. On call to x-ray in AM
UGI (Upper gastrointestinal tract)	1. n.p.o. after midnight 2. On call to x-ray in AM
BE (Barium enema)	1. Clear liquid diet day before examination 2. Four (4) tablespoons iced castor oil with fruit juice at 7:00 PM 3. n.p.o. after midnight 4. On call to x-ray in AM
Complete GI Series	1. First day, barium enema as above 2. Second day, UGI as above
IVP (Intravenous pyelogram)*	1. Four (4) tablespoons castor oil at 7:00 PM 2. May have liquids as desired 3. No solid foods after midnight 4. On call to x-ray in AM
IVC (Intravenous cholengiogram; bile ducts)*	1. n.p.o. after midnight 2. On call to x-ray
T-Tube Cholangiogram*	1. No preparation necessary 2. On call to x-ray
KUB (Kidney, Ureter, Bladder; do before an IVP)	1. No preparation necessary 2. On call to x-ray

Combined studies may be ordered without conflict of orders as follows:

1. Gallbladder series, UGI
2. Gallbladder series, BE
3. Gallbladder series, IVP
4. IVP, BE, Gallbladder series

*A contrast medium is used in these x-rays. Find out if the patient has ever had a reaction to any x-ray procedure or is allergic to seafood or iodine.

Nursing Tips

- Never give castor oil to a weak, debilitated, or elderly patient without first discussing this with the physician. There are less-severe bowel preparations.
- It is necessary to obtain a laxative or enema order following barium x-rays.

BIBLIOGRAPHY

CENTRAL VENOUS PRESSURE
BOOKS
Krueger J: Monitoring CVP. New York, Springer 1973

JOURNALS
Fischer R: Measuring central venous pressure. Nursing 79 9(10):74, October, 1979

Houghey B: CVP lines: Monitoring and maintaining. Am J Nurs 78(4):635, April, 1978

CHEST TUBE DRAINAGE
Byrne N: Critical care of the thoracic surgical patient. Cancer Nursing 1:135, April, 1978

Cimprich B, Gaydos D, Langan R: A pre-operative teaching program for the thoractomy patient. Cancer Nursing 1:35, February, 1978

Cook S: Bronchogenic carcinoma: Pre-operative and post-operative care. RN Magazine 41:83, September, 1978

DeVries WC: Principles of drainage of wounds and body cavities. OR Tech 10:34, Nov/Dec, 1978

Kirsten L: Chest tube drainage. Heart Lung 3(1):97, 1974

ELECTROCARDIOGRAM (ECG/EKG) LEADS
Andreoli K, Fowkes VH, Zipes DP et al: Comprehensive Cardiac Care, 3rd ed, p 87. St Louis, CV Mosby, 1975

ELECTROENCEPHALOGRAM (EEG)
Ford RG, Clinical use of EEG. Professional Medical Assistant 11:16, November/December, 1978

ENDOSCOPIC PROCEDURES
Armstrong M, Patterson R: Arthroscopy: A new approach to knee surgery that affects patient care. RN Magazine 41:35–39, January, 1978

Carr-Locke DL: Gastrointestinal endoscopy (ERCP). Nursing Times 73:1443–49, 1977

Colwell CW, Oberle C: Arthroscopy. Official Journal Orthopedic Nurses Assn 6:54–57, February, 1979

Grossman MB: Gastrointestinal endoscopy. Clin Symp 32(3):2, 1980

GASTROINTESTINAL INTUBATION
BOOKS
Nursing Photobook: Performing GI Procedures. Horsham, Intermed Communications, 1981

Sorensen K, Luckmann J: Basic Nursing. Philadelphia, WB Saunders, 1979

Wood A: Nursing Skills for Allied Health Services, Vol 3. Philadelphia, WB Saunders, 1975

JOURNALS

Coyle N, Arbit E: How to protect your patients against aspiration pneumonia. Nursing 78 8(10):50–51, October, 1978

Griggs BA, Hoppe MC: Update: Nasogastric tube feeding. AM J Nurs 79(3):481–485, March, 1979

Hanson R: New approach to measuring adult nasogastric tubes for insertion. AM J Nurs 80(7):1334–1335, July, 1980

Kubo W et al: Fluid and electrolyte problems of tube fed patients. Am J Nurs 76(6):912–916, June, 1976

Letsou AP: Infusion control devices for parenteral and enteral administration. Aspects of enteral administration, the practical application of theory. Am J IV Therapy 5:36–40, Oct/Nov 1978

McConnell EA: All about gastrointestinal intubation. Nursing 75 5(9):30–37, September, 1975

McConnell EA: Ensuring safer stomach suctioning with the Salem sump tube. Nursing 77 7(9):54–57, September, 1977

Nursing 80. Giving Medication through a nasogastric tube. 10(5):71–73, May, 1980

Persons C: Why risk TPN when tube feeding will do? RN magazine 4(1):35–41, June, 1981

Shils ME: Infusion control devices for parenteral and enteral administration. Advances in the administration of parenteral and enteral solutions. Am J IV Therapy 5:51–52, May, 1978

Thomas S: Practical nursing. Passing tubes and catheters. Nursing Mirror 148:32–34, 1979

Volden C, Grinde J, Carl D: Taking the trauma out of nasogastric tube insertion. Nursing 80 10(9):64–67, September, 1980

Ziemer M, Carroll J: Infant gavage reconsidered. Am J Nurs 78(9):1543–1544, September, 1978

HYPOTHERMIA BLANKET

Bushnell S: Respiratory Intensive Care Nursing, pp 156–158. Boston, Little, Brown and Co, 1973

INTRAVENOUS THERAPY
BOOKS

Hamilton H: Monitoring Fluid and Electrolytes Precisely. Horsham, Intermed Communications, 1979

Metheny N, Snively W: Nurses Handbook of Fluid Balance, 2nd ed. Philadelphia, JB Lippincott, 1974

Plumer A: Principals and Practices of IV Therapy, 2nd ed. Boston, Little, Brown & Co, 1975

West R: Managing IV Therapy. Nursing Photobook 80. Horsham, Intermed Communications, 1980

JOURNALS

Allen SJ et al: IV fluid administration and the infusion pump. Hospital Formulary 13:769, October, 1978

Buickus B: Administering blood components. Am J Nurs 79(5)937, May, 1979

Crow S: Infection control and IV therapy. NITA 1:58, March/April, 1978

Gump D: Bugs along the lifeline. Emergency Medicine 10:57, April, 1978

Habel M: What you need to know about infusing plasma expanders. RN Magazine 43(8)30, August, 1980

Huxley V: Heparin lock: How, what, why. RN Magazine 42(10):36, October, 1979

Jeffrey LP, Johnson PN, Slonka DJ et al: IV fat emulsion. Hospital Formulary 12:772, November, 1977

Maki DG: Lifelines gone bad. Emergency Medicine 10:70, April, 1978

Miedzianowski S: Water and electrolytes: The rudiments of replacement. Am J IV Therapy 4:19, August/September, 1977

ISOLATION TECHNIQUE
BOOKS

Dept of HEW, Public Health Service, Atlanta Georgia: Isolation Techniques for Use in Hospitals, Washington, Government Printing Office, 1978

JOURNALS

Stamm W: Elements of an active, effective infection control program. Hospitals, JAHA 50(23):60, December, 1976

Steere A, Allison G: Handwashing practices for the prevention of nosocomial infections. Ann Intern Med 83(5):683, November, 1975

NASOPHARYNGEAL OR OROPHARYNGEAL SUCTIONING

Kiriloff L, Maskiewicz R: Guide to respiratory care in critically ill adults. Am J Nurs 79(10):2005, November, 1979

Sandham G, Reid B: Some Q^s and A^s about suctioning and a guide to better techniques. Nursing 77 7(10):60, October, 1977

OSTOMIES, FISTULAS, AND DRAINING WOUNDS
BOOKS

Brunner L, Suddath D: Textbook of Medical–Surgical Nursing, 4th ed. Philadelphia, JB Lippincott, 1980

Mahoney JM: Guide to Ostomy Nursing Care. Boston, Little, Brown & Co, 1976

JOURNALS

Broadwell D, Sorrells S: Loop transverse colostomy. Am J Nurs 78(6):1029–1031, June, 1978

Geels W, Bagley K: The enterocutaneous fistula: Supplanting surgery with meticulous nursing care. Nursing 78 8(4):52–55, 1978

Leibowitz RE, Stuver L, Wagner D et al: Wound management: How teamwork and innovation met a dying patient's needs. Nursing 79 9(6):38–43, June, 1979

Mahoney JM: What you should know about ostomies: Guidelines for giving better post-op care. Nursing 78 8(5):74–84, May, 1978

Manson H: Exorcising excoriation from fistulae and other draining wounds. Nursing 76 6(3):57–60, March, 1976

Taylor: Meeting the challenge of fistulas and draining wounds. Nursing 80 10(6):45–51, June, 1980

UNPUBLISHED WORKS

Weatherby, V: Ostomy Handbook for Suburban Hospital, Bethesda, MD, 1979

OXYGEN ADMINISTRATION

Fuchs P: Getting the best out of oxygen delivery systems. Nursing 80 10(12):34, December, 1980

Moody A: Oxygen therapy. Emergency Nursing 5(4)5, July /August, 1979

Promisloff R: Administering oxygen safely. Nursing 80 10(10):55, October, 1980

ROTATING TOURNIQUETS

Andreoli K, Fowkes VH, Zippes DP et al: Comprehensive Cardiac Care, 3rd ed, pp 52 St Louis, CV Mosby, 1975

Freitag J, Miller, L: Manual of Medical Therapeutics, 23rd ed, pp; 427. Boston, Little, Brown & Co, 1980

SCANS

Devey G, Wells P: Ultrasound in medical diagnosis. Sci Am 238:98, May, 1978

Eymontt M, Eymontt D: Preparing your patient for nuclear medicine: The safe diagnostic tool. Nursing 77 7(12):46, December, 1977

Gordon R, Herman GT, Johnson SA et al: Image reconstruction from projections. Sci Am 233(4):56, October, 1975

Kunkel J, Wiley J: Acute head injury: What to do when and why. Nursing 79 9(3):23, March, 1979

Reeves K: This CAT is a revolutionary scanner. RN Magazine 39(8):40, August, 1976

Traska MR: Ultrasound. Healthcare 7:24, December, 1977

TRACHEOSTOMY CARE

Grossbach–Landis I, McLane A: Tracheal suctioning: A tool for evaluation and learning needs assessment. Nurs Res 28(4):237, July/August, 1979

Kirilloff L, Maskiewicz R: Guide to respiratory care in critically ill adults. Am J Nurs 79(10):2005, November, 1979

O'Donnell B: How to change tracheotomy ties easily and safely. Nursing 78 8(3):66, March, 1978

Pagana K: Teaching your tracheostomy patients to cope at home. RN Magazine 41(12):63, December, 1978

Recommendations for the Disinfection and Maintenance of Respiratory Therapy Equipment. Bureau of Epidemiology, Center for Disease Control, Atlanta, Georgia, 1977

The Control of Pulmonary Infections Associated with Tracheostomy. Bureau of Epidemiology, Center for Disease Control, Atlanta, Georgia, 1979

URINARY BLADDER CATHETERIZATION AND DRAINAGE
BOOKS

Brunner L, Suddath D: Textbook of Medical–Surgical Nursing, 4th ed. Philadelphia, JB Lippincott, 1980

Nursing Photobook: Implementing Urologic Procedures. Horsham, Intermed Communications, 1981

Wood LA: Nursing Skills for Allied Health Services, Vol 3. Philadelphia, WB Saunders, 1975

JOURNALS

Bates P: A troubleshooter's guide to indwelling catheters. RN Magazine 44(3):62–68, March, 1981

Bielski M: Preventing infection in the catheterized patient. Nurs Clin North Am 15(4):703–713, December, 1980

Burke J, Garibaldi R, Britt M et al: Prevention of catheter associated urinary tract infections—efficacy of daily meatal care regimens. Am J Med 70:655–658, March, 1981

DeGroot J: Catheter-induced urinary tract infections: How can we prevent them? Nursing 76 6(8):34–37, August, 1976

Kinney A, Blount M, Dowell M et al: Urethral catheterization. Geriatric Nursing 1(4):258–263, November/December, 1980

Maizels M, Schaeffer AJ: Decreased incidence of bacteriuria associated with periodic instillations of hydrogen peroxide into the urethral catheter drainage bag. J Urol 123(6):841–845, June, 1980

Stamm W: Guidelines for prevention of catheter associated urinary tract infections. Ann Intern Med 82(30):386–390, March, 1975

Woodrow M, Wilsey G: Suprapubic catheters Part I: A direct line to better drainage. Nursing 76 6(10):40–45, October, 1976

4

Pharmacology (PH)

MATHEMATICS OF DOSAGE
METRIC SYSTEM

- In the hospital situation three types of metric measurement are of main concern: length, volume, and weight.
- The basic unit for length is a *meter,* for volume is a *liter,* and for weight is a *gram.*
- There are larger and smaller units of measurement for each basic unit. They will always contain the name of the basic unit (*e.g.,* milli*liter* refers to volume, milli*gram* refers to weight). The larger and smaller units are designated by the following prefixes: kilo, milli, micro.
  1. *Kilo* indicates a quantity larger than the basic unit and multiplies it by 1000 (*e.g.,* 1000 meters = 1 kilometer; 1000 grams = 1 kilogram).
  2. *Milli* indicates a quantity smaller than the basic unit and divides it by 1000 (*e.g.,* 1 liter = 1000 milliliters; 1 gram = 1000 milligrams).
  3. *Micro* indicates a quantity smaller than milli and divides a milli by 1000 (*e.g.,* 1 milligram = 1000 micrograms).
- Abbreviations are commonly used. Official abbreviations (from the National Bureau of Standards) are as follows:
  1. Basic units use the first initial in small letters: meter = m, liter = 1, gram = g.
  2. Larger unit: kilo = k.
  3. Smaller units: centi = c, milli = m, micro = mc.
  4. Unofficial abbreviations commonly used are: gram = Gm, milligram = mgm, microgram = mcgm.
  5. The following are some official examples: kilogram = kg, milliliter = ml, microgram = mcg.
- To ensure accuracy and avoid misunderstanding when using the metric system, always observe the following:
  1. Use Arabic numbers (*e.g.,* 1, 2, 3).
  2. The number is placed in front of the abbreviation (*e.g.,* 2 ml, 4 mg).
  3. A part of a whole is expressed in decimals (*e.g.,* 0.5 ml).
  4. If a whole number is not present in front of the decimal point, place a zero there to emphasize the decimal point (*e.g.,* 0.4 ml, 0.2 mg).
  5. Omit unnecessary zeros to the right of the decimal point (*e.g.,* 0.4 ml, not 0.40 ml).
- The metric system is a decimal system. To *convert* from larger to smaller units of measure or from smaller to larger, you simply move the decimal point.

1. The following units of weight commonly used are listed from highest to lowest value: kg, g, mg, mcg.
2. The units of volume (highest to lowest): 1, ml/cc. (1 ml is considered equivalent to 1 cc, and the abbreviations can be used interchangeably).
3. Each of the above units differs from the next by 1000, so when converting from one "neighbor" to another you move the decimal point three places.
4. When converting from a higher to a lower value, move the decimal point three places to the *right* (*e.g.,* 4.1 g = 4100 mg, 0.132 l = 132 ml).
5. When converting from lower to higher value, move the decimal point three places to the *left* (*e.g.,* 200 mcg = 0.2 mg, 600 ml = 0.6 l).

APOTHECARY SYSTEM

- In the hospital situation two types of apothecary measurement are of main concern: volume and weight
- The units for volume are *ounce, dram,* and *minim.* The unit for weight is a *grain.*
- The abbreviations and symbols used are as follows: ounce = ℥ , dram = ʒ , minim = m, grain = gr
- To ensure accuracy and avoid misunderstanding when using the apothecary system, always observe the following:
  1. Use Roman numerals (*e.g.,* I, II, III)
  2. The abbreviation or symbol is placed in front of the numeral (*e.g.,* gr **V, ʒii,℥** iv).
  3. A part of a whole is expressed in fractions (*e.g.,* gr 1/4; gr 1/2).
  4. s̄s̄ may be used for 1/2 (*e.g., gr ss*).

Nursing Tips

- The following measures and abbreviations are also used:

  tablespoon = T or tbs   drop = gtt
  teaspoon = t or tsp   unit = u
- A unit is an expression of biological action rather than weight. Insulin, heparin, and some antibiotics are measured in units.

CONVERSION TABLE: METRIC–APOTHECARY

- At times it will be necessary to convert between the metric and apothecary systems. The *safest* way to do this is to refer to a conversion table (see Table 4-1). The conversions presented are *equivalents.* Therefore you would find discrepancies if you figured out the same problem mathematically.

TABLE 4-1. **Apothecary Doses with Approximate Metric Equivalents**

Liquid			Weight		
			Grains	*Milligrams*	*Grams*
1 fl oz	= 30	ml	30	= 2000	= 2
1/2 fl oz	= 15	ml	15	= 1000	= 1
2 1/2 fl dr	= 10	ml	10	= 600	= 0.6
2 drams	= 8	ml	7 1/2	= 500	= 0.5
1 1/4 drams	= 5	ml	5	= 300	= 0.3
1 dram	= 4	ml	4	= 250	= 0.25
45 minims	= 3	ml	3	= 200	= 0.2
30 minims	= 2	ml	2 1/2	= 150	= 0.15
15 minims	= 1	ml	2	= 120	= 0.12
12 minims	= 0.75	ml	1 1/2	= 100	= 0.1
10 minims	= 0.6	ml	1	= 60	= 0.06
8 minims	= 0.5	ml	3/4	= 50	= 0.05
5 minims	= 0.3	ml	1/2	= 30	= 0.03
4 minims	= 0.25	ml	3/8	= 25	= 0.025
3 minims	= 0.2	ml	1/3	= 20	= 0.02
1 1/2 minims	= 0.1	ml	1/4	= 15	= 0.015
1 minims	= 0.06	ml	1/6	= 10	= 0.01
3/4 minims	= 0.05	ml	1/8	= 8	= 0.008
1/2 minims	= 0.03	ml	1/10	= 6	= 0.006
			1/15	= 4	= 0.004
			1/20	= 3	= 0.003
			1/30	= 2	= 0.002
			1/40	= 1.5	= 0.0015
			1/60	= 1	= 0.001
			1/100	= 0.6	= 0.0006
			1/120	= 0.5	= 0.0005
			1/150	= 0.4	= 0.0004
			1/200	= 0.3	= 0.0003
			1/250	= 0.25	= 0.00025
			1/500	= 0.12	= 0.00012
			1/600	= 0.1	= 0.0001
			1/1000	= 0.06	= 0.00006

NOTE: 1 ml = approx. 1 cc
       1 Kilogram = 2.2 pounds (lbs)
       1 Liter = 1000 ml

HOUSEHOLD EQUIVALENTS

60 drops (gtt) = 1 teaspoonful (t.)
3 teaspoonfuls = 1 tablespoonful (T.)

CALCULATING DRUG DOSAGE

- The following formula can be used to solve all drug dosage problems. Using a consistent approach helps eliminate errors.

$$\frac{D}{H} \times Q = X$$

D = the *d*osage you *d*esire to give, the *D*r's order
H = the dosage you *h*ave on *h*and, what the pharmacy sent
Q = quantity; for solid preparations the drug usually comes in a tablet or capsule; for liquid preparations the drug is usually in ml (cc) or ounces.
X = the unknown; what you must actually give to administer the desired dose.

Examples

Doctor's order reads: Lanoxin 0.25 mg p.o.
Label on tablet reads: 0.5 mg per tab

$$\frac{(D)\ 0.25\ mg}{(H)\ 0.5\ mg} \times (Q)\ 1\ tab = X \qquad X = 1/2\ tab$$

Doctor's order reads: Keflex 0.5 g p.o.
Label on capsule reads: 250 mg per capsule

$$\frac{(D)\ 0.5\ g}{(H)\ 250\ mg} \times (Q)\ 1\ capsule = X \qquad X = 2\ capsules$$

- Change g to mg in the numerator before working the problem. Numerator and denominator must be in the *same* measurement, and it is usually easier to change the larger quantity (*e.g.*, easier to change the grams in the numerator to milligrams)

$$\frac{0.5\ g}{250\ mg} \times 1\ cap = X$$

$$\frac{500\ mg}{250\ mg} \times 1\ cap = 2\ capsules$$

Doctor's order reads: Aspirin gr x p.o.
Label on tablet reads: Aspirin 325 mg

$$\frac{(D)\ gr\ x}{(H)\ 325\ mg} \times (Q)\ 1\ tab = X \qquad X = 2\ tablets$$

- This problem contains both the apothecary system and the metric system. Use the conversion table to change the gr to mg *before* working the problem. Remember, the two systems are equivalents,

not equals. You will find that gr x = 600 mg. When dividing 325 mg into 600 mg, you must round off the answer to two tablets.
Doctor's order reads: Talwin 30 mg IM
Label on ampule reads: 50 mg per 2 ml

$$\frac{(D)\ 30\ mg}{(H)\ 50\ mg} \times (Q)\ 2\ ml = X \qquad X = 1.2\ ml\ or\ cc$$

- Don't forget to consider that the quantity is 2 ml when calculating the dose.

PEDIATRIC DRUG DOSAGES

- *There are no average dosages for infants and children.* Safe dosages are usually based on the weight or body surface area of the child. The following formula can be used if the medication label does not specify a child's dosage.

$$\frac{average\ adult\ dose\ \times\ weight\ of\ child\ in\ pounds}{150} = estimated\ safe\ dose$$

Example

How much ampicillin should a 2-year-old child weighing 30 pounds receive if the average adult dose is 250 mg?

$$\frac{250\ mg\ \times\ 30\ lbs.}{150} = X \qquad X = 50\ mg$$

Nursing Tips

- Most oral drugs are liquids for ease of swallowing, and many are suspensions that must be mixed thoroughly before administering.
- Doses are usually much smaller than those administered to adults, especially if you are dealing with infants or small children.

CALCULATING IV FLOW RATES

- Solutions are ordered by the physician in ml per hr, but the nurse regulates flow rates in drops (gtt) per minute.
- The following is the formula needed to convert from the ml/hr to the gtt/min.

$$gtt/min\ (flow\ rate) = gtt/ml\ (calibration\ of\ set) \times \frac{ml/hr}{60}$$

- Size of drop varies according to the calibration of the set. Standard or *macrodrip sets* are calibrated at 10 gtt = 1 ml, 15 gtt = 1 ml, or 20 gtt = 1 ml. *Microdrip sets* are calibrated at 60 gtt = 1 ml. This information is found on the package of the IV tubing.

Examples

- Administer an IV at 125 ml/hr, using a set calibrated at 10 gtt/ml.

$$\text{gtt/min} = 10 \text{ gtt/ml} \times \frac{125 \text{ ml/hr}}{60}$$

$$\text{gtt/min} = \frac{125}{6} = 21 \text{ gtt/min}$$

- If tubing calibrated at 10 gtt/min is consistently used you will always divide the 10 into 60 to get 6. Therefore, you can figure out the flow rate in one step by dividing 6 into the ml/hr.
- Administer an IV at 100 ml/hr, using a microdrip set.

$$\text{gtt/min} = 60 \text{ gtt/ml} \times \frac{100 \text{ ml/hr}}{60}$$

$$\text{gtt/min} = \frac{100}{1} = 100 \text{ gtt/min}$$

- When using microdrip tubing, you will always divide the 60 into 60 to get 1. Therefore, the gtt/min will always *equal* the ml/hr.
- Administer an IV at 3000 ml in 24 hr, using a set calibrated at 15 gtt/ml. First you must find out how much fluid to give in *one* hour.

$$24 \sqrt{3000} = 125 \text{ cc/hr}$$

$$\text{gtt/min} = 15 \text{ gtt/ml} \times \frac{125 \text{ ml/hr}}{60}$$

$$\text{gtt/min} = \frac{125}{4} = 31 \text{ gtt/min}$$

- If tubing used is always calibrated at 15 gtt/ml, you will always divide 15 into 60 to get 4. Therefore, just divide the ml/hr by 4 to get the gtt/min. If using tubing calibrated at 20 gtt/ml, you simply divide the ml/hr by 3.

DRUG THERAPY
ADMINISTRATION OF MEDICATIONS

Distributing medications is a crucial and often time-consuming responsibility. You *cannot* underestimate the importance of this task or allow careless habits or distractions to endanger the safety of your patients.

The following are some facts and safety guidelines to consider. For complete "how to" details, consult a nursing fundamentals textbook.

When administering medications, you aim to achieve either a *local* effect (confined to the site of application) or a *systemic* effect (distributed by the blood and diffused into one or more body tissues), although drugs given for a local effect (*e.g.*, eye drops, skin preparations) can be absorbed by the body and produce systemic effects. To achieve systemic effects, the following routes are used:

- *Oral:* safest route, most economical, most convenient, slower onset, at times more prolonged but less potent effects than the parenteral route.
- *Sublingual:* drug is placed under patient's tongue and is retained until dissolved and absorbed by way of the venous capillaries. This route prevents drug destruction by the digestive juices and enzymes of the liver.
- *Rectal:* used when stomach is nonretentive or when the patient is unconscious. Rectum should be free of feces in order to promote optimal absorption.
- *Parenteral:* refers to all forms of drug injection into the body tissues or fluids. Drugs must be sterile and nonirritating. Usually a more rapid onset of action than with the oral route, but duration is shorter. There are four main categories of parenteral injection.
  1. *Intravenous:* direct injection into the blood stream; most rapid acting but least safe. Carefully consider the purpose of the IV when choosing the site and equipment. For example, emergency situations usually require a large vein and one of the plastic cannulas rather than a butterfly needle. You are then prepared to deliver large volumes of fluid rapidly if this is necessary.
     a. *Heparin locks* are a popular means for delivering intermittent IV medications. The butterfly-type needle has a rubber stopper on the end that can receive repeated injections. The vein is kept open by flushing the tubing with a small amount of a dilute heparin preparation after each medication. This allows the patient much greater freedom of movement than the traditional IV setup.
  2. *Intramuscular:* injection into muscular tissue. Sources differ as to the safe maximum amount to be injected into a single site. Factors to consider are the drug, the site used, and the disease state. An injection of 3 ml is considered safe by most sources. These injections are given at a 90° angle, using a 1 to 1½-inch needle with a gauge of 20 to 23 (the larger the gauge, the finer the needle). Commonly used sites are the ventrogluteal muscle, the upper outer quadrant of the buttocks, the midlateral and midanterior thigh, and the deltoid muscle (see Fig. 4-1). These sites are chosen to avoid nerves and major blood vessels. Using the ventrogluteal muscle is often preferable to using the upper outer quadrant because it keeps the injection further away from the sciatic nerve. When charting the medication, always chart the site given, and rotate sites whenever possible.

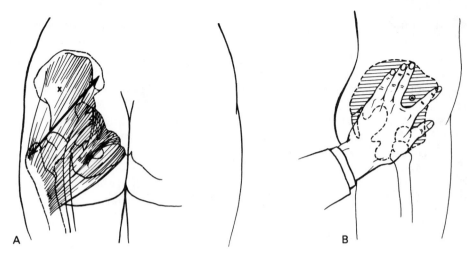

FIG. 4-1. *Two sites for intramuscular injections.* (A) *The upper outer quadrant of the buttocks;* (B) *the ventrogluteal muscle.* (Wolff L, Weitzel MH, Fuerst EV: Fundamentals of Nursing, 6th ed, p 616. Philadephia, JB Lippincott, 1980)

    a. Some intramuscular injections are given using the Z-track technique (*e.g.,* to administer iron dextran; see Fig. 4-2).
       1. Draw up solution and then change to a fresh needle. Usually a 19 to 20 gauge, 2 to 3 inch needle is used.
       2. Draw up 0.5 cc of air into the syringe.
       3. Choose injection site (*e.g.,* upper outer quadrant of the buttocks) and firmly displace skin, fat, and muscle to one side.
       4. Clean area, insert needle, check for blood return.
       5. Inject solution slowly, followed by the air in the syringe.
       6. Wait 10 seconds, pull the needle straight out, and release the tissues. Apply direct pressure.
  3. *Subcutaneous:* injection under the layers of the skin. Amount usually ranges from 0.5 to 2 ml in one site. Needle length ranges from 1/2 to 5/8 inch with a gauge of 25. Because of the needle length, injection should be given at a 90° angle. Extremely thin patients may require the 45° angle.
    a. *Hypodermoclysis:* introduction of large amounts of fluid (500 to 1000 ml) into subcutaneous tissue (*e.g.,* under breasts or upper thighs). Used for dehydrated patients when IV therapy cannot be done.
  4. *Intradermal:* injection into upper layers of the skin. Amount is

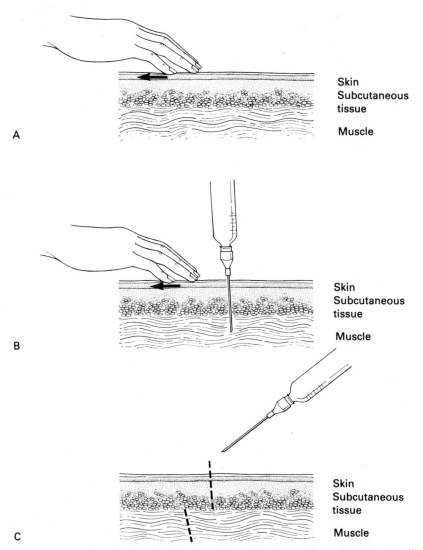

FIG. 4-2. *Z-track technique for injections. Tissue is retracted laterally* (A) *as needle is inserted* (B). *After needle is withdrawn* (C), *tissue returns to normal. The track of needle is thus broken, so medication cannot leak out.*

small (measured in minims) and absorption is slow. Needle length ranges from 1/2 to 3/4 inch and 26 or 27 gauge. Usually a 10° to 15° angle is used. This method is used for skin testing for allergic reactions and for administering tuberculosis tests.

Nursing Tips

- In order to avoid errors you must concentrate on what you are doing. This means working alone, without interruptions, whenever possible.
- Do not give a medication if you can't read the label. Many medications are similar in color and shape. Return it to the pharmacy to be relabeled. If a patient is being discharged with medications, the pharmacist must relabel them appropriately for home use. Planning ahead for this can avoid delays at departure time.
- Be sure you have correctly identified your patients. Check the ID bracelet. Some patients (especially if confused) will respond to a name other than their own. Therefore it is best to ask the patient to tell you his or her name.
- Never chart medications before giving them. Never chart a medication given by another person unless it is clearly stated who administered the drug (*e.g.,* the physician). Chart all medications as soon as possible after giving them, especially p.r.n.'s or STAT drugs. Otherwise the patient may receive a double dose.
- Never administer drugs prepared by another person—you will be responsible for any errors. If you wish to help a busy co-worker, make a bed or give a bath!
- If a patient has any symptoms of an allergic reaction, report it immediately.
- If the patient indicates that a drug is different from what he has been taking, recheck before giving it. Patients can help you prevent errors too.
- When drugs are omitted intentionally for OR or diagnostic testing, record the omission and the reason on the patient's chart.
- It is very important to maintain therapeutic blood levels of most medications. The physician may want the drug given even if the patient should not eat or drink prior to a diagnostic test. If you have any questions, check with the physician before withholding the drug.
- Report drug errors or omissions immediately, and for your own protection fill out an incident report.
- Never give any medication, even a placebo, without a physician's written order. If you are in a position where you must accept phone or verbal orders, be sure the physician signs the order as soon as possible.
- You should have a physician's written order before leaving any medication at a patient's bedside (*e.g.,* nitroglycerin or eye drops).
- When drawing up some medications, double-check your results with another qualified person. When administering such drugs as

heparin and insulin, small differences can be crucial to the patient.
- Preparations for internal use should be kept separate from those used externally.
- Never crush enteric-coated tablets. Your patient may experience gastric irritation, and the effectiveness of the drug may be affected.
- Never divide tablets, suppositories, and so forth unless they are clearly scored. Return the preparation to the pharmacist and obtain the correct dosage, or have the pharmacist prepare it.
- In order to prevent toxic reactions from some drugs, physicians order blood levels of the drug checked. Timing is important to ensure accurate results. The blood should be drawn *before* the drug is given, and the nurse is responsible for coordinating drug administration with the laboratory. Examples of drug levels frequently checked are digoxin, gentamicin, heparin, and aminophylline.
- Eye drops are sterile and must not be contaminated. They should be instilled only in the lower conjunctival sac, never dropped directly on the cornea.
- To help reduce systemic absorption of eye drops, apply gentle pressure on the inner canthus (near the nose) for a few minutes after the drops are administered.
- If you feel a medication order is wrong, question it!

PHARMACOKINETICS

This term refers to the processes by which the body absorbs, distributes, metabolizes, and removes drugs. Also considered are the variables that influence drug action in the body.
- *Absorption:* the drug is transferred from the site of entry to the circulating fluids of the body (*e.g.,* blood and lymphatics). Absorption is affected by the following: route of administration (*e.g.,* IV produces immediate absorption), the solubility of the drug and how it is influenced by pH, local conditions at site of administration (*e.g.,* poor circulation or edema can delay absorption), drug concentration or dosage, and enteric coating.
- *Distribution:* the drug is transferred to its sites of action, metabolism, and excretion. Drugs will diffuse faster to areas of greater blood perfusion (*e.g.,* brain, liver, kidneys). Drugs can combine with plasma proteins and thus remain longer in the circulating fluids. Circulatory problems (*e.g.,* atherosclerosis) may slow drug distribution.
- *Biotransformation:* the drug is metabolized, usually in the liver. The drug is converted into products that are generally less active and more easily excreted. The metabolism is usually accomplished by the body's enzyme systems. Factors that depress enzyme function

(*e.g.*, hepatic disease or advanced age) will depress metabolism and may allow drugs to accumulate to toxic levels in the body.

- *Excretion:* the drugs, both metabolized and unchanged, leave the body by a variety of routes. Gaseous substances like anesthetics are excreted by way of the lungs. The majority of drugs and drug products are excreted by way of the kidneys.

VARIABLES INFLUENCING DRUG ACTION

- Neonates and the elderly often have particular problems with drug action because they lack or have diminished enzyme systems.
- The dosage of a drug is frequently calculated on the basis of the ratio of milligrams of the drug to the patient's weight (as expressed in pounds or kilograms).
- Pregnancy is a factor because many drugs easily cross over the placental barrier and can cause malformations and other problems with the fetus.
- Sex itself is a variable because body weight, percentage of body fat, and hormonal changes can affect drug action.
- Because of the body's biologic or diurnal rhythms, drugs can be affected by time of administration. They may also react with food in the stomach.
- Pathological states, especially of the kidneys and liver, interfere with drug action.
- Genetic differences can produce differences in drug metabolism (usually because of effects on the enzymes).
- A patient's belief in the effectiveness of a drug and the manner in which it is administered can influence drug action.
- Occasionally a patient's immune system produces antibodies against a drug. Subsequent administration of the drug can produce serious problems for the patient.
- Tolerance—a decreased physiologic response to repeated administration of a drug—develops in some people.
- Cumulation (drug is excreted more slowly than absorbed) can lead to toxic levels of a drug in the body (*e.g.*, digoxin, lead).
- Interactions between drugs can interfere with the desired effects of a drug. Both prescription and over-the-counter medications can cause problems in this manner.

DRUGS AND THE ELDERLY

- The elderly frequently take more medications on a regular basis than other patient populations. This includes both prescription and over-the-counter drugs.
- The elderly are usually at a higher risk for experiencing side-effects because of normal aging changes that can affect drug action.

They frequently have one or more acute or chronic illnesses that can also alter drug action. And finally, they are more likely to be taking multiple medications that increase the risk of drug interactions.

- Aging changes can alter sensitivity to drug action. Drug receptor sites may be affected, and the person may experience a decrease in homeostatic mechanisms. However, altered pharmacokinetics appear to cause the main changes in drug action.
- The action of drugs can also be affected by bed rest, dehydration, diet, fever, humidity, malnutrition, stress, and temperature.

ABSORPTION

- Most drugs are absorbed by passive diffusion, which appears to be unchanged by the aging process. The mucosa in the aging intestine may actually be less of a barrier to drugs than that of a younger person.
- Absorption of drugs in the elderly may be delayed or reduced for the following reasons:
  1. Decreased fluid volume and decreased gastric acidity may influence pH and affect the solubility of the drugs.
  2. Decreased peristalsis and gastric emptying could increase local gastric adverse effects.
  3. Decreased blood flow to the intestine
  4. Concurrent administration of other drugs

DISTRIBUTION

- The elderly may experience a decrease in plasma proteins to bind with drugs. Both kidney and liver disease may further decrease plasma proteins.
- Increased levels of unbound drugs can enhance drug action and lead to an increase in adverse reactions and toxicity.
- The blood–brain barrier may become more permeable in the elderly, increasing the chance of central nervous system toxicity.
- A decreased cardiac output, increased circulation time, and cardiovascular disease will also alter distribution.
- Multiple drug use may affect distribution by affecting the protein binding. Drugs may compete for binding sites, and some drugs may be capable of displacing others. Again, the elderly may be left with increased amounts of free drug and the increased risk of toxicity.

BIOTRANSFORMATION

- Aging changes may depress enzyme function and metabolism in the elderly.

- Decreased blood flow to the liver (*e.g.,* from congestive heart failure) may reduce the rate of metabolism.
- Vitamin deficiency may alter enzyme activity.
- Drugs themselves may either increase or decrease enzyme activity, and again we are concerned with a population that frequently uses multiple drugs.

EXCRETION

- With aging there is a reduction in blood flow to the kidneys and therefore a reduction in the glomerular filtration rate. There may also be a reduction in the number of functioning tubules.
- Renal impairment is increased by arteriosclerosis, infections, and hypertension.

DRUGS IN RELATION TO SYSTEMS AND SPECIALTIES
ANALGESIC ANTIPYRETICS, ANTI-INFLAMMATORY AGENTS, DRUGS FOR GOUT

ACETAMINOPHEN, U.S.P. (TYLENOL, TEMPRA)
Actions

- Analgesic; antipyretic.

Indications

- Relieves mild to moderate pain.
- May be preferred to aspirin
    1. when patients easily experience gastrointestinal irritation
    2. for gout patients receiving drugs to promote excretion of uric acid
    3. for patients on anticoagulants or those with hemorrhagic disorders
    4. for patients who are allergic to the salicylates

Adverse Effects, Contraindications

- Few side-effects from ordinary doses.
- Rarely, renal damage, hemolytic anemia, and methemoglobinemia (a part of hemoglobin is changed and oxygen cannot be transported) have occurred.
- Drug should be discontinued if skin redness, itching, or urticaria occur.
- Liver damage, especially in children, can occur with normal therapeutic doses.
- Massive overdose may lead to death from acute hepatic necrosis, hypoglycemia, or metabolic acidosis.

Dosage, Administration

- Usual adult dosage is 300 to 600 mg p.o. q 4 hr. It is available in tablets, syrups, and drops.

Nursing Tips

- Some over-the-counter (OTC) preparations that contain acetaminophen are Bromo-Seltzer, Excedrin, Medache, and Vanquish.
- Acetylcysteine (Mucomyst) *(see PH, Respiratory, Mucolytic agents)* is an antidote to acetaminophen toxicity when given orally if used within 24 hr of the poisoning.

ALLOPURINOL, U.S.P. (ZYLOPRIM)
Actions

- Reduces the production of uric acid by inhibiting the biochemical reactions immediately before its formation.

Indications

- Reduces hyperuricemia in both primary and secondary gout.
- Reduces the recurrence of uric acid stone formation.
- Prevents renal calculi, uric acid nephropathy, and tissue urate deposits in patients with leukemias, lymphomas, and malignancies who are receiving antineoplastic drugs or radiation therapy that elevate serum uric acid levels.

Adverse Effects, Contraindications

- Discontinue allopurinol at the first sign of skin rash or other adverse effects. Severe hypersensitivity reactions may follow a skin rash.
- Patients may experience nausea, vomiting, and diarrhea.
- Blood dyscrasias have occurred in patients receiving allopurinol. Concurrent administration of other drugs that have the potential of causing blood dyscrasias is usually involved.
- Drowsiness occurs occasionally.

Dosage, Administration

- Average adult dosage is 200 to 300 mg orally, daily for mild hyperuricemia and 400 to 600 mg orally, daily for more severe hyperuricemia.
- Patients receiving antineoplastic drugs may require 600 to 800 mg orally, daily for 2 or 3 days with a high fluid intake. Dosage should not exceed 800 mg daily.
- Allopurinol is usually administered in divided doses after meals.

Nursing Tips

- Serum uric acid levels are used to determine appropriate maintenance doses of allopurinol.
- Liver and kidney function should be monitored during therapy.
- Caution patients against driving if the medication causes drowsiness.
- Allopurinol may precipitate attacks of gout when treatment is started. Usually, maintenance doses of colchicine (0.5 mg b.i.d) are given as a prophylactic measure.
- Patients receiving allopurinol should drink enough fluid to produce two liters of urine daily. Another measure to prevent calculi is the use of urinary alkalinizers.
- Oral iron salts should not be taken with allopurinol because the iron may be deposited in the liver.
- Allopurinol can prolong the half-life of anticoagulants. Monitor prothrombin times carefully.
- The doses of mercaptopurine (antileukemic drug) and azathioprine (an immunosuppressant) should be reduced by $\frac{1}{3}$ to $\frac{1}{4}$ when allopurinol is added. Otherwise severe bone marrow depression results.

ASPIRIN, U.S.P. (ACETYLSALICYLIC ACID)

Actions

- Analgesic; antipyretic; anti-inflammatory; inhibits platelet aggregation and prolongs bleeding time.

Indications

- Reduces fever.
- Relieves mild to moderate pain (*e.g.,* in joints and muscles, with headache).
- Reduces inflammation.
- To prevent coronary thrombosis and cerebral or pulmonary embolism.
- Relieves pain associated with osteoarthritis.

Adverse Effects, Contraindications

- Nausea, vomiting, *gastrointestinal bleeding,* and ulceration.
- Mild toxicity produces tinnitus (ringing in ears), visual blurring, drowsiness, and mental confusion.
- Acute toxicity produces severe *acid–base imbalances* especially in children, *convulsions, coma,* and *respiratory failure.*
- May also produce skin rashes and wheezing.
- Patients with gout or hemorrhagic disorders should use aspirin cautiously.

Dosage, Administration

- Usual adult dosage is 600 mg (gr x) p.o. q. 3 to 4 hr.
- For rheumatic disorders, dosage ranges from 3.6 to 10 g q.d.
- Ecotrin is enteric-coated aspirin. Each tablet contains 325 mg (5 gr) of aspirin. The coating prevents disintegration in the stomach and minimizes the possibility of gastric irritation.
- Aspirin suppositories contain 2 gr, 5 gr, or 10 gr.

Nursing Tips

- To minimize gastrointestinal irritation, give aspirin with meals, milk or snacks.
- Some over-the-counter (OTC) preparations that contain aspirin are Alka-Seltzer, Anacin, A.P.C. Tablets, Bufferin, Empirin Compound, Excedrin, and Vanquish.
- In small doses aspirin can interfere with probenecid and uric acid excretion.
- Aspirin may potentiate the action of oral anticoagulants.
- Salicylates are the most common cause of accidental poisoning among children.
- Some surgeons recommend abstaining from the use of aspirin products for 2 weeks prior to elective surgery to minimize the risk of bleeding.

COLCHICINE, U.S.P.

Actions

- Inhibits the migration of granulocytes into the inflamed area.
- Thought to decrease lactic acid production by the leukocytes, thereby decreasing urate crystal deposits and subsequent inflammation.

Indications

- Prevents and treats acute attacks of gout.

Adverse Effects, Contraindications

- Nausea, vomiting, or diarrhea can occur with therapeutic doses.
- Prolonged therapy may cause bone marrow depression with agranulocytosis, thrombocytopenia and aplastic anemia. The drug is not indicated for more than 5 to 7 days.
- Use cautiously in the elderly and the debilitated, or in those with cardiovascular disease.

Dosage, Administration

- Usual adult dose is one to two tablets (0.6 mg/tab) orally at the first warning of an acute attack. This is followed by one tablet every 1 to 2 hr until pain is relieved or until nausea, vomiting, or diarrhea occurs.

- Number of tablets used ranges from 6 to 16.
- To prevent attacks, one tablet may be taken one to four times a week for mild or moderate cases and one to two times daily for severe cases.

Nursing Tips

- Monitor blood counts for signs of bone marrow depression.

IBUPROFEN U.S.P. (MOTRIN)

Actions

- Reduces inflammation.
- Possesses analgesic and antipyretic activities.

Indications

- Relieves symptoms of rheumatoid arthritis and osteoarthritis.
- Also relieves mild to moderate pain.

Adverse Effects, Contraindications

- Gastrointestinal effects are most frequent. They include nausea, heartburn, diarrhea, vomiting, and constipation.
- Dizziness, headache, nervousness, and tinnitus can occur.
- Patients have experienced rashes, decreased appetite, and fluid retention.
- Use cautiously for patients with a history of gastrointestinal disease because ulceration and bleeding have been reported in patients receiving ibuprofen.
- Patients with cardiovascular disease should use this drug cautiously because of the fluid retention that can occur.
- Ibuprofen inhibits platelet aggregation and prolongs bleeding time. Use cautiously for patients with hemostatic defects or those receiving anticoagulants.
- Blurred or diminished vision and changes in color vision have been reported.
- Anaphylactoid reactions have occurred in patients with aspirin hypersensitivity.

Dosage, Administration

- Rheumatoid arthritis and osteoarthritis: Usual adult dosage is 300 to 600 mg orally three or four times daily.
- Mild to moderate pain: 400 mg orally every 4 to 6 hr as needed.

- Gastrointestinal side-effects may be reduced by giving ibuprofen with meals or milk.
- Maximum dose per day is 2,400 mg.

Nursing Tips

- The incidence of epigastric distress with ibuprofen is reported to be only half that with aspirin.
- Periodic eye examinations are recommended to detect any adverse ocular effects.
- Ibuprofen can displace other drugs from the plasma proteins and thus increase their activity. These drugs include anticoagulants, antiepileptic drugs, oral hypoglycemics, and sulfonamides.

INDOMETHACIN, N.F. (INDOCIN)

Actions

- Relieves inflammation.
- Possesses analgesic and antipyretic activities.

Indications

- Relieves symptoms of rheumatoid arthritis and osteoarthritis.
- Also relieves symptoms of ankylosing spondylitis and acute gouty arthritis.

Adverse Effects, Contraindications

- Gastrointestinal reactions include anorexia, nausea, vomiting, epigastric distress, abdominal pain, and diarrhea.
- Gastrointestinal bleeding, ulceration, and possible perforation have occurred.
- Headache, drowsiness, dizziness, and light-headedness have been reported.
- Tinnitus and blurring of vision are possible.
- Indomethacin may aggravate epilepsy, parkinsonism, and psychiatric disturbances.
- Inhibits platelet aggregation and prolongs bleeding time. Use cautiously for patients with hemostatic defects or those receiving anticoagulants.

Dosage, Administration

- Always give the drug with food, immediately after meals, or with antacids. The smallest, effective dose should be determined for each patient.
- Usual adult dosage initially is 25 mg orally two or three times daily.

Daily dosage may be increased 25 or 50 mg at weekly intervals. Maximum total daily dose is 150 to 200 mg.
- Acute gouty arthritis is treated with 50 mg orally, t.i.d. After pain relief is obtained, the dose should be rapidly reduced and then the drug discontinued.

Nursing Tips
- Indomethacin may mask signs and symptoms of infection.
- Prolonged, high doses of aspirin decrease indomethacin blood levels.
- Plasma levels of indomethacin usually increase when probenecid is given concurrently.
- Indomethacin may interfere with the action of furosemide.

PHENYLBUTAZONE, U.S.P. (BUTAZOLIDIN)
Actions
- Anti-inflammatory; analgesic; antipyretic; uricosuric.

Indications
- Relieves symptoms of rheumatoid arthritis when the patient is unresponsive to salicylates.
- Relieves acute gout attacks not controlled by colchicine.

Adverse Effects, Contraindications
- This drug produces a *high* incidence of side-effects.
- Edema, nausea, stomatitis, rash, and dizziness occur.
- Hemorrhage and peptic ulcer are possible.
- Bone marrow depression has occurred, leading to serious blood dyscrasias (*e.g.,* leukopenia, thrombocytopenia, and agranulocytosis).
- Patients with a history of cardiac, liver, or renal disorders, peptic ulcer, or blood dyscrasias should not receive this drug.
- Toxic effects may also include hepatitis, hypertension, or renal and liver necrosis.

Dosage, Administration
- Usual initial adult dosage is 300 to 600 mg q.d. in divided doses. The minimal effective dose is then determined. Should not be given for more than 10 days.

Nursing Tips
- Take immediately before or after meals or with milk.
- The following drug interactions occur with phenylbutazone:
  1. It potentiates the action of warfarin.

2. It potentiates the hypoglycemic effects of insulin and oral hypoglycemic drugs.
3. It potentiates penicillin and the sulfonamides.
4. It inhibits the action of barbituates, and the barbituates inhibit phenylbutazone.
5. It inhibits the action of steroids, sex hormones, and other anti-inflammatory drugs.

PROBENECID, U.S.P. (BENEMID)
Actions
- Inhibits tubular reabsorption of urate.
- Increases urinary excretion of uric acid.
- Inhibits tubular secretion of penicillin, and increases penicillin plasma levels.

Indications
- Hyperuricemia associated with gout and gouty arthritis.

Adverse Effects, Contraindications
- Nausea, vomiting, headache, and urinary frequency have occurred.
- Hypersensitivity reactions such as anaphylaxis, dermatitis, and fever have been reported.
- May precipitate attacks of gout and increase the formation of uric acid stones.

Dosage, Administration
- Therapy is begun *after* an acute gouty attack has subsided.
- Usual adult dosage is 0.25 g ($\frac{1}{2}$ tab) orally twice a day for 1 week, followed by 0.5 g (1 tab) twice a day thereafter.
- If necessary, dosage may be increased but should not exceed 2 g per day.
- Usual dosage for adults receiving penicillin therapy is 2 g daily in divided doses.

Nursing Tips
- Therapy with probenecid may precipitate an attack of gout. If this occurs colchicine is usually given.
- Uric acid tends to crystallize out of an acid urine. Patients should drink enough fluid to produce 2 liters of urine daily. Three to 7.5 g of sodium bicarbonate given daily can maintain an alkaline urine.
- Probenecid increases plasma levels of methotrexate. The dosage of methotrexate should be reduced, and serum levels should be monitored.

- Salicylates should not be used with probenecid because they antagonize the uricosuric action of probenecid.
- Probenecid may potentiate the action of oral hypoglycemics. Blood glucose should be monitored.
- Plasma levels of indomethacin usually increase when probenecid is given concurrently.

ZOMEPIRAC SODIUM (ZOMAX)
Actions

- Analgesic; anti-inflammatory agent; also possesses antipyretic properties.

Indications

- Relieves mild to moderately severe pain.

Adverse Effects, Contraindications

- Nausea is the most frequent adverse effect. Patients also experience diarrhea, vomiting, abdominal pain, constipation, flatulence, and dyspepsia.
- Dizziness, drowsiness, insomnia, and paresthesia have occurred.
- Edema and elevated blood pressure have been reported.
- Rash and urinary tract infection also occur.
- Therapy with zomepirac for longer than 6 months is not recommended because of possible kidney damage.
- Use cautiously in patients with fluid retention, hypertension, and heart failure.
- Patients with coagulation disorders should use this drug cautiously because it inhibits platelet function and prolongs bleeding time.
- Use cautiously for patients with a history of gastrointestinal disease because patients receiving zomepirac have developed peptic ulceration and bleeding.

Dosage, Administration

- Usual adult dosage is one tablet (100 mg) orally every 4 to 6 hrs as needed.
- In mild pain, one-half tablet (50 mg) every 4 to 6 hr may be sufficient.
- Maximum daily dose should not exceed 600 mg.

Nursing Tips

- If gastrointestinal symptoms occur, zomepirac may be given with antacids.
- The administration of aspirin with zomepirac is not recommended.

- Kidney function should be monitored especially for patients on long-term therapy.
- Periodic eye exams are recommended for patients receiving zomepirac. Eye changes have been reported with other nonsteroid anti-inflammatories.

ANTIMICROBIALS
Actions

- Antimicrobials exert either *bacteriostatic* or *bactericidal* activity (or a combination of both). Bacteriostatic drugs inhibit the growth of the organism, allowing the person's own defense mechanisms to function. Bactericidal drugs actually kill the organism. Antimicrobials can exert their activity in one of several ways:
  1. synthesis of bacterial cell walls is inhibited
  2. utilization of substances needed for growth and reproduction is reduced (antimetabolites)
  3. the permeability of the cell wall is altered so that essential components may leak out
  4. protein synthesis is impaired and genetic information is misread by the cells.
- The action of an antimicrobial is designated as either *narrow-spectrum* or *broad-spectrum.*
  1. narrow-spectrum drugs are effective against only a few microorganisms.
  2. broad-spectrum drugs are effective against a wide variety of microorganisms.
- The action of antimicrobials is complimented by the person's own defense mechanisms (*e.g.,* antibody production and phagocytosis).

Indications

- Antimicrobials are indicated when the problem is caused by a pathogen that will respond to these drugs, especially when the person's own defense mechanisms are depleted. Few drugs are effective against common viral diseases (*e.g.,* colds) and treatment with antimicrobials is not usually indicated in these cases.
- At times, antimicrobials are indicated to prevent infection (*e.g.,* recurrences of rheumatic fever or bacterial endocarditis). Because of the wide variety of antimicrobials available, proper drug selection is crucial. The pathogen causing the infection must be identified. Specimens for culture must be carefully obtained. *(See LAB, Cultures)*
- Certain drugs are known to be effective against certain pathogens. Otherwise, sensitivity testing is done to determine the cause of the infection. *(See LAB, Cultures)*

Adverse Effects, Contraindications

- *Allergic reactions* that can affect the skin, organs, blood, and bone marrow. These reactions range from simple skin rashes to anaphylactic shock.
- *Lack of selective toxicity* (the antimicrobials will exert their bacteriostatic and bactericidal activity upon normal cells as well as the pathogens). The kidneys, liver, nervous tissue, bone marrow, or gastrointestinal tract are frequently affected.
- *Superinfections:* the patient's own protective bacteria may be eliminated by the antimicrobials, allowing pathogens to grow where they normally would be restrained. The superinfection can be much more dangerous to the patient than the original problem.

Dosage, Administration

- It is extremely important that the antimicrobials be administered in high enough doses and for the proper duration. Otherwise, the infection may recur as a chronic problem, and resistance to the antimicrobial may develop. Though the patient may feel better he must be counseled to finish the entire prescription.
- Resistance may also be delayed or prevented by using two or more antimicrobials at the same time.
- Always check to determine whether or not the antimicrobial should be given with food.

Nursing Tips

- Be alert for any changes in your patient's condition or behavior in order to identify any allergic reactions or toxic effects that may be occurring. Further administration of the drug could greatly intensify the reaction. Withhold the medication and notify the physician *immediately* if you suspect a reaction.
- Because allergic reactions are relatively common with antimicrobials, taking a complete drug history is crucial.
- Some antimicrobials, especially the liquid preparations for children, contain additives for coloring and flavoring. The additives, rather than the medication itself, may cause adverse effects (*e.g.,* CNS stimulation).
- Cultures must be obtained *before* the antimicrobial therapy is begun for accurate results. If therapy cannot be delayed until culture results are returned, a broad-spectrum antimicrobial is used.

AMINOGLYCOSIDES
Actions

- These drugs are both bacteriostatic and bactericidal.
- They cause a misreading of genetic information, thereby altering protein synthesis in the bacteria.

Indications

- Used mainly to treat severe infections caused by gram-negative bacteria (*e.g.,* bacteremia, meningitis, peritonitis, urinary infections).
- These drugs are not usually indicated to treat gram-positive infections (though they are effective) because less toxic antimicrobials are available.

Adverse Effects, Contraindications

- Ototoxicity—damage to the eighth cranial nerve. May cause permanent deafness and ataxia. Damage is most likely when the medication is given parenterally but can also occur with oral and topical preparations.
- Nephrotoxicity—damage to the kidneys. Again, damage is most likely to occur with the parenteral forms given in long-term therapy.
- If patient has received a neuromuscular-blocking drug (*e.g.,* during surgery), skeletal muscle paralysis can occur.
- Resistance to these drugs develops easily, especially when administered topically.

Nursing Tips

- Question patients concerning ringing in ears, vertigo, dizziness, and persistent, severe headache. Patients on long-term therapy should have periodic tests of hearing.
- Perform laboratory determinations of renal function. Creatinine clearance rates are a good indication of the kidneys' ability to eliminate the drugs. *(See LAB)*

GENTAMICIN SULFATE, U.S.P. (GARAMYCIN)

(See PH, Aminoglycosides: actions, indications, adverse effects, nursing tips)

- Most frequently used to treat serious urinary tract infections, meningitis, and septicemia.
- Because of the synergistic activity that occurs, gentamicin is combined with ampicillin to treat endocarditis and with carbenicillin to destroy the Pseudomonas bacteria.
- Gentamicin may be used topically to treat both skin and eye infections.
- Do not administer with other drugs that are also nephrotoxic (*e.g.,* polymyxins, cephaloridine, potent diuretics).
- Topical use may lead to overgrowth of fungi and resistance.
- Usual daily dosage is 3 mg/kg IV or IM (but may range from 0.8 to 5 mg/kg) divided equally and given every 8 hr.
- Frequently, gentamicin blood levels are drawn to determine the

effectiveness and toxicity of the drug. Blood should be drawn $\frac{1}{2}$ to 1 hr *before* the next dose is administered.

- Frequency of administration may be reduced to every 12, 18, 24, 36, or 48 hr if kidney function is compromised. Duration of therapy is usually 7 to 10 days.
- Cream or ointment is usually applied three or four times daily.
- Ophthalmic ointment is usually applied two or three times daily.

KANAMYCIN SULFATE, U.S.P. (KANTREX)

(See PH, Aminoglycosides: actions, indications, adverse effects, nursing tips)

- The parenteral form is employed mainly in *short-term* therapy in severe systemic infections (*e.g.*, septicemia, gram-negative urinary infections, some pneumonias).
- The oral form is used to control infections in the gastrointestinal tract and to destroy normal intestinal flora prior to surgery and in the management of hepatic coma.
- Ototoxicity from parenteral administration can occur as early as day five of therapy. Do not administer with other ototoxic drugs (*e.g.*, potent diuretics).
- Do not administer with nephrotoxic drugs such as the polymyxins and gentamicin.
- Usual dosage range is 250 to 500 mg every 6 hr IM (seldom given IV, and maximum daily dose is usually limited to 1.5 g).
- Usual oral dosage is 1 g every 4 hr, but patients in hepatic coma may receive 8 to 12 g daily.

NEOMYCIN SULFATE, U.S.P. (MYCIGUENT)

(See PH, Aminoglycosides: actions, indications, adverse effects, nursing tips)

- *Seldom* used systemically because of its toxicity.
- Used orally to suppress the normal bacterial flora of the bowel in hepatic coma and prior to abdominal surgery.
- May also be used to treat some types of infectious diarrhea.
- Topically, it is used to prevent and treat skin infections and, in solution, to irrigate urinary bladders of patients with indwelling catheters.
- Nausea, vomiting, and diarrhea occur frequently with oral administration.
- A reversible malabsorption syndrome is a rare occurrence.
- Overgrowths of bacteria and fungi may cause superinfections.
- Do not give to patients with large ulcers or intestinal obstruction because of the danger of systemic absorption.

- Neomycin easily reaches toxic levels in patients with impaired kidney function.
- Topical administration can lead to hypersensitivity reactions (*e.g.,* skin rashes).
- For preoperative bowel preparation, 1 g is given orally every hour for 4 hours, then 1 g every 4 hr for the rest of the 24 hr.
- Usual oral dosage range for hepatic coma is 4 to 12 g per day for 5 to 6 days.
- Daily oral dose for infectious diarrhea is 3 g.

STREPTOMYCIN SULFATE, U.S.P.

(See PH, Aminoglycosides: actions, indications, adverse effects, nursing tips)

- Used mainly with other antitubercular drugs in the treatment of tuberculosis, especially for cases with large lung cavities or for extrapulmonary tuberculosis.
- May be combined with other antimicrobials to treat urinary tract infections, nocardiosis, and tularemia.
- Vertigo is the most frequent side-effect.
- Optic and peripheral nerves are occasionally affected.
- Allergic reactions (*e.g.,* skin eruptions) occur both in patients receiving the drug and persons administering it.
- Blood dyscrasias can develop.
- Patients with compromised kidney function are susceptible to kidney damage.
- Usual dosage is 1 to 2 g daily, deep IM, divided into two equal parts at 12-hr intervals.

ANTIFUNGALS
AMPHOTERICIN B, U.S.P. (FUNGIZONE)
Actions

- This is a systemic antifungal agent.
- This antimicrobial is both fungistatic and fungicidal.

Indications

- Used parenterally to treat serious systemic fungal infections (*e.g.,* histoplasmosis or blastomycosis).
- May be used topically on the skin, nails, and mucous membranes of the mouth to treat infections caused by candidal species.

Adverse Effects, Contraindications

- Intravenous administration frequently causes chills, fever, vomiting, and headache.

- Kidney and liver toxicity and anemia may occur.
- Severe hypotension and electrolyte imbalances can result.
- Allergic reactions from topical application are infrequent.

Dosage, Administration

- Maximum dosage is usually 1 mg/kg per day or 1.5 mg/kg every other day given IV.

Nursing Tips

- Intravenous solutions should be used as soon as possible after preparation and should be protected from light.
- Alkalinization of the urine will promote excretion of the drug and thereby help prevent toxic reactions.
- Patient's blood count and kidney and liver function should be closely monitored during therapy. *(See LAB)*
- Concurrent administration of antipyretics *(see PH, Analgesic antipyretics),* antihistamines, and antiemetics *(see PH, Gastrointestinal system)* may decrease adverse reactions.
- Amphotericin should not be mixed with other drugs.

GRISEOFULVIN, U.S.P. (FULVICIN, GRISACTIN, GRIFULVIN)
Actions

- A fungistatic drug that binds with keratin and is deposited in diseased hair, nails, and epidermis. New growth of the fungi is prevented.

Indications

- Used to treat tinea (ringworm) infections of skin, hair, and nails (*e.g.,* tinea pedis—athlete's foot, tinea capitis—scalp ringworm, tinea cruris—groin ringworm, and tinea unguium—nail fungi).
- More effective for chronic fungal infections.
- Should not be used for systemic fungal infections.

Adverse Effects, Contraindications

- Skin rashes and photosensitivity reactions may occur.
- Headache (severity usually decreases during course of therapy), dizziness, and mental confusion are possible.
- Oral thrush can result from monilial overgrowths.
- The leukopenia that can occur usually reverses itself during the course of therapy.
- Patients with liver damage or acute porphyria should not receive this drug.

Dosage, Administration

- Usual oral daily dosage is 500 mg to 1 g in divided doses after meals. Duration of therapy ranges from several weeks to several months.
- Fulvicin-U/F consists of microsize crystals offering a greater and more effective surface area for increased gastrointestinal absorption.

Nursing Tips

- Milk and other fatty foods enhance absorption of the drug.
- This drug antagonizes warfarin anticoagulants, and the dosage of the anticoagulant may need to be increased.
- Barbiturates antagonize griseofulvin, and dosage of the antimicrobial may need to be increased.
- Patients should be encouraged to shampoo hair and cut hair and nails frequently *to assist the drug therapy.*
- Blood counts and renal and hepatic function tests should be done periodically. *(See LAB)*

NYSTATIN, U.S.P., (MYCOSTATIN)
Actions

- Both fungistatic and fungicidal against a wide variety of yeasts and yeastlike fungi.

Indications

- Used topically to treat monilial infections of the skin, mucous membranes of the mouth (thrush), and the vagina.
- Used orally to prevent superinfections (from increased fungi of the intestine) when tetracyclines or other broad-spectrum antimicrobials are taken. High-risk patients (*e.g.,* diabetics or patients on steroids or antineoplastic drugs) may benefit from this type of prophylactic use.

Adverse Effects, Contraindications

- Diarrhea and epigastric distress may occur after large oral doses.
- Hypersensitivity reactions to topical application are rare.

Dosage, Administration

- To suppress intestinal fungi, 0.5 to 1 million units are given orally t.i.d.
- Vaginal infections are treated with 100,000 to 200,000 units daily inserted in the vagina.

• To treat thrush in infants and children, an oral suspension is dropped in the mouth q.i.d.

Nursing Tips

• Nystatin should be kept in light-resistant containers.
• Fixed dosage combinations (nystatin and another antibiotic contained in the same tablet or capsule) are not usually as effective in preventing intestinal moniliasis as when the drugs are taken separately because the dosage of nystatin is too small.

ANTITUBERCULOSIS DRUGS

Overview

• A variety of drugs are now available that are effective against *Mycobacterium tuberculosis. (See SS, Respiratory system)*
• Long-term chemotherapy (often up to 2 years) is necessary.
• Usually a combination therapy, using two or three drugs concurrently, is necessary to prevent resistant forms of the bacteria from developing.
• The most common reason for treatment failure is that the patients do not take their medication for the prescribed length of time.
• The following individuals may need drug therapy (usually isoniazid) on a preventive basis:
  1. infants born to mothers with active tuberculosis
  2. other household members where tuberculosis has been diagnosed
  3. individuals whose skin tests have recently changed from negative to positive (recent converters); and those who have had an inactive, untreated infection for many years
  4. Patients who have a *positive skin test* and a *low resistance* to infection may also receive isoniazid, for example,
     a. those on prolonged therapy with corticosteroids
     b. those treated for leukemia or Hodgkin's disease
     c. patients with poorly controlled diabetes
     d. children with measles or whooping cough
• Antituberculosis drugs are available free of charge from most health departments throughout the country.

AMINOSALICYLIC ACID, U.S.P. (PAS)
Actions

• Has a relatively weak bacteriostatic effect when used alone.
• However, when used with other drugs (*e.g.,* isoniazid or strepto-

mycin) it can decrease the rate at which resistance develops and can potentiate the effects of the other drugs.

Indications

- Used in combination with other drugs (*e.g.*, isoniazid or streptomycin) to treat: pulmonary tuberculosis, miliary tuberculosis, tuberculous meningitis, renal tuberculosis, and bone and joint tuberculosis.

Adverse Effects, Contraindications

- Frequently causes anorexia, nausea, vomiting, cramps, and diarrhea.
- Patients with peptic ulcer should not receive PAS.
- Occasionally, skin eruptions, sore throat, fever, and blood dyscrasias occur.
- Liver damage and goiter are rare.

Dosage, Administration

- Usual adult dosage is 12 g daily p.o. in four divided doses after meals.

Nursing Tips

- Food and antacids may help reduce the gastrointestinal irritation.
- Sodium, potassium, and calcium salts of this drug are available. These derivatives may cause less gastric irritation. Avoid the sodium derivative if the patient is on a sodium-restricted diet.

ETHAMBUTOL HCL, U.S.P. (MYAMBUTOL)

Actions

- Has a good bacteriostatic effect but is also used in combination because resistance develops rapidly.

Indications

- Used in combination with other drugs (*e.g.*, isoniazid or streptomycin) to treat: pulmonary tuberculosis (both primary and chronic relapsing cases), miliary tuberculosis, tuberculous meningitis, renal tuberculosis, and bone and joint tuberculosis.
- Frequently replaces the use of aminosalicylic acid because it causes less gastric irritation. (*See PH, Antimicrobials, antituberculosis drugs*)

Adverse Effects, Contraindications

- Optic neuritis, resulting in loss of visual acuity, peripheral vision, and color discrimination, is the most serious side-effect.

- Skin eruptions, joint pains, headache, gastric distress, mental confusion, and anaphylactoid reactions also occur.
- Patients with impaired kidney function should receive a reduced dose.
- Do not give to children under 13 years old.

Dosage, Administration

- Usual adult oral dosage is 15 mg/kg in a single daily dose. 25 mg/kg per day is given to treat relapses.

Nursing Tips

- Patients on long-term therapy should have their vision checked before beginning treatment and at monthly intervals. If changes are significant the drug must be discontinued.
- Decreased ability to distinguish red and green is an early indication of optic toxicity.

ISONIAZID, U.S.P. (INH)
Actions

- Single, most effective bacteriostatic drug for treating and preventing tuberculosis.
- Resistance develops when used alone.

Indications

- Used in combination with other drugs (*e.g.,* PAS or streptomycin) to treat: pulmonary tuberculosis (both primary and chronic relapsing cases), miliary tuberculosis, tuberculous meningitis, renal tuberculosis, and bone-and-joint tuberculosis.
- This is also the drug of choice for preventing tuberculosis. *(See PH, Antituberculosis drugs: overview for list of individuals who would receive INH for this reason)*

Adverse Effects, Contraindications

- Patients most likely to experience toxic effects are those who take high doses, inactivate the drug slowly, or are hypersensitive to it.
- Severe and sometimes fatal hepatitis may develop.
- Peripheral neuropathy occurs (*e.g.,* muscle weakness, numbness, tingling).
- Blood dyscrasias have been reported.
- Central nervous system effects include convulsive seizures, hallucinations, and mental depression.
- Patient may experience postural hypotension and difficulty in urinating.

- Use cautiously in patients with convulsive disorders, diabetes, active liver disease, and impaired kidney function.

Dosage, Administration

- Usual adult dosage is 5 mg/kg/day p.o. (up to 300 mg), and children receive 10 to 30 mg/kg depending on severity of infection.
- For prevention, adults receive 300 mg/day p.o., and children receive 10 mg/kg/day (up to 300 mg total).

Nursing Tips

- Monitor liver function at monthly intervals, and observe for nausea, vomiting, and jaundice. *(See LAB)*
- This drug may cause a deficiency of pyridoxine (vitamin B_6). A supplement is recommended for adolescents and malnourished patients.

RIFAMPIN, U.S.P. (RIFADIN, RIMACTANE)
Actions

- Bacteriostatic against *Mycobacterium tuberculosis.*
- Resistance develops easily when used alone.

Indications

- Used in combination with other drugs (*e.g.,* isoniazid or ethambutol) to treat pulmonary tuberculosis. Also used to treat miliary tuberculosis, tuberculous meningitis, renal tuberculosis, and bone and joint tuberculosis.
- Asymptomatic carriers of meningococci are treated with this drug to prevent spreading the meningitis in high-risk situations.

Adverse Effects, Contraindications

- Causes abnormalities in liver-function tests, high serum bilirubin, and jaundice.
- Use cautiously in patients with liver disease.
- Nausea, vomiting, cramps, diarrhea, and anorexia can occur.
- Thrombocytopenia and leukopenia may develop.

Dosage, Administration

- Usual adult daily dose is 600 mg p.o. on an empty stomach.
- Children receive 10 to 20 mg/kg (maximum 600 mg/day).

Nursing Tips

- Liver function studies should be done periodically. *(See LAB)*
- Rifampin interacts with anticoagulant drugs *(see PH, Cardiovascular*

system). Prothrombin times should be checked daily because the dose of the anticoagulant may need to be increased. *(See LAB)*

- Rifampin–isoniazid combination drugs are available, but they are usually more expensive than the use of the drugs separately. However, the combinations provide greater convenience for the patients.

STREPTOMYCIN SULFATE, U.S.P.

(See PH, Aminoglycosides)

- Usually administered by deep IM injection in daily doses of 1 to 2 g (divided into two equal parts at 12-hr intervals).

CEPHALOSPORINS

Actions

- These drugs are bactericidal and interfere with bacterial cell-wall synthesis.

Indications

- May be used to treat infections from many gram-positive cocci and gram-negative bacilli because they have a broad-spectrum of activity.
- However, the penicillins are usually the first choice in treating gram-positive infections because they are safer and less expensive. *(See PH, Penicillins)*
- One advantage that cephalosporins have over many of the penicillins is that they are not inactivated by penicillinase (a bacteria that destroys some penicillins). But they are inactivated by cephalosporinase—a closely related enzyme.

Adverse Effects, Contraindications

- A positive Coombs' test may develop when large doses are given, and hemolytic anemia can occur.
- Reversible renal tubular necrosis has occurred.
- Pain and sterile abscesses at injection sites may result; also thrombophlebitis following IV administration.
- Skin rashes may occur in patients with a history of penicillin allergy.

Dosage, Administration

- Cephalexin, U.S.P., (Keflex): Usual adult dosage is 1 to 4 g, q.d., p.o., given in divided doses of 250 mg to 500 mg.
- Cephalothin sodium, U.S.P. (Keflin): Usual adult dosage is 500 mg to 1 g every 4 to 6 hr, IV. However, severe infections may require

up to 2 g every 4 hr. The medication may be given intermittently or by continuous infusion.

Nursing Tips

- At times, cephalosporins are used to treat infections when the patient is allergic to the penicillins. However, these drugs are similar in chemical structure to penicillin, and it is possible that the patient could be cross-sensitive. Observe very carefully for adverse effects.
- Anaphylactic reactions to cephalosporins are rare.
- For long-term therapy, for use of large doses, or for patients with impaired kidney function, blood counts should be monitored.
- Cephalosporins may produce false positives when certain agents are used for testing (*e.g.,* Clinitest).

ERYTHROMYCIN

Actions

- This drug can be either bacteriostatic or bactericidal depending on the size of the dose and the infecting pathogen. It interferes with protein synthesis.

Indications

- Safe substitute for penicillin in patients who are allergic to it.
- Effective against gram-positive cocci, and used to treat such problems as: streptococcal pharyngitis; pneumococcal pneumonia and meningitis; subacute bacterial endocarditis.
- Because the incidence of toxicity is very low, erythromycin is frequently given to children.
- Also used for some gram-negative urinary tract infections when the urine is kept alkaline (by administering sodium bicarbonate).

Adverse Effects, Contraindications

- Occasionally causes nausea, vomiting, diarrhea, abdominal discomfort, and cramps.
- The estolate ester of erythromycin has produced an allergic hepatitis characterized by jaundice, fever, and abdominal pain.
- Skin and other hypersensitivity reactions have occurred.
- Superinfection by resistant bacteria and fungi can develop. The drug is then discontinued.
- Patients with impaired liver function or a history of hepatic disease should use these drugs cautiously.

Dosage, Administration

- Erythromycin, U.S.P. (Erythrocin): Adult oral dosage is usually 250 mg q. 6 hr but may be increased to 4 g per day.

- Erythromycin Estolate, N.F. (Ilosone): Adult oral dosage is 250 mg q. 6 hr.
- Erythromycin Ethylsuccinate, U.S.P. (Pediamycin, EES): Usual dosage is 100 mg q. 4 to 8 hr deep IM. Very irritating and should not be used for small children.
- Erythromycin gluceptate, U.S.P. (Ilotycin gluceptate): Usual dosage is 500 mg to 1 g q. 6 hr IV or by continuous infusion.
- Erythromycin lactobionate, U.S.P.: Usual dose is 1 to 4 g daily by continuous IV infusion or divided every 4 to 6 hr.
- Erythromycin stearate U.S.P. (Erythrocin stearate):
  1. Usual adult dosage is 250 mg orally every 6 hours.
  2. When administering IV erythromycin, dilute each 250 mg in at least 100 ml of NS or D_5W. Run in slowly, over 20 to 60 min.

Nursing Tips

- Patients on long-term therapy, especially those receiving the estolate, should have periodic tests of liver function.
- The erythromycin base is usually administered before meals. The acid-resistant coatings keep the drug from being inactivated.

PENICILLINS

Actions

- The penicillins are bactericidal drugs that inhibit the synthesis of the bacterial cell wall.
- Because the cell walls of the bacteria differ from those of mammalian cells, the penicillins exhibit a high degree of selective toxicity (*e.g.*, they are not toxic to the human cells).

Adverse Effects, Contraindications

- Allergic or hypersensitivity reactions are very common with the penicillins. They range from all types of skin eruptions and rashes to *anaphylactic shock*.
- Phlebitis and thrombophlebitis have resulted from intravenous administration of the penicillins.
- Muscular twitching or convulsions may result from large doses.
- Intravenous forms of penicillin are either sodium or potassium salts. When large doses are used, electrolyte imbalances can occur. Particular care should be used if the patient's kidney function is impaired.

Nursing Tips

- Taking a complete drug history is of crucial importance because of the high incidence of allergic reactions.

- Most forms of penicillin are affected by gastric acid. (Penicillin V Potassium, U.S.P. Pen-Vee-K is an exception). Therefore, most oral penicillins should be given at least 1 hour before meals or 2 to 3 hours after meals.
- The kidneys efficiently filter out, excrete, and secrete the penicillins into the tubules. Probenecid, U.S.P. (Benemid) blocks the secretion of the penicillin into the tubules and keeps the drug in the blood and tissues for longer periods.
- Intravenous forms of penicillin can be very irritating to the veins and can cause phlebitis or thrombophlebitis. The medication should be well diluted and run in slowly.
- Carbenicillin and gentamycin are frequently used together to fight serious infections. The two drugs should never be mixed together because they may inactivate each other.

PENICILLIN G PREPARATIONS: PENICILLIN G BENZATHINE, U.S.P. (BICILLIN); PENICILLIN G POTASSIUM, U.S.P.; PENICILLIN G PROCAINE, U.S.P. (WYCILLIN)

(See PH, Penicillins: actions, adverse effects, nursing tips)
- Used to treat streptococcal infections such as acute pharyngitis, tonsillitis, scarlet fever, and subacute bacterial endocarditis. Also used in patients on a prophylactic basis if they have mitral valve disease and will be undergoing such procedures as dental extractions or surgery, or cystoscopy.
- Used to treat *staphylococcal* infections but only after the laboratory has indicated that the organism is more sensitive to it than to one of the other types of penicillins (see below).
- *Pneumococcal pneumonia* responds to penicillin G, especially if treatment is begun early. Usually the IM route is used (penicillin G procaine).
- *Meningococcal meningitis* responds to large doses given intravenously.
- Although resistant strains of gonorrhea have developed, penicillin G is still effective when given in large doses. (4.8 million units of penicillin G procaine given IM—this dose is usually divided into 2 or more sites).
- *Syphilis* is usually responsive to penicillin G benzathine.

Dosage, Administration

- Penicillin G benzathine U.S.P. (Bicillin): usual dosage is 500,000 units orally or 600,000 units IM at various intervals. This is the longest-lasting form of penicillin and may be administered only every 2 to 4 weeks.
- Penicillin G potassium, U.S.P.: Usual dosage is 400,000 units q. 6

hr orally or IM. Intravenously, 10 million units may be given daily in divided doses.

- Penicillin G procaine, U.S.P. (Wycillin): This long-lasting form is given IM, 300,000 units every 12 to 24 hr.

ACID RESISTANT PENICILLINS: PENICILLIN V POTASSIUM, U.S.P. (PEN-VEE-K)

(See PH, Penicillins: actions, adverse effects, nursing tips)

- Achieves higher plasma levels than oral penicillin G because it is more resistant to destruction by stomach acids.
- Used to treat the same types of mild to moderate infections for which oral penicillin G is employed.
- It is *not* indicated for the acute phase of meningitis, endocarditis, pneumonia (in these cases high doses of penicillin G are given IM or IV).

Dosage, Administration

- Usual adult dosage ranges from 200,000 units to 500,000 units every 6 to 8 hr.

PENICILLINASE-RESISTANT PENICILLINS: METHICILLIN SODIUM, U.S.P. (STAPHCILLIN); OXACILLIN SODIUM, U.S.P. (PROSTAPHLIN)

(See PH, Penicillins: actions, adverse effects, nursing tips)

- Used to treat penicillinase-producing staph infections.
- If the laboratory indicates that the organism is not a penicillinase-producing staphylococcus, the less expensive penicillin G preparations can be used.
- Bone marrow depression has been reported with methicillin.

Dosage, Administration

- Methicillin sodium, U.S.P. (Staphcillin): Usual dosage is 1 to 1.5 g every 4 to 6 hr IM or IV. Intramuscular injections are painful.
- Oxacillin sodium, U.S.P. (Prostaphlin): Usual dosage is 500 mg q 4 to 6 hr for 5 or more days. When given orally it should be taken on an empty stomach. For serious infections, the IM or IV routes are usually preferred.

BROAD-SPECTRUM PENICILLINS: AMOXICILLIN (AMOXIL); AMPICILLIN, U.S.P. (OMNIPEN); CARBENICILLIN DISODIUM (GEOPEN)

(See PH, Penicillins: actions, adverse effects, nursing tips)

- Effective against all organisms for which the penicillin G preparations are used (see above). However, penicillin G preparations are less expensive and are the drug of choice when they are shown to be effective.

- Used to treat *Hemophilus influenzae,* which frequently causes acute otitis media in children.
- Infections caused by *E. Coli, Proteus mirabilis* and some strains of shigella and salmonella respond to these drugs.
- Amoxicillin rather than ampicillin may be indicated for some infections because it achieves higher blood levels and is excreted in the urine in larger amounts (therefore, it may be more effective for urinary tract and systemic infections). Also, less of the drug reaches the intestinal flora, so there is less chance of drug-induced diarrhea.
- Carbenicillin is also effective against serious infections caused by *Pseudomonas aeruginosa* and some proteus strains.
- Intramuscular carbenicillin occasionally causes local inflammation and pain.
- When carbenicillin is administered to patients with impaired kidney function, their prothrombin time (PT) and partial thromboplastin time (PTT) should be monitored because bleeding episodes can occur. *(See LAB)*
- Ampicillin usage is most frequently linked with the development of superinfections. These resistant organisms cause stomatitis, glossitis (black, "hairy" tongue), nausea, vomiting, and diarrhea.

Dosage Administration

- Amoxicillin (Amoxil): Usual dosage is 250 to 300 mg orally t.i.d.
- Ampicillin U.S.P. (Omnipen): Usual dosage is 250 to 500 mg q. 6 hr p.o. May be given IM or IV every 4 hr for serious infections.
- Carbenicillin disodium (Geopen): Daily dosage IM or IV is usually 25 to 30 g in divided doses.

SULFONAMIDES

Actions

- When administered in the usual dosage range, these drugs are primarily bacteriostatic.
- They prevent bacterial cells from using one of the B complex vitamins, para-aminobenzoic acid (PABA), that inhibits the formation of folic acid. Therefore, the bacteria cannot grow and reproduce.
- These drugs are divided according to the duration of their action: short acting, intermediate, long acting, and ultra long acting.

Indications

Because more effective bactericidal drugs are available (*e.g.*, penicillins and aminoglycosides), the sulfonamides are not used as frequently to treat common infections. Sensitivity testing should be done because many organisms have become resistant to the sulfonamides. However, they continue to be useful when patients are allergic to the first-choice antibiotics and in the following conditions:

- Acute and chronic urinary tract infections (UTI) caused by gram-negative bacteria (*e.g.*, *E. coli*). Usually, a short-acting sulfonamide (*e.g.*, sulfisoxazole) is used to treat uncomplicated acute UTIs and an intermediate-acting sulfonamide (*e.g.*, sulfamethoxazole with trimethoprim) may be used for chronic UTIs.
- Sulfamethoxazole with trimethoprim is used for patients with chronic obstructive pulmonary disease (COPD) when they develop infections of the respiratory tract and, at times, to prevent these infections.
- Patients with a history of rheumatic fever who are allergic to penicillin use sulfisoxazole to prevent recurrences of the rheumatic fever.
- Ulcerative colitis may be treated with sulfasalazine. It is also used to prevent relapses.
- Occasionally used to treat shigella and salmonella infections, but sensitivity testing must be done because many strains are now resistant to the sulfonamides.
- Topical preparations, silver sulfadiazine and mafenide acetate, are used adjunctly in the treatment of severe burns. The purpose is to prevent local sepsis and septicemia from such organisms as *Staphylococcus, Streptococcus* and *Pseudomonas.*
- Sulfonamides may be combined with other drugs to treat malaria, nocardiosis, actinomycosis, and histoplasmosis.
- Some strains of gonorrhea and chancroid are sensitive to the sulfonamides.

Adverse Effects, Contraindications

- Nausea, vomiting, and abdominal discomfort are the most frequent side-effects.
- Crystalluria (especially from the long-acting sulfonamides) can result in hematuria, oliguria, anuria, and uremia. This precipitation of crystals of the drug out of the urine in the kidneys is less frequent now because many of the available preparations are highly soluble in acid urine.
- Rarely, blood dyscrasias occur (*e.g.*, agranulocytosis, thrombocytopenia, aplastic anemia, and hemolytic anemia).

- Allergic reactions range from skin rashes and eruptions to ana-phylactic shock. Drug fever and Stevens-Johnson syndrome have occurred.
- Some patients may become photosensitive.
- Mafenide acetate, when applied to burns covering over 50% of body surface, may cause metabolic acidosis. Toxic reactions and subsequent damage can involve almost every organ and system in the body.
- Used cautiously for patients with impaired kidney or liver function and those with blood dyscrasias.
- Pregnant women near term, nursing mothers, and infants less than one month old should not receive sulfonamides.

Dosage, Administration

- Mafenide acetate, U.S.P. (Sulfamylon): Apply topically once or twice daily in a layer 1/16 inch thick.
- Silver sulfadiazine (Silvadene): Apply the 0.1% ointment topically once or twice daily in a layer 1/16 inch thick.
- Sulfamethoxazole, N.F. (Gantanol): This is an intermediate-acting sulfonamide. Initial adult dose is usually 2 g p.o., followed by main-tenance doses of 1 g b.i.d. or t.i.d.
- Sulfamethoxazole with trimethoprim *(Bactrim, Septra)*: Tablets con-tain 400 mg sulfamethoxazole and 80 mg of trimethoprim. Double-strength (DS) tablets contain 800 mg sulfamethoxazole and 160 mg trimethoprim. Usual adult dosage is two tablets or one DS tablet every 12 hr p.o. for 10 to 14 days.
- Sulfasalazine *(Azulfidine)*: Initial adult dose is usually 4 g p.o., fol-lowed by maintenance doses of 1 g q.i.d.
- Sulfisoxazole, U.S.P., *(Gantrisin)*: This is a short-acting sulfona-mide. Initial adult dose is usually 4 g p.o., followed by maintenance doses of 1 g four to six times daily.
- Sulfisoxazole with phenazopyridine hydrochloride, N.F. (Azo-Gan-trisin): Tablets contain 0.5 g sulfisoxazole and 50 mg phenaxopyr-idine hydrochloride. Usual adult dosage is four to six tablets ini-tially, followed by two tablets q.i.d. for up to 3 days. The phenazopyridine reduces the burning, urgency, and frequency that occurs with urinary infections. After pain relief is achieved, patient may be treated with sulfisoxazole alone.

Nursing Tips

- Though crystalluria occurs less frequently now, the patient should be instructed to force fluids while taking sulfonamides. Urine out-put should be measured, and the patient should take enough fluids to produce a minimum of 1200 ml of urine in 24 hr.

- Observe the patient for skin and mucosal blisters with bleeding centers that could indicate the development of Stevens-Johnson syndrome.
- Monitor the patient for clinical indications of blood dyscrasis (*e.g.*, rash, sore throat, purpura, paleness, jaundice).
- Patients receiving a sulfonamide with phenazopyridine (*e.g., Azo-Gantrisin*) should be informed that their urine will become orange red in color.
- When the sulfonamides are given with other drugs that also deplete the bacteria's sources of folic acid, a synergistic effect occurs that increases the antibacterial activity. Trimethoprim is such a drug. Bactrim and Septra are commonly used combinations.
- Sulfonamides and some oral hypoglycemics (the sulfonylurea type) interact and can cause severe hypoglycemia.
- Sulfonamides potentiate *oral anticoagulants* and may produce hemorrhage.
- Antacids can decrease the absorption of sulfonamides.

TETRACYCLINES

Actions

- When administered in the usual dosage range, these drugs are primarily bacteriostatic.

Indications

Because many tetracycline-resistant bacteria have emerged, these broad-spectrum drugs are generally not the first choice for treating common bacterial infections. However, when sensitivity studies indicate that the tetracyclines are effective, and if the patient is sensitive to the penicillins, these drugs may be employed. They are also used to treat the following:

- Recommended for prevention of acute respiratory infections in patients with chronic obstructive pulmonary disease (COPD). *(See SS, Respiratory)*
- Effective for treating "viral" pneumonia caused by *Mycoplasma pneumoniae* (this organism is not a true virus).
- Common urinary tract and venereal infections may be sensitive to the tetracyclines. However, these drugs are especially useful for treating the chlamydiae infections (*e.g.*, lymphogranuloma venereum; psittacosis—parrot fever; and trachoma—a chronic eye infection).
- Rickettsial diseases such as Rocky Mountain fever and typhus respond to the tetracyclines (usually large doses given IV).

- Cholera and brucellosis can be effectively treated with these drugs.
- Used systemically and topically to treat acne.
- Inner eye infections may be treated with the tetracyclines.

Adverse Effects, Contraindications

- Frequently causes nausea, and occasionally diarrhea and vomiting.
- May discolor children's teeth because the tetracyclines bind with calcium in bones and teeth. Also, fetal skeletal development may be retarded, and bone growth may be slowed temporarily in young children. Pregnant women and young children should avoid the tetracyclines, especially for long-term use.
- Patients taking these drugs can experience photosensitivity, especially if they have a history of it. Skin rashes do occur but less frequently than with the penicillins.
- Tetracyclines are hepatotoxic and can cause fatty degeneration of the liver. Patients with impaired kidney function should receive a reduced dose.
- Outdated or degraded drugs have caused kidney tubule impairment with acidosis, proteinuria, and glycosuria.
- Superinfections are fairly common and range from moniliasis to severe staphylococcal enterocolitis.
- Prolonged IV use may lead to thrombophlebitis.

Dosage, Administration

- Doxycycline hyclate, U.S.P. (Vibramycin): Usual adult oral dosage is 200 mg on the first day (100 mg q. 12 hr), followed by 100 mg q.d. Requires smaller doses and is less frequently administered than Terramycin or Achromcyin. Usual IV dosage is 200 mg the first day, followed by 100 mg to 200 mg q.d. depending on the severity of the infection. The infusions last from 1 to 4 hours depending on the dose. Do not give IM or SC.
- Minocycline, HCl, U.S.P. (Minocin): Usual oral adult dosage is 200 mg initially, then 100 mg q. 12 hr.
- Oxytetracycline HCl, U.S.P. (Terramycin): Usual oral adult dosage is 250 mg q.i.d. Usual IV adult dosage is 500 mg daily.
- Tetracycline HCl, U.S.P. (Achromycin): Usual oral adult dosage is 500 mg q.i.d. Usual IV adult dosage is 500 mg b.i.d.

Nursing Tips

- Age, exposure to light, extreme heat, and humidity can cause the tetracyclines to undergo toxic changes. Always store properly and check for expiration dates.

- Patients receiving these drugs should avoid direct sunlight and keep their skin covered.
- Do not administer the tetracyclines with antacids or iron because the drugs will combine with metal ions and will not be absorbed.
- Avoid giving the tetracyclines (except doxycycline and minocycline) with milk or other dairy products because the drug will join with the calcium. Giving tetracyclines 1 hr before meals or 2 to 3 hr after meals will prevent the possibility of drug–food interactions.
- The tetracyclines may delay blood coagulation.
- Superinfections such as candidiasis occur most often in diabetic, debilitated, or pregnant patients and in those receiving corticosteroids.

URINARY TRACT ANTISEPTICS
METHENAMIDE MANDELATE, U.S.P. (MANDELAMINE);
METHENAMINE HIPPURATE (HIPREX)
Actions
- When the urine is acid, formaldehyde is released and exerts a bactericidal effect.
- Contributes to the acidification of the urine.

Indications
- Used to suppress or eliminate bacteria in the urine in cases of pyelonephritis, cystitis, and other chronic urinary tract infections.
- May be used on a long-term basis because there is a low incidence of resistance and it is low in toxicity.

Adverse Effects, Contraindications
- Occasionally, patients experience gastrointestinal distress.
- Rarely, skin rashes occur.
- High doses may cause dysuria.
- Do not give to patients with renal insufficiency.
- Do not give if the patient's urine cannot be acidified.

Dosage, Administration
- Usual adult oral dosage is 1 g q.i.d.

Nursing Tips
- It may be necessary to acidify the patient's urine by using such drugs as ascorbic acid, sodium acid phosphate, or ammonium chloride.
- Because the bactericidal effects depend on the release of formaldehyde in the urine, it is questionable whether a patient with a

Foley catheter would benefit from the use of this drug since the cathether keeps the bladder empty.

- When Mandelamine is given with the sulfonamides, an insoluble precipitate forms in the urine.
- The gastrointestinal distress may be alleviated by giving the drug after meals or by using the enteric-coated form.

NITROFURANTOIN, U.S.P. (FURADANTIN, MACRODANTIN)
Actions

- This drug exerts bactericidal effects in the urine.

Indications

- Used to treat cystitis, pyelitis, and pyelonephritis.
- Frequently used in cases of chronic urinary tract infections because resistance seldom develops.

Adverse Effects, Contraindications

- When used to treat acute infections the large doses can cause nausea and vomiting.
- Headache, dizziness, and drowsiness may occur.
- May produce various types of skin rashes.
- Pregnant women (especially near term) and young infants should not receive this drug.
- Do not give to patients with impaired kidney function because the drug accumulates to toxic levels in nervous tissue.
- Hemolytic anemia has occurred in patients who lack the enzyme glucose 6-phosphate dehydrogenase and in young infants whose enzyme systems are immature.

Dosage, Administration

- Usual adult oral dosage is 50 to 100 mg q.i.d. with food for at least 7 days.
- Usual IM or IV dose is 180 mg if patient is over 120 lb., or 3 mg/lb for patients weighing less.

Nursing Tips

- Nitrofurantoin causes a yellow brown discoloration of the urine.
- When taken on a long-term basis, the patient may take a single daily dose at bedtime. He should empty his bladder before taking the drug because the urine stored during the night will have a higher concentration of the drug.
- The absorption of Macrodantin is slower, and its excretion somewhat less, than Furadantin.

PHENAZOPYRIDINE HYDROCHLORIDE, N.F. (PYRIDIUM)

Actions

- Weak bacteriostatic action, but it is used for its topical anesthetic effects.

Indications

- Used to relieve bladder irritation and to reduce the burning, urgency, and frequency that occurs with urinary tract infections and following endoscopic procedures.

Adverse Effects, Contraindications

- Occasionally causes gastrointestinal discomfort.
- Overdoses may lead to kidney and liver toxicity and blood dyscrasias.
- Patients with impaired kidney function should not receive this drug.

Dosage, Administration

- Usual adult dosage is 200 mg p.o., t.i.d.

Nursing Tips

- Patients should be told that their urine will become orange red in color.

ANTINEOPLASTICS

Overview

Chemotherapy—the use of drugs to treat cancer—can accomplish three things: regression of the neoplasm, prolongation of life, and palliation (alleviation of symptoms without curing). This mode of therapy has limitations: long-term remissions are not possible in many instances; resistance to drugs emerges; and the drugs lack selective toxicity (they also damage normal cells). Choice of drugs and dosage is highly individualized. The aim is to destroy the maximum number of cancer cells with minimal toxicity to normal tissues. Normal cells most susceptible to damage are those with a naturally high rate of proliferation (*e.g.,* bone marrow, mucosal lining of the gastrointestinal tract, hair-follicle cells of the scalp).

Combinations of two or more drugs are frequently used. The advantages over single-dose therapy are that resistance can be delayed or prevented, and that the combinations are frequently more effective. It is common to give the drugs intermittently, in high doses, rather than in small, daily doses. This allows time for the bone marrow to recover. Individual dosages are usually computed according to total body surface. Therefore, accurate weights are very important.

Drug dosages must be checked carefully because some are ordered in micrograms, others in milligrams. Drug names may also be similar.

The patient receiving antineoplastic drugs should not use any over-the-counter preparations without the approval of his physician. Unwanted drug interactions must be avoided.

Patients who are still in their reproductive years should understand that these medications can cause permanent sterility and could be damaging to a developing fetus.

Nursing Tips

Bone marrow toxicity results in thrombocytopenia, leukopenia and anemia.

- Baseline blood and platelet counts should be done before chemotherapy is started.
- If granulocytes fall below 1,000 per cubic millimeter, or if platelets fall below 50,000 per cubic millimeter, the drugs are usually discontinued or changed. At these levels the patient is exposed to life-threatening infections and hemorrhage.
- When platelet production is depressed, IM and SC injections are avoided as much as possible. When IVs are removed, pressure should be applied to the site for 5 minutes. Observe the patient carefully for signs of bleeding.
- When white blood cell production is depressed, the patient must be protected from all sources of infection. Strict aseptic technique must be observed for dressing changes, injection, IVs, and Foley catheter insertion and care. Reverse isolation may be indicated.

Gastrointestinal toxicity frequently causes anorexia, nausea, vomiting, and diarrhea.

- Administration of an antiemetic or antidiarrhea medication before the chemotherapy is started, and again in 4 hours, often controls these symptoms.
- Chemotherapy given in the evening may be better tolerated by some patients.
- Frequent, small meals of soft, bland foods may be more acceptable.
- The gastrointestinal tract is also subject to mucosal inflammation, stomatitis, and proctitis. Meticulous oral care can reduce the incidence and severity of the stomatitis.
- Mucosal inflammation and stomatitis may require that drugs be discontinued or changed. Report these symptoms to the physician. Ulceration and perforation of the GI tract are possible.

Alopecia (hair loss) may have distressing effects on a person's self-image.

- Hair-follicle cells of the scalp are damaged, and hair frequently falls out in clumps.

- Wigs, scarves, and short haircuts obtained before chemotherapy is started can help in the adjustment. Hair will usually grow back in 8 to 10 weeks.
- The drugs that consistently result in alopecia are cyclophosphamide, dactinomycin, doxorubicin, methotrexate, and vincristine.
  High serum uric acid levels frequently occur because of the high turnover of neoplastic cells.
- Allopurinol may be administered to prevent kidney damage.
- Fluid intake should be increased to 2 liters per day beginning the day before therapy and continuing through one day following treatment.
- Kidney and liver function studies should be done.
  Severe tissue necrosis can occur if intravenous medications infiltrate.
- Watch closely for signs of extravasation (infiltration), and if seen, stop the infusion immediately.
- Specific protocols for dealing with infiltration do exist. Check ahead of time to determine what should be done.
- Four drugs that can cause severe tissue damage are mechlorethamine, doxorubicin, daunorubicin and vincristine sulfate.

ALKYLATING AGENTS
CYCLOPHOSPHAMIDE, U.S.P. (CYTOXAN)
Actions

- Cyclophosphamide is chemically related to the nitrogen mustards—alkylating agents which inactivate DNA.
- Onset of action is slower and more prolonged than with other alkylating agents because the drug must first be metabolized to biologically active alkylating metabolites in the liver.

Indications

- Malignant lymphomas (*e.g.,* Hodgkin's disease), multiple myeloma, leukemias, and mycosis fungoides frequently respond to cyclophosphamide.
- Such solid malignancies as neuroblastoma, adenocarcinoma of the ovary, and retinoblastoma are frequently responsive.
- Patients with bronchogenic carcinoma, carcinoma of the breast and cervix, and ovarian malignancies have responded favorably.

Adverse Effects, Contraindications

- Anorexia, nausea, and vomiting are common.
- Alopecia is a frequent side-effect.
- Secondary malignancies (*e.g.,* of the urinary bladder) have developed.
- Bone marrow depression leads primarily to leukopenia.

- A severe, even fatal complication is sterile hemorrhagic cystitis, which may necessitate interruption of therapy.
- Pregnant and nursing women should not use this drug.
- Sterility can result and may be permanent.
- Pulmonary fibrosis has occurred with prolonged therapy.
- Cyclophosphamide may interfere with normal wound healing.
- Use cautiously in patients with impaired liver and kidney function.

Dosage, Administration

- Usual initial intravenous loading dosage is 40 to 50 mg/kg given in divided doses over 2 to 5 days.
- Usual oral maintenance therapy is 1 to 5 mg/kg daily.
- Intermittent dosage schedules may call for IV administration of the drug twice a week or once every 7 to 10 days.

Nursing Tips

- See *PH, Antineoplastics: nursing tips* for general information common to most chemotherapy.
- Because of the possiblity of cystitis, the patient should drink plenty of fluids and empty his bladder frequently.
- High doses of phenobarbital may increase cytotoxicity.

CHLORAMBUCIL, U.S.P. (LEUKERAN)
Actions

- Chlorambucil is a derivative of nitrogen mustard. It binds with the DNA molecules of both cancer and normal cells. The cells are damaged in any phase of the cell cycle.

Indications

- Chronic lymphocytic leukemia and malignant lymphomas (*e.g.* Hodgkin's disease).

Adverse Effects, Contraindications

- Bone marrow depression is frequent.
- Do not use within 4 weeks of a full course of radiation therapy or chemotherapy.
- Avoid using this drug during the first trimester of pregnancy.

Dosage, Administration

- Usual daily dosage is 4 to 10 mg orally in one dose. The dose is given 1 hour before breakfast or 2 hours after the evening meal. Duration of therapy is 3 to 6 weeks.
- If white blood cell count (WBC) falls, dose may be decreased.

Nursing Tips

- See *PH, Antineoplastics: nursing tips* for general information common to most chemotherapy.
- Monitor blood counts once or twice weekly. Close observation is needed to avoid irreversible bone marrow damage.

ANTIBIOTICS
BLEOMYCIN SULFATE, U.S.P. (BLENOXANE)
Actions

- Inhibits the synthesis of DNA and, to a lesser extent, RNA and protein synthesis.

Indications

- Squamous cell carcinomas of the head and neck, tongue, tonsils, and palate.
- Tumors of the cervix, vulva, scrotum, and penis.
- Lymphomas such as Hodgkin's disease and lymphosarcoma are responsive to this drug.
- Remissions of testicular carcinoma are high when bleomycin is combined with vinblastine.

Adverse Effects, Contraindications

- Pulmonary side-effects are most serious. Pneumonitis occasionally progresses to pulmonary fibrosis.
- Idiosyncratic reactions occur that resemble anaphylaxis (*e.g.*, hypotension, mental confusion, fever, chills, and wheezing).
- Frequent side-effects include skin and mucous membrane reactions. Redness, rash, blistering, and hyperpigmentation occur. Nail changes, alopecia, and stomatitis have been reported.
- Fever, chills, and vomiting are also common side-effects.
- Use cautiously for patients with impaired pulmonary or renal function.

Dosage, Administration

- Usual dosage range is 0.25 to 0.5 units/kg (or 10 to 20 units/m^2) IV, IM, or SC, weekly or twice weekly.
- Lymphoma patients should receive 2 units or less for the first two doses because of the increased danger of an anaphylactoid reaction.

Nursing Tips

- See *PH, Antineoplastics, nursing tips* for general information common to most chemotherapy.

- Patients over the age of 70 or those who have received over 400 units of bleomycin are at greatest risk for developing pulmonary complications.
- Chest x-rays should be done on all patients every 1 to 2 weeks to monitor pulmonary reactions.
- Assess patients for dyspnea and fine rales.
- The skin reactions are most likely to occur in the second or third weeks of therapy.
- Patients with Hodgkin's disease or testicular tumors usually demonstrate improvement within 2 weeks if they are responsive to bleomycin.
- Improvement is slower in squamous cell carcinomas and may not be seen until the third week.

DOXORUBICIN HYDROCHLORIDE, U.S.P. (ADRIAMYCIN)
Actions
- Binds to DNA and inhibits synthesis of the molecule.

Indications
- Acute lymphoblastic and myeloblastic leukemias; Wilms' tumor; neuroblastoma; soft tissue and bone sarcomas; breast, ovarian, bladder, and lung carcinomas; Hodgkin- and non-Hodgkin-type lymphomas, and some solid tumors.

Adverse Effects, Contraindications
- Cardiac toxicity leading to heart failure can occur and is frequently unresponsive to therapy.
- Bone marrow depression frequently causes leukopenia and thrombocytopenia.
- Gastrointestinal effects commonly experienced are nausea, vomiting, diarrhea, stomatitis, and esophagitis.
- Complete alopecia occurs in most patients.
- Occasionally fever, chills, and urticaria have been reported. Anaphylaxis may occur.
- Patients with pre-existing bone marrow depression or heart disease should not receive doxorubicin.
- Extravasation during administration causes severe cellulitis, blistering, and tissue necrosis.

Dosage, Administration
- Usual dosage range is 60 to 75 mg/m^2 as a single intravenous injection, at 21-day intervals.
- May also be administered at 30 mg/m^2 on each of 3 successive days, repeated every 4 weeks.

- The lower dosage range or a reduced dosage should be used for patients with decreased marrow reserves (*e.g.*, from old age or prior therapy) or if liver function is impaired.

Nursing Tips

- See *PH, Antineoplastics: nursing tips* for general information common to most chemotherapy.
- Patients who receive more than 550 mg/m^2 (the recommended limit) are prone to cardiac toxicity.
- Other cardiotoxic drugs (*e.g.*, cyclophosphamide) given with doxorubicin increase the chance of cardiac toxicity.
- Cardiac problems (*e.g.*, congestive heart failure) may occur several weeks after doxorubicin has been discontinued.
- The following is one method used to prevent tissue necrosis if extravasation occurs. Always check with the physician *ahead* of time so that treatment can be instituted immediately.
  1. Stop the flow of the doxorubicin.
  2. Inject 5 ml (5 mEq) of sodium bicarbonate through the existing infusion needle.
  3. Inject hydrocortisone sodium succinate (Solu-Cortef) 100 mg, SC, into the area of infiltration.
  4. Apply hydrocortisone cream 1% topically, and cover with a sterile 4 × 4.
  5. Apply an ice pack for 24 hours.

ANTIMETABOLITES
FLUOROURACIL, U.S.P. (5-FU)
Actions

- Blocks the synthesis of thymidylic acid, a precursor of thymine. Therefore, DNA synthesis is also prevented.

Indications

- Produces temporary remission of carcinomas of the colon, rectum, pancreas, stomach, and breast.

Adverse Effects, Contraindications

- Stomatitis and esophagopharyngitis are common and can lead to sloughing and ulceration.
- Patients frequently experience diarrhea, anorexia, nausea, and vomiting.
- Leukopenia follows almost every course of therapy.
- Alopecia and dermatitis occur frequently.
- Acute cerebellar syndrome occurs occasionally and may persist after treatment is stopped.
- Fluorouracil should not be given to patients with potentially serious

infections or bone marrow depression, or to those with malnutrition.

- Use cautiously in patients with impaired liver and kidney function.

Dosage, Administration

- Usual dosage is 12 mg/kg, intravenously, for 4 days. Dosage should not exceed 800 mg/day.
- If no toxicity occurs, give 6 mg/kg on the 6th, 8th, 10th, and 12th days.
- Poor-risk patients receive lower doses, which should not exceed 400 mg/day.

Nursing Tips

- See *PH, Antineoplastics: nursing tips* for general information common to most chemotherapy.
- Therapy with fluorouracil should be discontinued if any of the following occur: stomatitis or esophagopharyngitis; leukopenia (WBC under 3500) or rapidly falling WBC; severe vomiting or diarrhea; gastrointestinal ulceration and bleeding; thrombocytopenia (platelets under 100,000); hemorrhage from any site.
- Monitor WBC after each dose.
- The stomatitis that occurs consists of white, patchy membranes that can ulcerate and become necrotic.

METHOTREXATE, U.S.P. (AMETHOPTERIN)
Actions

- Inhibits the conversion of dietary folic acid to the coenzyme needed for synthesis of DNA.

Indications

- Produces lasting remissions in choriocarcinoma and hydatidiform mole.
- Commonly used to maintain induced remissions of acute lymphoblastic leukemia in children.
- Carcinomas of the breast, tongue, pharynx, and testes and mycosis fungoides respond to methotrexate.
- High-dose methotrexate followed by leucovorin "rescue" has caused regression of tumors in carcinoma of the lung and osteogenic sarcoma.
- Methotrexate is also used to treat severe psoriasis.
- Effective in treating advanced stages of lymphosarcoma.

Adverse Effects, Contraindications

- Produces severe bone marrow depression with anemia, leukopenia, thrombocytopenia, and bleeding.

- May be toxic to the liver. Use cautiously if patient has liver damage or impaired hepatic function.
- Diarrhea and ulcerative stomatitis occur frequently. Death from intestinal perforation may result; therefore, therapy is discontinued when these symptoms arise.
- Use cautiously if kidney function is impaired because methotrexate is excreted principally by the kidneys.
- Headache, drowsiness, blurred vision, aphasia, and convulsions have occurred.
- Rashes, photosensitivity, and alopecia have been reported.

Dosage, Administration
- Usual dosage range for leukemia is 2.5 to 5 mg/kg/day orally or parenterally.
- Usual dosage range in choriocarcinoma is 15 to 30 mg orally or IM for 5 days.

Nursing Tips
- See *PH, Antineoplastics: nursing tips* for general information common to most chemotherapy.
- Kidney and liver function tests, chest x-rays, and blood counts should be done before, during, and after therapy with methotrexate. The potential for toxicity is very high and is usually dose related.
- In the plasma, portions of the methotrexate are bound to serum albumin. The following drugs can displace methotrexate and increase its potential for toxicity: salicylates (aspirin and aspirin products), sulfonamides, diphenylhydantoin (Dilantin), phenylbutazone, tetracycline, chloramphenicol, and para-aminobenzoic acid. They should not be given at the same time as the methotrexate.
- Response to methotrexate may be decreased by vitamin supplements containing folic acid.

PLANT ALKALOIDS
VINBLASTINE SULFATE, U.S.P. (VELBAN)
Actions
- Inhibits mitosis, arrests cell division, and prevents the synthesis of DNA

Indications
- Complete remissions have occurred when vinblastine is used in combination with bleomycin and cisplatin to treat metastatic testicular tumors.

- Lymphomas, including Hodgkin's disease, and Letterer-Siwe disease are frequently responsive to vinblastine.
- Remissions also occur in carcinoma of the breast and choriocarcinoma.

Adverse Effects, Contraindications

- Most frequent side-effect is leukopenia. This is usually temporary but may limit the amount of drug given.
- Neurologic side-effects occur, especially with high doses. The manifestations are numbness, tingling, mental depression (usually occurs the 2nd or 3rd day after treatment), loss of reflexes, headache, and convulsions.
- Alopecia is infrequent and usually not complete.
- Autonomic nervous system effects include constipation, urinary retention, paralytic ileus, tenderness of the parotid glands, and dry mouth.
- Nausea, vomiting, and diarrhea can occur.
- Extravasation during administration may cause cellulitis and phlebitis.

Dosage, Administration

- Initial therapy for adults is 3.7 mg/m^2 of body surface area (bsa). Dosages are given intravenously at weekly intervals and dosage is increased according to the patient's WBC.
- Duration of therapy depends on the type of cancer being treated and is limited by bone marrow toxicity.

Nursing Tips

- See *PH, Antineoplastics: nursing tips* for general information common to most chemotherapy.
- Blood counts, especially WBC, must be monitored carefully.
- Liver function should be determined before therapy because the drug is excreted by the liver into the bile.
- If extravasation occurs, injecting hyaluronidase into the area and applying heat may minimize damage.
- Vinblastine can be injected directly into the vein or into the tubing of a running intravenous infusion. The medication should not be diluted in large amounts of fluid (*e.g.,* 100 to 250 ml) or given for long periods (30 to 60 minutes) because this can cause vein irritation.

VINCRISTINE SULFATE, U.S.P. (ONCOVIN)
Actions

- Inhibits mitosis, arrests cell division, and prevents synthesis of DNA.

Indications

- Induces remissions in children with acute lymphoblastic leukemia when given with prednisone.
- Effective against Hodgkin's disease, especially when used with MOPP regimen (mechlorethamine, Oncovin, prednisone, and procarbazine).
- Produces remissions in non-Hodgkin's lymphomas, rhabdomyosarcoma, neuroblastoma, and Wilms' tumor.

Adverse Effects, Contraindications

- Alopecia is the most common side-effect, but it is usually reversible.
- Frequent neuromuscular abnormalities are noted. Tingling and numbness of extremities usually occur first. Dosage may be reduced or stopped to prevent loss of deep-tendon reflexes, muscle weakness and footdrop, hoarseness, headache, ptosis, and double vision. Convulsions are rare.
- Severe constipation may result in obstruction.
- Leukopenia occurs less frequently than when vinblastine is used, but it can occur.
- Hyperuricemia can be prevented by giving the patient allopurinol.

Dosage, Administration

- Administered intravenously at weekly intervals. Usual dose for children is 2 mg/m². Usual adult dose is 1.4 mg/m².

Nursing Tips

- See *PH, Antineoplastics; nursing tips* for general information common to most chemotherapy.
- Monitor white blood count (WBC) carefully.
- Liver function should be determined before therapy because the drug is excreted by the liver into the bile.
- If extravasation occurs, injecting hyaluronidase into the area and applying heat may minimize damage.
- Injection may be given over 1 minute, either directly into the vein or into the tubing of a running IV.

HORMONES
ADRENOCORTICOSTEROIDS

For a discussion of the use of steroids for conditions other then cancer, see *PH, Endocrine system.*

Actions

- Suppress mitosis (cell division) in lymphocytes.
- Have lymphocytic effects.

Indications

- When used with vincristine, prednisone effectively induces remissions in children with acute lymphocytic leukemia.
- As part of the MOPP combination, prednisone induces remissions in Hodgkin's disease.
- Also used in the treatment of lymphosarcoma and for palliative effects in lung and breast carcinomas.
- Reduce some cases of radiation edema.
- Restore appetite, strength, lost weight, and sense of well-being to patients with advanced carcinomas.
- Lower blood-plasma calcium levels in patients receiving estrogen or androgen therapy.
- Relieve cerebral edema secondary to central nervous system metastasis.

Adverse Effects, Contraindications

(See PH, Endocrine system)

Dosage, Administration

- Prednisone, U.S.P. (Meticorten): Daily dosage may range from 10 to 100 mg orally. To decrease the incidence of adverse effects, the lowest effective dosage is used.

Nursing Tips

- See *PH, Antineoplastics: nursing tips* for general information common to most nonhormonal chemotherapy.
  (See PH, Endocrine system: adrenocorticosteroids, nursing tips)

  ESTROGENS

Actions

- Interfere with the growth, function, and cell integrity of carcinomas of the reproductive organs by changing the hormonal environment.

Indications

- Metastatic prostatic carcinoma may respond to estrogens.
- Used to treat advanced mammary carcinoma when surgery and radiation are no longer feasible. Women should be at least 5 years past menopause.

Adverse Effects, Contraindications

- Nausea, vomiting, abdominal cramps, breast enlargement, and tenderness are common.

- Women may experience breakthrough bleeding or spotting and an increase in size of uterine fibroid tumors.
- Men may experience feminizing effects.
- Frequently, fluid retention leads to edema and weight gain.
- Headache, dizziness, mental depression, nervousness, fatigue, and irregular brown spots on skin (chloasma) also occur.
- Hypercalcemia in patients with breast cancer and bone metastases is a problem, especially when calcifications occur in the urinary tract.
- Exacerbation of the malignant process can result.
- Estrogens increase the risk of thromboembolic disorders, hypertension, gallbladder disease, and edometrial carcinoma. Contraindications to estrogen therapy must be weighed against the potential benefits for patients with advanced carcinomas.

Dosage, Administration
- Diethylstilbestrol, U.S.P. (DES): Daily dosage may range from 1.5 to 15 mg orally.

Nursing Tips
- See *PH Antineoplastics: nursing tips* for general information common to most nonhormonal therapy.
- Onset of hormonal action is slow. Eight to twelve weeks may be needed before the effectiveness of the treatment can be determined.
- Hypercalcemia should be treated with high fluid intake, possible discontinuation of the estrogen therapy, and administration of such drugs as diuretics and steroids.
- Monitor blood plasma calcium levels.

ANDROGENS
Actions
- Interfere with growth, function, and cell integrity of carcinomas of the reproductive organs by changing the hormonal environment.

Indications
- Used to treat advanced mammary carcinoma when surgery and radiation are no longer feasible. Both pre- and post-menopausal women receive androgens.

Adverse Affects, Contraindications
- Woman frequently experience masculinizing effects, such as growth of facial hair, acne, deepening of the voice, hair recession

at temples and thinning at crown, amenorrhea, and enlargement of the clitoris.
- Fluid retention leads to edema and weight gain.
- Hypercalcemia in patients with breast cancer and bone metastases is a problem, especially when calcifications occur in the urinary tract.
- Exacerbation of the malignant process can result.

Dosage, Administration

- Fluoxymesterone, U.S.P. (Halotestin): Usual dosage is 10 mg orally t.i.d.
- Calusterone, U.S.P. (Methosarb): Usual dosage is 50 mg orally q.i.d.

Nursing Tips

- See *PH, Antineoplastics: nursing tips* for general information common to most nonhormonal chemotherapy.
- Onset of hormonal action is slow. Eight to twelve weeks may be needed before the effectivness of the treatment can be determined.
- Hypercalcemia should be treated with a high fluid intake, possible discontinuation of the androgen therapy, and administration of such drugs as diuretics and steroids.
- Monitor blood plasma calcium levels.

RADIOACTIVE ISOTOPES

- A few radioactive elements are used in the treatment of selected neoplasms.
- The beta particles destroy living tissues, including some normal cells as well as the malignant cells.
- Radiogold (^{198}Au) solution, U.S.P. (Aurcoloid): Used to treat pleural effusion and ascites caused by cancer.
- Sodium iodide I-131 solution, U.S.P. (Iodotope): Used for the diagnosis and treatment of hyperthyroidism and thyroid carcinoma.
- Sodium phosphate P32 solution, U.S.P. (Phosphotope): Used to treat polycythemia vera.
- Use of radioactive isotopes requires special precautions for both hospital personnel and patients. Consult nuclear medicine departments and procedure books for the necessary information.

AUTONOMIC NERVOUS SYSTEM
OVERVIEW

- The autonomic nervous system is also called the involuntary nervous system. It has two main divisions, the sympathetic and parasympathetic branches. It regulates the function of internal organs to maintain homeostasis and controls the function of most bodily organs.

- The ends of the nerve fibers in this system release chemical substances called neurohormones that transmit their impulses to cardiac and smooth muscle and to the exocrine glands. The two principal neurohormones are acetylcholine (ACh) and norepinephrine (NE).
- Drugs that mimic the action of ACh are referred to as cholinergics. Drugs that function similarly to NE are called sympathomimetics.

CHOLINERGICS—MIOTICS

Actions

- Cause contraction of the ciliary muscle.
- Increase drainage of fluid into Schlemm's canal.

Indications

- Used to treat glaucoma.

Adverse Effects, Contraindications

- Initial use frequently causes stinging, redness, and lacrimation.
- Pupil constriction leads to dimming of vision.
- Contraction of the ciliary muscle causes blurring of vision and nearsightedness (myopia).
- Long-term use can result in iris cysts; lens opacities—which may progress to cataracts; obstruction of the nasolacrimal duct and canal; and allergic reactions.
- Use cautiously in patients with a history of retinal detachment.
- Significant systemic absorption is unlikely with normal dosages. However, systemic absorption could possibly produce the following effects:
    1. Reduced heart rate and lowered blood pressure. Use cautiously for patients with a recent myocardial infarction.
    2. Bronchoconstriction and wheezing. Use cautiously for patients with bronchial asthma and other types of chronic obstructive lung disease.
    3. Nausea, vomiting, cramps, and diarrhea can occur. Use cautiously for patients with peptic ulcers.
    4. Salivation and sweating.

Dosage, Administration

- Pilocarpine hydrochloride and nitrate, U.S.P. (Pilocar): Most commonly used solutions range from 0.5% to 4%.

1. Open-angle glaucoma: one or two drops instilled in the eye every 6 to 8 hr at first, and as frequently as every 2 hr later.
2. Acute narrow-angle glaucoma: one or two drops of a 4% solution every 10 minutes, three or more times.

- Ocusert Pilo-20 or Pilo-40: A plastic disc placed in either the upper or lower conjunctival sac, which diffuses the pilocarpine into the film of tears over the eye. Delivers either 20 or 40 micrograms (mcg) per hour for 7 days.
- Pilocarpine is the most commonly used of the miotics in treating glaucoma.
- Carbachol chloride, U.S.P. (Carcholin, Doryl): Usual dosage is 0.1 ml of a 0.75% to 3% solution, administered one to four times daily in the eye.

Nursing Tips

- To reduce systemic absorption of eye medications, apply gentle pressure on the inner canthus immediately after instilling the eye drops.
- For further details regarding the administration of eye medications, see *SS, Eye-patient care.*

ANTICHOLINERGICS

Actions

- Anticholinergics interfere with the action of acetylcholine and cholinergic drugs.
- They decrease gastrointestinal (GI) muscle tone and motility, and in large doses they decrease secretion of gastric acid and digestive enzymes (*e.g.,* pepsin).
- They reduce the tone and motility of the ureters and the bladder wall, and they increase bladder sphincter tone.
- Large doses may accelerate the heart rate; small doses may slow it.
- Ocular effects include mydriasis (dilation of pupil) and cycloplegia (paralysis of accommodation).
- Anticholinergics cause a decrease in sweating, salivation, and nasal and bronchial secretions, and abnormal skeletal muscle tone.

ATROPINE SULFATE, U.S.P.
Actions

(See PH, Anticholinergics: actions)

Indications

- Treats GI disorders such as peptic ulcer, gastritis, and spastic colitis.

- It counteracts bradycardia and partial heart block by causing an increase in heart rate.
- It is used in diagnostic eye exams.
- It is frequently included in preoperative medications to reduce salivation and bronchial secretions.

Adverse Effects, Contraindications

- Common side-effects include dryness of mouth and blurring of vision.
- The tachycardia often produced is undesirable in cardiac disorders.
- Constipation and urinary retention can occur.
- Do not give to patients with prostatic hypertrophy or narrow-angle glaucoma.

Dosage, Administration

- Usual adult dose is 0.4 to 0.6 mg IM.
- Atropine is also available as a sterile ophthalmic ointment.

PROPANTHELINE BROMIDE, U.S.P. (PRO-BANTHINE)
Actions

(See PH, Anticholinergics: actions)

Indications

- Effective as adjunctive therapy in the treatment of peptic ulcer.

Adverse Effects, Contraindications

- Dries salivary secretions and decreases sweating.
- Patients may experience blurred vision, mydriasis, cycloplegia, and increased ocular tension.
- Tachycardia and palpitations may adversely affect patients with cadiovascular problems.
- Constipation and urinary retention can occur.
- Do not give to patients with prostatic hypertrophy or narrow-angle glaucoma.
- Use cautiously in the elderly, and in patients with kidney or liver disease, ulcerative colitis, or hyperthyroidism.

Dosage, Administration

- Usual initial adult dose is 15 mg taken 30 min. before each meal, and 30 mg at bedtime.

Nursing Tips

- Excessive cholinergic blockade may occur if Pro-Banthine is given with phenothiazines, tricyclic antidepressants, quinidine, antihistamines, procainamide, or other anticholinergic agents.

TRIHEXYPHENIDYL HYDROCHLORIDE, U.S.P. (ARTANE)

Actions

(See PH, Anticholinergics: actions)

- Reduces skeletal muscle rigidity, decreases tremor and akinesia.
- Reduces excess sweating and drooling, and produces mild euphoria.

Indications

- Relieves symptoms of Parkinson's disease.
- Treats the parkinsonism-type symptoms produced by some drugs (*e.g.*, phenothiazines).

Adverse Effects, Contraindications

- About one-half of the patients using trihexyphenidyl experience minor side-effects.
- Frequent side-effects include dry mouth, nausea, vomiting, blurred vision, and constipation. These discomforts can be relieved by reducing the dosage.
- Tachycardia and hypotension may also occur.
- Overdose can produce mental confusion, excitement, disorientation, and psychosis.
- Use cautiously for patients with hypertrophy of the prostate, a tendency for gastrointestinal obstruction, cerebral arteriosclerosis, or cardiovascular disorders.
- Contraindicated for patients with narrow-angle glaucoma.

Dosage, Administration

- A total daily dose of 6 to 10 mg p.o. is common.
- Treatment is started initially with 1 mg and is increased by 2 mg every 3 to 5 days. The dosages are usually divided and given near meals and at bedtime.

Nursing Tips

- Dry mouth can be reduced by giving this drug with meals.

BETA ADRENERGIC BLOCKING AGENTS

Actions

- The cardiac effects include: reduction in heart rate (negative chronotropic); reduction in cardiac contractility (negative inotropic); slowing of atrioventricular (AV) conduction (negative dromotropic); and decrease in the automaticity of ectopic pacemakers. Some slight lessening of local blood flow can occur.
- Patients, especially those with asthma or COPD (chronic obstructive pulmonary disease) may experience bronchoconstriction.

- May potentiate hypoglycemic response in diabetics following insulin administration.

PROPRANOLOL HYDROCHLORIDE, U.S.P. (INDERAL)
Actions

(See PH, Beta adrenergic blocking agents: actions)

Indications

- Treats supraventricular and ventricular arrhythmias, angina pectoris, and essential hypertension.
- Also used to prevent migraine headaches. *(See SS, Cardiovascular)*

Adverse Effects, Contraindications

- May cause excessive slowing of heart rate, atrioventricular block, and reduced myocardial contractility.
- Patients with congestive heart failure (CHF) or second- and third-degree block should not receive propranolol.
- May mask symptoms of diabetic drug overdose.
- Rarely, psychiatric disturbances such as depression and hallucinations occur.

Dosage, Administration

- For arrhythmias, an average dosage is 10 to 30 mg, t.i.d. or q.i.d., orally.
- Usual dosage for angina pectoris initially is 10 to 20 mg, t.i.d. or q.i.d.
- Usual dosage for hypertension is 40 mg b.i.d.
- Usual initial dosage for migraine headache is 40 mg orally b.i.d.

Nursing Tips

- Check BP and apical and radial pulse before giving.
- Important to maintain the therapeutic blood levels; therefore if dosage calls for q.i.d., give q. 6 hr instead, and consult with the physician before witholding any dose (*e.g.,* if the patient is n.p.o. for a lab test).

TIMOLOL MALEATE (TIMOPTIC)
Actions

- Appears to reduce the formation of aqueous humor and to increase the outflow.

Indications

- Treatment of chronic open-angle glaucoma, secondary glaucoma, and ocular hypertension.

Adverse Effects, Contraindications

- Occasionally, mild irritation and rash have occurred.
- Some patients experience a slight reduction in heart rate.
- Bronchospasm is rare, but use cautiously in patients with bronchial asthma.
- Use cautiously in patients with severe heart block, heart failure, and sinus bradycardia.

Dosage, Administration

- Usual dosage is 1 drop of a 0.25% or 0.5% solution in each eye, twice daily.

Nursing Tips

- Monitor heart rate, especially if patient has a history of heart disease.
- To reduce systemic absorption of eye medications, apply gentle pressure on the inner canthus immediately after instilling the eye drops.
- Often better tolerated than pilocarpine, and does not cause the dimming and blurring of vision that occurs with the miotics.
- For further details regarding the administration of eye medications, see *SS, Eye-patient care.*

CATECHOLAMINES

Nursing Tips

- Because of an additive effect, ectopic pacemakers can occur when the catecholamines and digitalis are used concurrently, causing arrhythmias.
- Patients receiving catecholamines and monoamine oxidase (MAO) inhibiters may experience a hypertensive crisis.
- Diuretics and some antihypertensives can interfere with the effects of the catecholamines.
- Serious arrhythmias can occur if epinephrine and isoproterenol are administered at the same time.

DOBUTAMINE (DOBUTREX)

Actions

- Stimulates the beta receptors of the heart, and increases myocardial contractility and cardiac output.
- Produces mild increases in heart rate and blood pressure, and some vasodilation occurs.

Indications

- Used in short-term parenteral therapy to treat congestive heart failure resulting from organic heart disease or cardiac surgery.

Adverse Effects, Contraindications

- Tachycardia and hypertension occur in about 10% of patients.
- Dobutamine should never be used for patients with idiopathic hypertrophic subaortic stenosis (IHSS).
- Use cautiously for patients with atrial fibrillation, hypertension, continuing hypotension, or hypovolemia.
- There is still question as to whether dobutamine could increase the area of a myocardial infarction.

Dosage, Administration

- Patient's weight must be known to determine accurate dosage.
- Usual range is 2.5 to 10 mcg/kg/min IV.
- Toxic levels are about 15 mcg/kg/min.

Nursing Tips

(See PH, Catecholamines: nursing tips)
- Using a consistent method of mixing the dobutamine will minimize errors. One example is to mix a 250-mg vial in 250 ml of D_5W, giving one mg per ml. An IV pump with microdrip tubing should be used.
- The patient must be weaned from the medication gradually and must be watched carefully for signs of heart failure. *(See SS, Cardiovascular)*
- Drug interactions:
  1. The actions of dobutamine may be antagonized by beta-blocking drugs (dobutamine stimulates beta receptors).
  2. Dobutamine must be piggybacked to the main IV line because sodium bicarbonate (administered to treat metabolic acidosis) would inactivate it.

DOPAMINE HYDROCHLORIDE (INTROPIN)
Actions

- Strengthens cardiac contractility, and increases cardiac output.
- Blood flow to the peripheral vascular beds decreases; mesenteric flow increases.

Indications

- Treats cardiogenic shock following a myocardial infarction, septicemic shock, and shock from CHF.

- Dopamine has certain advantages over other vasoconstrictors. It dilates mesenteric and renal blood vessels and often increases urine output. It causes less peripheral vasoconstriction, and myocardial oxygen consumption is comparatively low.

Adverse Effects, Contraindications

- Hypertension and increased heart rate are common side-effects.
- Overdose can cause ectopic heartbeats, tachycardia, anginal chest pains, or dyspnea. Decreasing the infusion rate may correct these.
- Tachyarrhythmias and hypovolemia should be corrected before administering dopamine.
- Nausea, vomiting, and headache may also occur.

Dosage, Administration

- Patient's weight must be known to determine accurate dosage.
- Mix a 5-ml ampule (200 mg dopamine) in 500 ml of D_5W.
- Initial infusion rate is usually 2 to 5 mcg/kg/min and is adjusted according to the individual's blood pressure, urine flow, and cardiac output.

Nursing Tips

(See PH, Catecholamines: nursing tips)
- Blood pressure and apical and radial pulse should be monitored q 10 min. Because of the constant care required, these patients are usually placed in an intensive-care unit (ICU).
- An IV pump and microdrip tubing should be used.
- If extravasation occurs, infiltration of the area with phentolamine (Regitine) may dilate the constricted blood vessels and prevent tissue damage.
- Dopamine should be discontinued gradually.

EPINEPHRINE, U.S.P. (ADRENALIN)
Actions

- Imitates all actions of the sympathetic nervous system except those on the arteries of the face and sweat glands.

Indications

- Because of rapid bronchodilation and vasoconstriction effects, epinephrine is useful in treating acute asthmatic attacks and anaphylactic shock.
- In cardiac arrest and complete heart block, epinephrine can speed and strengthen cardiac contractions.
- When used topically it exerts a hemostatic effect in epistaxis.

- When combined with local anesthetics it prolongs local effect and delays systemic absorption.
- Nasal and ocular decongestion occur with topical preparations.

Adverse Effects, Contraindications

- Overdose causes rapid rise in blood pressure and may lead to severe headache and intracranial hemorrhage.
- Severe, rapid arrhythmias can occur.
- Smaller doses may cause tachycardia, dyspnea, pallor, palpitations, feelings of anxiety, fear, and dizziness.
- Usually not given to patients with diabetes, angina pectoris, hypertension, and hyperthyroidism.

Dosage, Administration

- Varies according to problem under treatment.
- Prepared in solutions of 1:1000 for SC or IM injection.
- Also comes in solutions for inhalation and in nose and eye drops.

Nursing Tips

(See PH, Catecholamines: nursing tips)
- Epinephrine is extremely potent. Draw up dosages with great care.

ISOPROTERENOL HYDROCHLORIDE, U.S.P. (ISUPREL)
Actions

- Increases cardiac output by increasing cardiac contractility and heart rate.
- Relaxes smooth muscle, especially that of the bronchi and gastrointestinal tract.

Indications

- Treats some cardiac arrhythmias, such as standstill, and excessively slow rhythms, such as that caused by digitalis toxicity.
- Because it dilates blood vessels, it is useful in treating septic shock when vasoconstriction is excessive.
- Relieves brochial spasms to provide symptomatic treatment of chronic bronchopulmonary disorders (*e.g.*, asthma and COPD). *(See SS, Respiratory)*

Adverse Effects, Contraindications

- Do not give in the presence of rapid arrhythmias because tachycardia and heart palpitations can occur.
- Headache, flushing, sweating, tremors, and nervousness may also occur.
- When administering to treat shock, slow or discontinue the infusion if the pulse goes above 110.

Dosage, Administration

- Varies according to problem under treatment.
- For IV infusion, mix 5 ml of 1:5000 solution in 500 ml of D_5W.
- Sublingual dosage is 10 to 15 mg q.i.d.
- Also available in solutions for nebulization and oral inhalation.

Nursing Tips

(See PH, Catecholamines: nursing tips)
- Check BP and apical and radial pulse during administration.
- For IV administration, an IV pump and microdrip tubing should be used.
- Saliva and sputum may appear pink after oral inhalation.

LEVARTERENOL BITARTRATE, U.S.P. (LEVOPHED BITARTRATE)

Actions

- Powerful peripheral vasoconstrictor.
- Increases cardiac contractility and dilates coronary arteries.

Indications

- Treats acute hypotension resulting from vasomotor depression, trauma, and shock.
- Effective in treating cardiogenic shock because it increases venous return to the heart and strengthens contractions without producing an excessive increase in myocardial oxygen consumption.

Adverse Effects, Contraindications

- Hypertension, bradycardia, ventricular tachycardia, and fibrillation can occur from too-rapid administration.
- Local leakage can cause severe vasoconstriction, leading to death of tissue with sloughing and gangrene.

Dosage, Administration

- Dosage is adjusted to the patient's response.
- Mix 4 ml of 0.2% solution of levarterenol in 1000 ml of D_5W.

Nursing Tips

(See PH, Catecholamines: nursing tips)
- Monitor blood pressure q 2 min when infusion is started and then q 5 min when BP is stabilized at low-normal levels.
- Phentolamine (Regitine) is used to infiltrate an area of levarterenol leakage.
- Patients must be weaned from this medication gradually,
- An IV pump and microdrip tubing should be used.

CARDIOVASCULAR SYSTEM
ANTIANEMICS
CYANOCOBALAMIN INJECTION, U.S.P. (VITAMIN B$_{12}$)
Actions

- Hematopoietic substance (forms blood cells)
- Counteracts glossitis (smooth, sore, ulcerated tongue).
- Decreases gastrointestinal (GI) symptoms such as constipation or diarrhea.
- Prevents damage to the spinal cord and other central nervous system (CNS) areas (*e.g.*, numbness, tingling, and muscle incoordination decreases).

Indications

- Treats pernicious anemia, a lack of intrinsic factor, and inability to absorb B$_{12}$.
- Replaces vitamin B$_{12}$ in patients who have had their entire stomach or portions of it removed.

Adverse Effects, Contraindications

- Toxic reactions to B$_{12}$ are rare, but thrombosis, hypokalemia, congestive heart failure, and pulmonary edema have been reported.
- Patients who have optic nerve damge or who are hypersensitive to cobalt should not receive B$_{12}$.

Dosage, Administration

- An average course of treatment would be 30 to 100 mcg, q.d. for 1 week, then one to three times weekly until remission is achieved. This is followed by 100 mcg per month for the rest of the patient's life.
- B$_{12}$ can be given SC or IM.

Nursing Tips

- Emphasize that the medication is treating, not curing, the anemia and that therefore the therapy cannot be discontinued.
- The patient or a family member should be taught to give the injections, which will result in the dual benefits of self-sufficiency and lower cost.

FOLIC ACID, U.S.P. (FOLVITE)
Actions

- A member of the vitamin B complex, folic acid is essential for cell division in all types of tissue.

Indications

- Used to treat individuals with deficiencies: for example, patients with malnutrition from alcoholism, advanced age, or poverty; food faddists; women with several successive pregnancies; and patients on long-term anticonvulsant therapy.

Adverse Effects, Contraindications

- Adverse effects are rare.
- Folic acid is contraindicated in patients with pernicious anemia because it masks the symptoms and makes diagnosis difficult.

Dosage, Administration

- A maintenance dose of 1 mg p.o. daily is usually adequate, but you may see up to 20 mg prescribed.

IRON
Actions

- Iron is needed by all body cells and is essential in the body's red blood cells to form the hemoglobin (Hb) responsible for oxygen and carbon dioxide transportation.

Indications

- Iron is used to prevent and treat iron-deficiency anemias in susceptible individuals: 6-month-old to 2-year-old infants, adolescents (especially female), pregnant women in the second and third trimesters, women with heavy menstrual flow, and GI bleeders.

Adverse Effects, Contraindications

- Iron can cause varying degrees of epigastric distress: nausea, vomiting, or abdominal cramps (with either diarrhea or constipation).
- Overdose can result in corrosion of the lining of the stomach and intestine, with black, tarry stools; weak, rapid pulse; and hypotension sufficient to produce shock.
- The IM preparation can result in *anaphylactic shock* and should be used very cautiously if liver function is impaired. Iron administration parenterally can also cause vomiting, chills, fever, headache, joint pain, and urticaria.
- Caution should also be used in the presence of GI disorders (*e.g.*, ulcers).

Dosage, Administration

- Ferrous sulfate, U.S.P. (Feosol): usual daily dose is one to four 300-mg tablets.

- Ferrous gluconate, U.S.P. (Fergon): usual daily dose is 1 capsule (435 mg), yielding 50 mg of elemental iron.
- Iron-Dextran injection, U.S.P. (Imferon): maximum adult daily dose is usually 250 mg (5 ml), IM.
- Iron dextran can be administered intravenously to avoid the pain and discoloration of IM injections. Use only the Imferon brand, the 2-ml and 5-ml ampules *without* preservatives. Mix with 500 to 1000 ml of normal saline. Observe for allergic reactions by running the solution in slowly (10 gtt/min) for about 10 to 15 minutes. Then increase the rate to no more than 60 gtt/min.

Nursing Tips

- Giving more iron than the situation warrants is useless and can also be harmful. The intestines regulate the amount absorbed, which is usually enough to replace daily loss (about 10% to 15% of ingested iron).
- Oral iron is absorbed best from an empty stomach, but this can be very irritating. Begin giving the medication on a full stomach, and gradually reduce the amount of food taken with it.
- Liquid preparations can stain teeth. Dilute the liquid and have the patient drink it through a straw.
- Iron given IM can produce staining, soreness, and inflammatin. It should be given deep IM using the Z-track technique. *(See PH, Drug Therapy)*
- Inform patients that their stools may be black and tarry even with normal doses. Otherwise they may think they are bleeding.
- To reduce the risk of phlebitis when giving the Imferon IV, do not mix with D_5W. If possible, do not let the infusion run over 5 hours.

ANTIARRHYTHMICS
QUINIDINE
Actions

- Quinidine preparations can be considered a prototype of other antiarrhythmic drugs.
- They depress automaticity, especially in the latent or ectopic (non-sinoatrial node) pacemakers, giving the sinoatrial node a chance to regain control, or at least causing a decrease in heart rate.
- They can delay conduction, which worsens heart block.
- Contractility may also be decreased but usually not to a serious extent.

Indications

- Prevents and treats both atrial and ventricular arrhythmias.
- One of its main uses is to prevent recurrences of atrial tachycardia,

fibrillation, or flutter following conversion to a normal sinus rhythm (NSR) by electric shock or other drugs.

Adverse Effects, Contraindications

- Gastrointestinal (GI) symptoms are very common, especially diarrhea.
- Hypotension can occur.
- A common toxic effect is the development of atrioventricular (AV) block. This can result in asystole, premature ventricular contractions (PVCs), ventricular tachycardia, or fibrillation.
- Quinidine can also cause or worsen congestive heart failure (CHF).
- Thrombocytopenia can occur as a hypersensitivity reaction.
- Quinidine is contraindicated in patients with heart block.

Dosage, Administration

- Quinidine sulfate, U.S.P. (Quinidex): usual maintenance dosage is 200 to 300 mg, p.o., t.i.d. or q.i.d. It is readily absorbed from the GI tract.
- Quinidine gluconate, U.S.P. (Quinaglute): usually given IM. Initial dose is from 300 to 500 mg.

Nursing Tips

- Always check patient's blood pressure (BP) and apical and radial pulse before giving. Notify physician of any significant decrease.
- Quinidine can prolong the patient's prothrombin time (PT) and potentiate anticoagulants. Observe for signs of bleeding.
- To maintain therapeutic blood levels, the drug should be evenly spaced (*e.g.*, q 6 hr rather than q.i.d.). Check with the physician before withholding *any* dosage.
- Quinidine can potentiate the effects of antihypertensives and diuretics and can cause excessive hypotension.
- Serum digoxin levels can more than double rapidly when quinidine is added. Digoxin levels should be checked, and it may be necessary for the physician to lower the dose of digoxin.
- Toxic reactions to quinidine are most likely to occur in patients with liver disease, renal insufficiency, or CHF.

DISOPYRAMIDE PHOSPHATE (NORPACE)
Actions

- Norpace decreases the rate of ectopic pacemakers and decreases the rate of impulse conduction in the atrial and ventricular muscle.
- It does not significantly alter conduction through the atrioventricular (AV) node.

Indications

- Used to suppress PVCs and ventricular tachycardia.

Adverse Effects, Contraindications

- Severe hypotension may develop.
- Not recommended for patients with heart block.
- Patients may also experience atropinelike side-effects, such as mouth dryness and blurred vision. May be unsafe for patients with glaucoma or prostatic hypertrophy.
- Use cautiously for patients with CHF because severe hypotension and cardiogenic shock could result.

Dosage, Administration

- Usual p.o. dosage is 100 to 150 mg, q.i.d.

Nursing Tips

- Always check patient's BP and apical and radical pulse before giving.
- This is a fairly new drug (as compared to other antiarrhythmics), and new adverse effects may be reported as use increases. A few cases of drug-induced ventricular arrhythmias have been reported, so be alert to your patient's reports of fainting, dizziness, weakness, and pulse changes.

LIDOCAINE, U.S.P. (XYLOCAINE)

Actions

- Depresses excessive automaticity and, therefore, PVCs.
- It does not depress conduction, so there is less likelihood of heart block or ventricular, ectopic rhythms.
- It does not depress contractility, so CHF is less likely.

Indications

- Lidocaine is useful for rapid control of PVCs in patients with myocardial infarction, and thus helps to prevent ventricular tachycardia.
- Ventricular arrhythmias resulting from digitalis toxicity also respond well to lidocaine.

Adverse Effects, Contraindications

- Lidocaine can produce bradycardia and hypotension.
- Drowsiness is usually the first central nervous system (CNS) effect but excitation may follow.
- Lidocaine should not be used with severe heart block.

Dosage, Administration

- To ensure accurate dosage, patient's weight must be known.
- The usual IV dose is 1 mg/kg.
- In emergency siuations a bolus of 50 to 100 mg is given IV push first. Then 1 g is mixed in 500 ml of D_5W for administration, piggyback to the main IV line.
- Because *fluid overload* is always a danger, mixing *2g* in *500 ml* may be indicated because the patient would receive less fluid. The use of microdrip tubing and an infusion pump is also indicated.

Nursing Tips

- Monitor BP and apical and radial pulse very carefully.
- Lidocaine must be administered by IV injection. It goes quickly to the myocardium and other organs with a rich blood supply, but the infusion must continue for relatively long periods to maintain effective levels. The patient must be weaned from it gradually.
- Anticonvulsants and barbituates can increase the metabolization of lidocaine. Therefore, higher doses of the lidocaine may be needed.
- The risk of congestive heart failure (CHF) is increased when the following drugs are used with lidocaine: phenytoin, procainamide, propranolol, quinidine, and disopyramide.

PHENYTOIN SODIUM, U.S.P. (DILANTIN)
Actions

(See PH, Central nervous system)

- Phenytoin's antiarrhythmic activity is similar to lidocaine.
- Suppresses automaticity in ectopic pacemakers and may actually increase the rate at which impulses are conducted through the atrioventricular (AV) node and Purkinje's fibers.

Indications

- Treats the arrhythmias caused by digitalis toxicity.
- Suppresses both premature atrial and ventricular beats, and improves AV block rather than increases it.

Adverse Effects, Contraindications

- Bradycardia and hypotension can occur.
- Should not be given in advanced heart block.
- Nausea, vomiting, and constipation occur.
- Gingival hyperplasia (overgrowth of gum tissue) is common.
- Hirsutism, skin rashes, and megaloblastic anemia occur.

- Excessive doses cause lethargy, slurred speech, and staggering gait. Patients also experience double vision, dizziness, and headache.
- Overdose results in coma, apnea, and death.
- Cardiac arrest can occur from rapid IV administration.

Dosage, Administration

- An average oral maintenance dosage is 200 to 400 mg, q.d.

Nursing Tips

- Monitor BP and apical and radial pulse carefully.
- Heart block or bradycardia may be reversed with IV administration of atropine.
- Patients metabolize phenytoin at different rates, so blood levels should be checked to monitor the drug for effectiveness and toxicity.
- Giving phenytoin during or after meals will minimize the gastric distress.
- Patients receiving this drug for long periods may need folic acid to prevent anemia.
- The following drug interactions occur with phenytoin:
  1. The action of phenytoin is potentiated by aspirin, estrogens, sulfonamides, and anticoagulants.
  2. The action of phenytoin is inhibited by alcohol, antihistamines, barbituates, and sedatives.
  3. Phenytoin potentiates the action of quinidine and antihypertensives.
  4. Phenytoin inhibits the action of steroids and digitalis.

PROCAINAMIDE HYDROCHLORIDE, U.S.P. (PRONESTYL HYDROCHLORIDE)

Actions

- Procainamide is similar to quinidine. Parenteral administration, though, is considered to be somewhat safer than with quinidine. *(See PH, Cardiovascular)*

Indications

- Controls PVCs and ventricular tachycardia, especially following myocardial infarction and digitalis toxicity.

Adverse Effects, Contraindications

- Hypotension can occur, especially following IV administration.
- Gastrointestinal disturbances, such as anorexia, nausea, and vomiting, occur.

- Prolonged oral administration can produce signs and symptoms resembling the syndrome of lupus erythematosus. If the antinucleur antibody test (ANA) becomes positive, the drug should be discontinued. Agranulocytosis and the lupus syndrome are rare but very serious.

Dosage, Administration

- An average range is 250 to 500 mg, p.o., q. 6 hr.

Nursing Tips

- Monitor BP, especially during IV administration. Apical and radial pulse should also be checked.
- Observe for clinical signs of lupus (*e.g.,* fever, arthritis, or pleuritic pain).
- Observe for clinical signs of decreased white blood count (WBC) *e.g.,* sore throat or upper respiratory infections.

PROPRANOLOL HYDROCHLORIDE, U.S.P. (INDERAL)

(See PH, Autonomic nervous system)

ANTICOAGULANTS

Nursing Tips

- Observe for bleeding (*e.g.,* in the stool, urine, nose, vagina, gums, or as indicated by any abnormal bruising). Patients may need soft tooth-brushes and stool softeners. Use an electric razor rather than a blade. Test urine and stool for occult blood.
- Patient should carry an ID card or wear a bracelet stating the medications he is receiving.
- Remind patients to inform their dentists that they are receiving anticoagulants when they go for treatment.

HEPARIN SODIUM

Actions

- Prevents the formation of new blood clots.
- Affects circulating factors in the blood stream in an immediate, rapid fashion to prevent clot formation. Has a short duration of action.
- Cannot dissolve pre-existing clots.

Indications

- Treats venous thromboembolism (from thrombophlebitis), pulmonary embolism, and thromboembolism from heart disease (*e.g.,* myocardial infarction, atrial fibrillation, CHF, and mitral-valve disease, which can produce cerebral emboli from intramural thrombi).

- Usually given in the acute stages when rapid effects are required.
- Also used for disseminated intravascular clotting (DIC).
- Heparin is usually given prior to oral anticoagulant therapy.

Adverse Effects, Contraindications

- *Hemorrhage* is the main adverse effect.
- Hypersensitivity reactions, such as chills, fever, and urticaria, have been reported.
- Patients have also experienced asthma, rhinitis, lacrimation, and anaphylactoid reactions.
- Intravenous doses of heparin have produced acute, reversible thrombocytopenia.
- Long-term therapy with high doses has produced osteoporosis and suppression of renal function.
- Heparin should not be used in the following conditions: history of blood disorders; peptic ulcer; ulcerative colitis; GI carcinoma; recent head injury; liver, kidney, or biliary disease; or following surgery on the CNS. Also, it should not be used with patients who cannot cooperate to take the proper dosages and receive the necessary follow-up care (*e.g.,* lab work).

Dosage, Administration

- Determined by lab results. A partial thromboplastin time (PTT) is usually used.
- The patient's PTT should be maintained at one and one-half to two times the control for the anticoagulation to be effective.
- Heparin must be administered parenterally. Three methods are used: continuous infusion—usually considered the most effective method because it maintains a constant blood level; intermittent IV injection through a heparin lock; and intermittent SC injection.

Nursing Tips

(See PH, Anticoagulants: nursing tips)
- A baseline PTT should be drawn before therapy is started.
- When a patient is receiving an intermittent form of heparin, blood samples to check PTT must be *carefully* timed. Usually the blood is drawn 30 min to 1 hr *before* the next dose. That dose of heparin is usually given; then the physician is notified of the lab results before other doses are administered. A change in dosage may be indicated.
- Heparin is considered most effective when administered through continuous infusion; however, this is also the most dangerous

method. Monitor the IV carefully, place on an IV pump, and use microdrip tubing.

- Heparin comes in prefilled tubexes. The size remains the same even though the doses differ (*e.g.*, a 100 unit tubex is the same size as a 10,000-unit tubex). Check *carefully*. Be very careful when mixing heparin in the IV bottle so that you will be administering the proper dose. The following is one method of mixing:

$$\frac{20,000 \text{ units heparin}}{500 \text{ ml D}_5\text{W}} = 40 \text{ units/ml}$$

- To maintain patency of the heparin lock: check for blood return; observe closely for signs of infiltration (*e.g.*, redness, swelling, pain); inject heparin slowly; and flush tubing completely.
- When removing a heparin lock be sure to apply firm pressure for 5 minutes. Then return to check for bleeding.
- To minimize bruising from heparin administered SC: do not draw back on syringe; do not massage area; apply firm pressure following injection; instruct patient not to scratch. Although the SC tissue of the abdomen has been the common site for injection, heparin can be given into any SC tissue.
- Heparin's antagonist is *protamine sulfate.*

WARFARIN SODIUM, U.S.P. (COUMADIN)
Actions

- Prevents the formation of new blood clots.
- Coagulation factors: Interferes with Factor II (liver synthesis of prothrombin) and Factors VII, IX, and X to prevent clot formation.
- Requires 1 to 4 days to become effective and is usually started while the patient is still receiving heparin.

Indications

- Treats venous thromboembolism (from thrombophlebitis), pulmonary embolism, and thromboembolism from heart disease (*e.g.*, myocardial infarction, atrial fibrillation, CHF, and mitral-valve disease, which can produce cerebral emboli from intramural thrombi).
- Use for long-term therapy when rapid action not required.

Adverse Effects, Contraindications

- *Hemorrhage* is the main adverse effect.
- Other side-effects are infrequent but include the following: alopecia, urticaria, dermatitis, fever, nausea, diarrhea, and a reaction consisting of hemorrhagic infarction and necrosis of the skin.

- Warfarin should not be used in the following conditions: history of blood disorders; peptic ulcer; ulcerative colitis; GI carcinoma; recent head injury; liver, kidney, or biliary disease; or following surgery on the CNS. Also, it should not be used with patients who cannot cooperate to take the proper dosages and receive the necessary follow-up care (*e.g.,* lab work).

Dosage, Administration

- Determined by lab results. A prothrombin time (PT) is usually used.
- A patient's PT should be maintained at two to two and one-half times the control (control is usually 11 to 13 seconds).
- The average initial loading, or priming, dose is 40 to 60 mg, p.o. The maintenance dosage range is usually 5 to 10 mg, p.o., q.d.

Nursing Tips

(See PH, Anticoagulants nursing tips)

- Drug interactions: Chloral hydrate, Atromid S, Butazolidin, quinidine and salicylate (*e.g.,* aspirin and aspirin products), oral hypoglycemics, sulfonamides, and broad-spectrum antibiotics can potentiate oral anticoagulants. Antacids, barbiturates, estrogens (*e.g.,* birth control pills), thiazides, and other diuretics can reduce the patient's response to oral anticoagulants.
- Oral anticoagulants should be taken at the same time each day. This aids in maintaining consistent blood levels. In the hospital situation, 6 PM is a convenient time because the PT is usually drawn in the morning. This gives the nurse adequate time to contact the physician with the results in case a dosage change is indicated.
- Warfarin's antagonist is vitamin K. *(See PH, Cardiovascular, hemostatic)*

ANTIHYPERTENSIVES

Nursing Tips

- Monitor BP daily (more frequently if patient's condition indicates).
- To help patients avoid orthostatic hypotension, instruct them to rise slowly from a sitting or lying position. They should not stand perfectly still for long periods of time because blood may pool in the legs. Weakness or dizziness can usually be alleviated by having them lie down for a few minutes.
- Sudden omissions of medications can cause rapid rise in BP and as a result severe crises for the patient.
- Antihypertensives are often administered with a diuretic because this enhances the hypotensive effects. The dosage of the antihypertensive, then, can be reduced, thus reducing side-effects.

DIAZOXIDE, U.S.P. (HYPERSTAT)

Actions

- Directly dilates the arterioles by relaxing vascular smooth muscle.

Indications

- Treats hypertensive crisis.

Adverse Effects, Contraindications

- Diazoxide causes sodium and water retention, hypotensive reactions, hyperglycemia, and tachycardia.

Dosage, Administration

- Usually 300 mg is given by rapid IV bolus injection (within 30 seconds). This usually lowers BP within 5 min.
- A second dose may be repeated in 1/2 hr. Subsequent doses are given at 4- to 24-hr intervals.

Nursing Tips

- Monitor blood pressure (BP) at frequent intervals.
- Patients may also receive a diuretic to prevent CHF from the sodium and water retention. However, potent diuretics can potentiate the antihypertensive, hyperglycemic, and hyperuricemic effects of diazoxide.
- Diazoxide should be given only into a peripheral vein, and extravasation will be irritating to the tissues.
- Monitor serum glucose levels, especially in diabetic patients.
- Diazoxide can displace coumarin from the blood proteins and cause higher blood levels of the coumarin.
- Drugs such as hydralazine and the nitrites are also direct peripheral dilators and can potentiate the antihypertensive effects of diazoxide.

HYDRALAZINE HYDROCHLORIDE, U.S.P. (APRESOLINE HCL)

Actions

- Directly dilates the arterioles by relaxing vascular smooth muscle.

Indications

- Treats essential hypertension both alone and in combination with other antihypertensives.

Adverse Effects, Contraindications

- Patients may experience headache, tachycardia, anginal chest pain, nausea, vomiting, and diarrhea.
- Discontinue if patient develops signs and symptoms of systemic lupus erythematosus (*e.g.*, fever and joint pains).

- Patients with coronary artery or mitral valve disease should not receive hydralazine.

Dosage, Administration

- Depending on the severity of the patient's problem, dosage can range from 40 to 200 mg, p.o., daily.
- A usual IV dose is 20 to 40 mg, repeated as necessary.

Nursing Tips

(See PH, Antihypertensives: nursing tips)

METHYLDOPA, U.S.P. (ALDOMET)

Actions

- Reduces transmission of impulses by adrenergic nerves.
- Decreases peripheral resistance, but does not decrease kidney perfusion or cardiac output.

Indications

- May be used alone for moderate hypertension, but is usually given with a diuretic.
- This drug is preferred for patients with renal insufficiency.

Adverse Effects, Contraindications

- Drowsiness is common, especially when therapy is begun.
- Mouth dryness, depression, and nightmares may occur.
- Hypersensitivity reactions involving liver, blood, and skin (*e.g.,* hepatitis and hemolytic anemia) have been reported.
- Patients may experience a drug-induced fever within about 3 weeks of starting the drug.
- Patients with active live disease should not receive methyldopa.

Dosage, Administration

- Usual adult dosage is 500 mg to 2 g, p.o., q.d., in divided doses.

Nursing Tips

(See PH, Antihypertensives: nursing tips)
- A baseline blood count should be done before therapy is begun to detect the presence of anemia. Blood counts should be repeated periodically to monitor the patient for hemolytic anemia.
- A direct Coombs' test should be done before therapy, and then at 6 months and 12 months. Patients with a positive direct Coombs' may develop hemolytic anemia.

- Monitor liver function during therapy, especially when unexplained fever occurs, to detect hypersensitivity reactions.

PROPRANOLOL HYDROCHLORIDE, U.S.P. (INDERAL)

(See PH, Autonomic nervous system and PH, Antihypertensives: nursing tips)

RESERPINE, U.S.P. (SERPASIL)
Actions

- Partially blocks transmission of impulses from sympathetic (adrenergic) nerves.
- Produces gradual drops in blood pressure (BP).
- Also slows the heart rate and reduces cardiac output.

Indications

- Used for chronic essential hypertension (mild to moderate severity). Usually combined with a diuretic.

Adverse Effects, Contraindications

- Patients may experience nasal congestion and stuffiness, drowsiness, weakness, fatigue, and severe mental depression.
- Do not give if there is a history of suicidal tendencies or epilepsy.
- Use cautiously for patients with history of peptic ulcer or ulcerative colitis.

Dosage, Administration

- Usual adult dosage is 0.25 to 0.5 mg, p.o., q.d.

Nursing Tips

(See PH, Antihypertensives: nursing tips)

THIAZIDES

(See PH, Urinary system: actions, adverse effects)

Indications

- May be used alone for mild hypertension but, should be used in combination with other antihypertensives for moderate hypertension.

Nursing Tips

(See PH, Antihypertensives: nursing tips)
- Observe for electrolyte imbalance, especially hypokalemia (decreased potassium).

DIGITALIS PREPARATIONS

Actions

- Digitalis increases the strength of myocardial contraction (positive inotropic effect) and slows the heart rate (negative chronotropic effect).

Indications

- Treats congestive heart failure (CHF). The increased contractility allows the ventricles to empty more completely, and the slower heart rate allows for more complete filling.
- In atrial fibrillation, digitalis does not usually convert the heart to a normal sinus rhythm (NSR), but it does keep the ventricles from being overstimulated.
- Treats atrial flutter and paroxysmal atrial tachycardia (PAT) and in some cases may convert the heart to a NSR.
- For elderly or cardiac patients digitalis may be given prophylactically before the stress of major surgery.

Adverse Effects, Contraindications

- Digitalis toxicity is the main problem with this drug.
- Early signs of digitalis toxicity are anorexia followed by nausea and vomiting.
- Drowsiness, fatigue, and headache are also common.
- Vision may be blurred, and patients may see colors (*e.g.,* yellow and green).
- The most serious effects are the *cardiac effects;* digitalis can produce almost any type of *arrhythmia.* Examples are partial or complete heart block, premature atrial contractions (PACs), PVCs, and ventricular fibrillation.

Dosage, Administration

- It has been common practice to begin a patient on digitalis therapy by the process called *digitalization.* This refers to giving priming, or loading, doses first, followed by a daily maintenance dose to replace what the body excretes.
- Rapid digitalization (especially IV) is dangerous and should be reserved for patients with severe CHF (specifically, pulmonary edema) and very rapid ventricular rates from atrial arrhythmias.
- Slower digitalization is safer and more common now. This method employs smaller doses at longer intervals (may take about a week to digitalize a patient).

Nursing Tips

- The following are predisposing factors to digitalis toxicity: a low serum potassium (K^+), especially from concurrent use of diuretics (therefore, a patient's electrolytes should always be checked both before he is started on digitalis and during the course of the therapy); pathological conditions, especially of the kidneys, liver, and heart (interferes with metabolism and excretion); old age (slower body functions); IV administration of digitalis and rapid digitalization; and drug interactions.
- The following drugs exert a synergistic effect when given with digitalis and increase the risk of toxicity: quinidine; diuretics that cause potassium loss (*e.g.*, thiazides and furosemide); amphotericin B; intravenous calcium and glucose; and propantheline.
- The following drugs could interfere with the action of digitalis: barbiturates; antacids; phenytoin; phenylbutazone; rifampin; sulfasalazine; kaolin-pectin mixtures; cholestyramine; colestipol; meto-clopramide; and neomycin.
- Correct dosage is extremely important because there is only a small range between therapeutic and toxic dosages.
- Check apical rate for a full minute before giving each dose. If the rate is below 60, hold the dose and notify the physician.
- Digitalis toxicity can be diagnosed partially by lab results. Safe levels are considered to be 0.8 to 1.6 nanograms per milliliter of serum (a nanogram, ng, is one-billionth of a gram). Patients usually experience symptoms if the level of digitalis is over 2 ng.
- Digitalis toxicity can easily occur while the patient is at home. Good teaching in the hospital can help prevent this.

DIGITOXIN, U.S.P. (CRYSTODIGIN)

(See PH, Digitalis: actions, indications, adverse effects, dosage, nursing tips)

Dosage, Administration

- An example of a digitalization dosage is 0.2 mg, p.o., b.i.d. for 4 days. This would be followed by a maintenance dosage of 0.15 mg, p.o., q.d.

Nursing Tips

- Digitoxin is absorbed almost totally from the GI tract.
- It binds to serum albumin and is slowly released. Therefore, it takes longer to become effective and stays in the body longer.
- It is metabolized in the liver, but most is reabsorbed into the blood-

stream. Therefore, digitoxin may be considered preferable if the patient has kidney disease.

DIGOXIN, U.S.P. (LANOXIN)

(See PH, Digitalis: actions, indications, adverse effects, dosage, nursing tips)

Dosage, Administration
- Average maintenance dosage is 0.125 to 0.25 mg, p.o., q.d. This range is usually effective enough to digitalize a person in about a week.
- The maintenance dose may be decreased for the elderly or for patients with poor renal function.
- Usual initial IV dose is 0.25 to 0.5 mg followed by 0.25 mg at 4- to 6-hr intervals.
- Dilution is not required, but mixing the appropriate dose in 10 ml of sterile 0.9% sodium chloride and running it in piggyback over 5 to 10 min increases the safety of administration.

Nursing Tips
- Digoxin is usually 55% to 75% absorbed from the GI tract.
- It circulates freely and diffuses easily, and therefore becomes effective quickly.
- It is relatively unchanged by the liver and excreted unchanged by the kidneys; therefore, kidney disease can drastically reduce excretion.
- Be sure digoxin blood levels are drawn *before* the daily dose is given.

HEMOSTATIC
PHYTONADIONE, U.S.P. (VITAMIN K, MEPHYTON, AQUA MEPHYTON)
Actions
- Controls bleeding and is involved in the synthesis of Factors II (prothrombin), VII, IX, and X in the liver.

Indications
- Antidote to oral anticoagulant therapy.
- Treats newborns who may lack vitamin K, patients with liver disease, and those who cannot absorb vitamin K.

Dosage, Administration
- Usual oral adult dose is 2.5 to 10 mg.
- Usual IM or SC dose is 0.5 to 10 mg.
- Usual IV dose is 0.5 to 10 mg given at a rate of 1 mg/min.

POTASSIUM SUPPLEMENTS

Actions

- Potassium, a predominately intracellular ion, maintains the excitability of nerves and muscles.
- Potassium is also necessary to maintain a normal acid–base balance.

Indications

- Treats hypokalemia (low serum potassium) resulting from the following: vomiting, diarrhea, and suction drainage; use of potassium-excreting diuretics and corticosteroids; diabetic ketoacidosis; uremia; cardiac arrhythmias due to digitalis toxicity; and administration of potassium-free IV fluids.

Adverse Effects, Contraindications

- Patients can experience nausea, vomiting, diarrhea, and abdominal discomfort from oral potassium supplements.
- Hyperkalemia (high serum potassium) can result from treatment with both oral or intravenous preparations. Symptoms include paresthesias of extremities; flaccid paralysis; listlessness; mental confusion; weakness; hypotension; and cardiac arrhythmias, including heart block and cardiac arrest.

Dosage, Administration

- Potassium bicarbonate, U.S.P. (K-Lyte)
  1. Each effervescent tablet contains 25 mEq of potassium.
  2. The tablets should be dissolved in 4 ounces of cold water, and the solution should be sipped slowly (over 5 to 10 minutes).
  3. A usual adult dosage is one tablet taken one to two times daily with meals.
- Potassium chloride, U.S.P. (Kay Ciel)
  1. Fifteen milliliters of the elixer contains 20 mEq of potassium. Each powder packet contains 20 mEq of potassium.
  2. Both the elixer and the powder should be mixed with 4 ounces of cold water or juice and taken after meals.
  3. A usual adult dosage is 20 mEq twice daily.
- Potassium chloride injection, U.S.P.
  1. Potassium is very irritating to the veins and should never be given IV push. No more than 40 mEq is usually added to 1 liter of fluid. Avoid adding the medication to partially-empty bottles.
  2. Usual adult dosage is 50 to 100 mEq per 24 hr.
- Potassium gluconate (Kaon)
  1. Each sugar-coated (not enteric-coated) tablet contains 5 mEq of potassium.

2. A usual adult dosage is two tablets, four times a day (after meals and at bedtime).

Nursing Tips

- Frequent serum potassium levels must be done to determine if adequate and safe dosages of potassium are being administered.
- Slow-release tablets (*e.g.*, Slow-K) have been associated with intestinal and gastric ulceration and bleeding. They should be used only when patients cannot tolerate the other preparations or refuse to use them.

VASODILATORS
NITRATES (CORONARY VASODILATORS)
Actions

- Relaxes all types of smooth muscle, which leads to vasodilation.
- Vasodilation increases blood flow but may also decrease blood pressure. Blood flow increases only to the *collateral* circulation because diseased coronary vessels cannot dilate.
- Nitrates also reduce the work load on the heart because blood can pool in the extremities.

Indications

- Used to treat angina pectoris (*see SS, Cardiovascular*). The nitrates may stop an existing attack, prevent an attack just before physical activity, or reduce the total number of attacks per day.

Adverse Effects, Contraindications

- Nitrates can cause postural hypotension (*e.g.*, dizziness, weakness, and fainting), throbbing headache, flushing, nausea, and vomiting.
- Nitrate syncope, a severe shocklike reaction, can also occur.
- These drugs are usually not given during the acute phase of a myocardial infarction.
- Use cautiously with glaucoma because the drug can cause an increase in intraocular pressure.

Dosage, Administration

- Isosorbide dinitrate, U.S.P. (Isordil, Sorbitrate): Sublingual dosage range is 2.5 to 10 mg; oral dosage range is 5 to 30 mg, t.i.d. or q.i.d. Peaks in 2 to 5 minutes (sublingually), and action lasts 1 to 2 hours.
- Nitroglycerin, U.S.P.: Dosage range is 0.15 to 0.6 mg sublingual— may repeat every 5 minutes for a total of three doses. This is a rapid-acting nitrate and should peak in 2 to 3 minutes. Prophylactic effect lasts 5 to 15 minutes.

- Nitroglycerin, topical (Nitro-Bid, Nitrol): Ointment applied to the skin, usually 1 to 2 inches. Can use the chest, abdomen, arms, and legs.
  1. The ointment should be spread and then covered with a 4 × 6-inch piece of plastic wrap. Taping all sides increases water content of skin, and increased hydration promotes absorption of the ointment. Wipe off old ointment before applying the new dose.
  2. Effective up to several hours for sustained prophylaxis.

Nursing Tips

- If the patient has not obtained relief from his angina in 15 minutes when using a rapid-acting nitrate, notify his physician.
- When applying topical preparations, do not touch the ointment with your fingers. Spread it with the measuring paper provided. Your fingers could absorb it, and you could experience drug effects.
- Tablets should be kept in the original dark bottle, tightly closed, in a relatively cool place. Remove the cotton from the bottle because it may absorb some of the drug. A potent tablet should produce a brief stinging or burning sensation when placed under the tongue.
- The patient should sit or lie down after taking the tablet to counteract the postural hypotension.
- Taking alcohol with a nitrate can intensify the hypotension and bring on nitrate syncope.
- Patients can develop tolerance to nitrates. Be sure to determine if a patient is obtaining the same degree of relief.
- Patients usually keep nitroglycerin at the bedside, but you are still responsible for recording the time, the number of tablets, and the relief obtained.

PROPRANOLOL HYDROCHLORIDE, U.S.P. (INDERAL)

(See PH, Autonomic nervous system)

- May be used to treat angina when the nitrates are ineffective.
- May also be used along with the nitrates for the synergistic effects.

CENTRAL NERVOUS SYSTEM
ANTICONVULSANTS

Nursing Tips

- Status epilepticus can result if anticonvulsant therapy is abruptly discontinued. Gradual weaning is necessary.

- Combinations of two or more drugs may be necessary to provide adequate control of seizures.
- Most drugs are started at low doses and are gradually increased until seizures are controlled or side-effects develop.
- The patient's understanding of his illness and the drug therapy is extremely important because failure to take the drugs is the most frequent cause of treatment failure.

DIAZEPAM, U.S.P. (VALIUM)

(See PH, Psychotropics, minor tranquilizers)

Indications

- Drug of choice for treating status epilepticus (given IV).
- May also be used to treat pure petit mal seizures.

Nursing Tips

(See PH, Anticonvulsants: nursing tips)

PHENOBARBITAL, U.S.P. (LUMINAL)

(See PH, Central nervous system: hypnotics)

Actions

- Reduces the number and severity of epileptic attacks.

Indications

- Treats grand mal, focal motor, and psychomotor epilepsy, often in combination with phenytoin. *(See PH, anticonvulsants phenytoin sodium)*
- Considered safer than other drugs for long-term management of chronic epilepsy.

Nursing Tips

(See PH, Anticonvulsants: nursing tips)

PHENYTOIN SODIUM, U.S.P. (DILANTIN)

(See PH, Cardiovascular system, antiarrhythmics)

Actions

- Reduces the number and severity of epileptic attacks.

Indications

- The oral form is used to treat grand mal and other major motor seizures and psychomotor epilepsy.

- Parenterally, phenytoin may be used to treat status epilepticus and to control rapid cardiac arrythmias, and it may be used prior to neurosurgical procedures to prevent seizures during surgery.

Adverse Effects, Contraindications
- Nausea, vomiting, and constipation occur.
- Gingival hyperplasia (overgrowth of gum tissue) is common.
- Hirsutism, skin rashes, and megaloblastic anemia may occur.
- Excessive doses cause lethargy, slurred speech, and staggering gait. Also, double vision, dizziness, and headache occur.
- Overdose results in coma, apnea, and death.
- Cardiac arrest can occur from rapid intravenous administration.
- Phenytoin may be gradually withdrawn before or during a pregnancy for patients with mild, infrequent seizures. However, the danger of hypoxia to the fetus following a major seizure may be indication for continuing the drug.

Dosage, Administration
- Usual initial p.o. dosage is 100 mg, t.i.d., but it may be increased to 600 mg per day.
- Intravenous phenytoin is injected slowly (maximum 50 mg/min) in doses of 150 to 250 mg. It should be given IV push because it is not soluble when mixed.
- May also be given IM (100 to 200 mg) but can cause tissue necrosis and sterile abcesses.

Nursing Tips
(See PH, Anticonvulsants: nursing tips)
- Patients metabolize phenytoin at different rates, so blood levels should be drawn to monitor the drug for effectiveness and toxicity.
- Giving phenytoin during or after meals will minimize the gastric distress.
- Patients receiving this drug for long periods may need folic acid to prevent anemia.
- The following drug interactions occur with phenytoin:
  1. The action of phenytoin is potentiated by aspirin, estrogens, sulfonamides, and anticoagulants.
  2. The action of phenytoin is inhibited by alcohol, antihistamines, barbiturates, and sedatives.
  3. Phenytoin potentiates the action of antihypertensives and quinidine.
  4. Phenytoin inhibits the action of steroids and digitalis.

ANTIPARKINSON DRUGS
DIPHENHYDRAMINE HYDROCHLORIDE, U.S.P. (BENADRYL)
(See PH, Central nervous system, hypnotics)

Indications
- Treats mild parkinsonism in elderly patients.

Dosage, Administration
- Usual adult dosage is 50 mg, orally, three or four times daily.

Nursing Tips
- The antihistaminic activity dries secretions and may assist in reducing drooling.
- Patients who are nervous or who experience insomnia may benefit from the sedative action.

LEVODOPA, U.S.P. (LARODOPA, DOPAR)
Actions
- Levodopa is converted to dopamine in the blood, peripheral tissues, and central nervous system (CNS).
- Only the levodopa that passes the blood–brain barrier intact can form dopamine in the CNS where it is needed.
- When dopamine deficiency in the CNS is relieved, many patients experience improvement in their parkinsonism symptoms. *(See SS, Neurological system)*

Indications
- Treats the symptoms of Parkinson's disease. *(See SS, Neurological system)*

Adverse Effects, Contraindications
- Nausea is most common and may be accompanied by anorexia and vomiting.
- Use cautiously for patients with a history of peptic ulcer because levodopa has caused hemorrhage and ulceration.
- Postural hypotension and cardiac arrhythmias occur. Use cautiously for patients with a history of heart disease.
- Involuntary movements of the mouth, face, and head occur. The drug may produce spasms of the trunk and limbs. The "on–off" syndrome (sudden slowing of movement and muscle weakness) occurs with long-term therapy.
- Mental changes occur and may take the form of either hyperac-

tivity and euphoria or depression and drowsiness. Patients with a history of psychiatric problems are especially at risk.
- Contraindicated for patients with narrow-angle glaucoma or a history of melonoma, or for those who are taking adrenergic bronchodilators. *(See PH, Respiratory system)*

Dosage, Administration
- Initial dosage is usually 0.5 to 1 g, p.o., q.d. in divided doses taken with food. Every 3 to 7 days, dosage may be increased by a maximum of 0.75 g—usually not more than 8 g taken daily.
- May take 6 to 8 weeks for the patient to achieve optimum benefits from the drug (*e.g.,* maximum improvement of symptoms with side-effects he can tolerate).

Nursing Tips
- The anorexia, nausea, and vomiting usually disappear after a few months. However, they can be reduced by giving the levodopa with meals, milk, or antacids and by gradually increasing the dosage.
- The effectiveness of levodopa will be increased by reducing the total amount of protein in the diet.
- The postural hypotension usually disappears. Caution the patient to rise slowly. Elastic stockings may help. Monitor blood pressure and apical and radial pulses. *Antihypertensive* medications may need to be reduced.
- Many of the extrapyramidal symptoms may be relieved by reducing the dosage of levodopa *(for extrapyramidal symptoms, see PH, Psychotropics, phenothiazines: adverse effects).* If the parkinsonism symptoms return, it may be possible to gradually increase the dosage without the return of these neurological side-effects.
- Observe for depression, suicidal tendencies, hallucinations, and delusions.
- Urine, saliva, and perspiration may darken in color, but this is not harmful.
- Other drug interactions
  1. The use of pyridoxine (vitamin B_6) with levodopa may cause its conversion to dopamine to occur *before* the drug reaches the brain, rendering it ineffective. A multivitamin preparation without B_6 is available.
  2. Antipsychotic drugs such as the phenothiazines *(see PH, Psychotropics)* may antagonize the effects of levodopa. If it is necessary to administer both drugs, the patient must be observed for the return of parkinsonism symptoms.

LEVODOPA–CARBIDOPA COMBINATIONS (SINEMET)
Actions

- The carbidopa inhibits conversion of levodopa to dopamine outside the CNS.
- Therefore, more levodopa reaches the CNS, where it is converted to dopamine and can be used to relieve dopamine deficiencies.

Indications

(See PH, Levodopa: indications)

Adverse Effects, Contraindications

(See PH, Levodopa: adverse effects)
- Anorexia, nausea, and vomiting usually occur less with a combination drug than with levodopa alone because the dosage of levodopa can be decreased.
- The adverse mental and extrapyramidal symptoms may be increased with a combination drug and may occur sooner and last longer. *(For extrapyramidal symptoms, see PH, Psychotropics, phenothiazines: adverse effects)*

Dosage, Administration

- Initial and maximum dosages are usually about one-quarter of the dosage for levodopa alone. *(See PH, Levodopa: dosage)*
- Tablets contain 10 mg of carbidopa and 100 mg of levodopa (10:100), 25 mg carbidopa and 250 mg levodopa (25:250), or 25 mg carbidopa and 100 mg levodopa (25:100). Maximum total daily dose is eight 25:250 tablets.

Nursing Tips

(See PH, Levodopa: nursing tips)
- Remember that the involuntary movements and mental changes are more common than with levodopa alone and the patient must be observed accordingly.
- The pyridoxine (vitamin B_6) enters the brain in greater concentrations than with the levodopa alone and assists in its conversion to dopamine. Therefore, the B_6 produces a synergistic effect with the combination drug, though it produces an antagonistic effect with the levodopa.

TRIHEXYPHENIDYL HYDROCHLORIDE, U.S.P. (ARTANE)

(See PH, Autonomic nervous system, anticholinergics)

HYPNOTICS AND SEDATIVES
BARBITURATES
Actions

- Barbiturates depress all parts of the central nervous system (CNS). Small doses produce sedation and a reduction in nervousness and irritability. Larger doses produce hypnosis or sleep.
- Barbiturates also have anticonvulsant action and in large doses produce anesthesia.
- When administered with an analgesic *(see PH, Central nervous system, analgesics)* the barbiturate reduces the patient's emotional response to pain.
- Barbiturates may also reduce inhibitions and produce amnesia.

Indications

- Relieve anxiety and restlessness; relieve insomnia; used as a preoperative medication; control epileptic seizures and other convulsions; with analgesics, relieve pain; used as an induction anesthetic; and used in psychiatry.

Adverse Effects, Contraindications

- Usual adult dosages can produce drowsiness, dizziness, and headache. Some patients (especially the elderly) experience excitation.
- Allergic skin reactions (rashes) and blood dyscrasias (*e.g.,* leukopenia, thrombocytopenia, and agranulocytosis) occur occasionally.
- *Chronic toxicity* (from excessive, long-term dosage): dizziness, slurred speech, impaired thought and judgment, and disturbances of vision.
- *Acute toxicity* (massive overdose): confusion, stupor, coma, shock and circulatory collapse, shallow respirations, and respiratory failure.
- Contraindicated for patients with acute intermittent porphyria and chronic obstructive pulmonary disease (COPD).
- Dependence and tolerance do develop.
- Overdose produces respiratory depression and hypotension.

Nursing Tips

- Patients should be cautioned against driving or operating machinery because these drugs reduce alertness.
- Other CNS depressants (*e.g.,* alcohol and analgesics) taken concurrently will potentiate the effects of these drugs. Life-threatening CNS depression can result.
- Barbiturates can alter a person's normal sleep patterns, and this

in itself can cause side-effects. The alterations may persist 3 to 5 weeks after the medication is discontinued.

- Barbiturates stimulate liver enzymes and will produce an increase in metabolism of other drugs. These drugs may require a *temporary* increase in dosage to maintain their effectiveness.
- Patients with reduced kidney and liver function and the elderly may require lower dosages to reduce the chance of toxicity.
- Patients receiving oral anticoagulants should use barbiturates cautiously.

PENTOBARBITAL SODIUM, U.S.P. (NEMBUTAL SODIUM)

(See PH, Central nervous system, barbiturates, for actions, indications, adverse effects, and nursing tips)

Dosage, Administration

- Usual adult sedative dosage is 20 to 30 mg, p.o., t.i.d. or q.i.d.
- Usual adult hyponotic dose is 100 mg, p.o., at bedtime. For hypnotic effects, 200-mg suppositories are available.
- Pentobarbital may also be given IM or IV. Intramuscular injections should be made into a large muscle, such as the gluteus maximus.

PHENOBARBITAL, U.S.P. (LUMINAL)

(See PH, Central nervous system, barbiturates, for actions, indications, adverse effects, and nursing tips)

Dosage, Administration

- Usual adult sedative dosage is 30 mg, p.o., t.i.d. or q.i.d.
- Usual adult hypnotic dose is 100 mg, p.o., at bedtime.
- For convulsive disorders the adult dosage range is 50 to 200 mg, p.o., q.d. Phenobarbital is the preferred barbiturate for preventing grand mal seizures. *(See PH, Anticonvulsants)*
- *Phenobarbital sodium (Sodium Luminal)* can be administered parenterally, but phenobarbital cannot.

SECOBARBITAL SODIUM, U.S.P. (SECONAL)

(See PH, Central nervous system, barbiturates, for actions, indications, adverse effects, and nursing tips)

Dosage, Administration

- Usual adult hypnotic dose is 100 mg, p.o., at bedtime. Hypnotic dose by way of rectal suppository is 120 mg or 200 mg.
- Intravenous dosage ranges from 50 mg to 250 mg (no faster than 50 mg in 15 seconds). May also be given IM.

NONBARBITURATES
CHLORAL HYDRATE, U.S.P. (NOCTEC)
Actions
- Depresses the central nervous system (CNS), and produces sedation and hypnosis (sleep).

Indications
- Relieves insomnia.

Adverse Effects, Contraindications
- Gastric irritation is common and may lead to nausea and vomiting.
- Alcohol and other CNS depressants potentiate the action of chloral hydrate and may produce serious respiratory depression and cardiac arrhythmias.
- Patients with severe heart, liver, or kidney disease should not use this drug. May irritate peptic ulcers.
- Patients receiving anticoagulants should use chloral hydrate cautiously because altered metabolism could precipitate bleeding.
- Physical and psychic dependence and tolerance do develop.

Dosage, Administration
- Adult oral dosages for sedation are 250 to 500 mg, t.i.d., p.c.
- Adult oral hypnotic doses are 500 mg to 1 g at bedtime. Chloral hydrate is also available as a suppository.

Nursing Tips
- If patient is receiving anticoagulants, observe carefully for signs of bleeding. *(See PH, Cardiovascular, anticoagulants)*
- Capsules should be taken with a full glass of fluid.

DIPHENHYDRAMINE, U.S.P. (BENADRYL)
Actions
- Antihistamine that has the following effects: sedative, antiemetic, antiparkinsonism, antitussive.

Indications
- Produces sedation and hypnosis in the elderly and may be better tolerated than other hypnotics.
- Treats mild parkinsonism in elderly patients.
- Relieves the extrapyramidal symptoms caused by antipsychotic drugs.
- Prevents and treats motion sickness.

- Relieves allergic reactions from food and pollens and from blood and plasma.
- Parenteral forms are used to treat anaphylaxis (as an adjunct to epinephrine), blood reactions, and other allergic reactions when oral therapy is not possible.

Adverse Effects, Contraindications

- Frequently causes drowsiness.
- Overdoses produce restlessness and confusion. Coma, convulsions, and death occur in children.
- Can cause dryness and thickness of pulmonary secretions, and should be used cautiously by patients with chronic obstructive pulmonary disease (COPD).
- Because of diphenhydramine's atropine-type effects, it is contraindicated for patients with narrow-angle glaucoma and obstructions of the gastrointestinal or genitourinary systems.

Dosage, Administration

- Usual adult oral dosage is 50 mg, three or four times q.d. May be given IM or IV, maximum of 400 mg q.d.

Nursing Tips

- Because of the drug's sedative effect, driving and operating machinery may be dangerous to the patient.
- Diphenhydramine has additive effects with alcohol and other CNS depressants.
- Monoamine oxidase (MAO) inhibitors *(see PH, Psychotropics, antidepressants)* potentiate the anticholinergic (drying) effects of antihistamines.

ETHCHLORVYNOL, N.F., (PLACIDYL)
Actions

- Depresses the CNS and produces sedation and hypnosis (sleep).

Indications

- Relieves insomnia if pain and anxiety are not present. Also used if patient cannot tolerate barbiturates.

Adverse Effects, Contraindications

- Headache, dizziness, confusion, nausea, and vomiting occur.
- Hypotension and excitation are possible.
- Physical and psychic dependence and tolerance do develop.

Dosage, Administration

- Usual adult hypnotic dose is 500 mg, p.o., at bedtime.
- For sedative purposes and for the elderly, doses are lower.

Nursing Tips

- Because this drug may cause confusion, patients (especially the elderly) should be observed carefully and protected (*e.g.*, by use of side rails).
- Blood pressure (BP) should be monitored to detect hypotension.

FLURAZEPAM, N.F. (DALMANE)
Actions

- Depresses the CNS and produces hypnosis.

Indications

- Relieves all types of insomnia.

Adverse Effects, Contraindications

- Drowsiness, dizziness, and motor incoordination (resulting in falls) occur frequently in the elderly.
- Alcohol and other CNS depressants potentiate the action of flurazepam and can result in serious respiratory depression.
- Physical and psychic dependence and tolerance do develop.

Dosage, Administration

- Usual adult hypnotic dose is 30 mg, p.o., at bedtime.
- Elderly or debilitated patients should be started on 15 mg.

Nursing Tips

- Elderly patients and those with reduced liver and kidney function will have difficulty metabolizing this drug. Observe carefully for signs that the drug is accumulating in the patient (*e.g.*, daytime drowsiness, sedation, and confusion).

NARCOTIC ANALGESICS
OPIATES
Actions

- Relieve pain; produce euphoria; may induce sleep; depress respirations; constrict pupil of the eye; depress cough center; decrease motility and muscle tone of the gastrointestinal (GI) tract and the genitourinary tract.
- Opiates are CNS depressants.

Indications

- Control moderate to severe pain.
- Relieve apprehension and facilitate induction preoperatively.

Adverse Effects, Contraindications

- Frequently causes *constipation;* occasionally causes nausea and vomiting.
- Urinary retention may occur (especially if patient already has problems with his prostate gland).
- Postural hypotension has been reported.
- *Respiratory depression* occurs, and the patient may need a narcotic antagonist to counteract the depression.
- Patients experience behavioral changes, such as restlessness, excitement, and insomnia.
- Opiates may also produce drowsiness, dizziness, sweating, and flushing.
- Allergic reactions, such as rash and itching, occur.
- *Tolerance* develops but at different rates for each individual.
- Can produce *physical* and *psychic dependency.*
- Patients with *head injuries* or postoperative *craniotomies* should not receive opiates. Respirations can be depressed, intracranial pressure can increase, and decreased responsiveness resulting from the drug can mask changes in the patient's condition.
- The increased excitation that can occur makes opiates unsafe for patients suffering from *convulsive disorders* and *acute alcoholism.*
- Patients with severe *chronic obstructive pulmonary disease* (COPD) may not be able to tolerate the decreased respirations.
- Patients with *liver disease* may not be able to metabolize these drugs.

Nursing Tips

- When opiates are given before the pain becomes too severe they are usually more effective.
- Because of decreased ability to metabolize drugs, the elderly will be more susceptible to adverse effects and may require less than the usual adult dosage.
- Combining opiates with sedatives or tranquilizers causes a synergistic effect and may allow for a decreased dosage of the opiate.

CODEINE PHOSPHATE, U.S.P.

(See PH, Opiates for actions, indications, adverse effects, and nursing tips)

- Compared to morphine, codeine causes less respiratory depression, has less dependency potential, and usually causes fewer side-effects.
- Codeine is the most effective of the opiates for relieving coughing and is used in many cough preparations.

- Codeine is often combined with aspirin and used to relieve mild to moderate pain.

Dosage, Administration

- Usual adult dosage is 30 mg (gr 1/2) p.o., SC or IM, q. 3 to 4 hr.
- For cough relief, 8 to 15 mg, p.o. several times daily, is given.

HYDROMORPHONE HYDROCHLORIDE, N.F. (DILAUDID)

(See PH, Opiates for actions, indications, adverse effects, and nursing tips)
- Compared to morphine, hydromorphone is more potent, but its effects are shorter.

Dosage, Administration

- Usual adult dosage is 2 mg IM every 3 to 4 hours.
- May also be given orally or SC, and by rectal suppository.

MORPHINE SULFATE, U.S.P.

(See PH, Opiates for actions, indications, adverse effects, and nursing tips)
- Morphine is the prototype of the narcotic analgesics.
- Frequently the drug of choice to relieve chest pain following an acute myocardial infarction.
- The sedative effects and the peripheral vasodilation make it very effective when used to treat acute pulmonary edema.

Dosage, Administration

- Usual adult dosage range is 10 to 15 mg, SC or IM, every 3 to 4 hours. Peaks in about 1 hour.
- For faster action, smaller doses may be given IV.

SYNTHETIC ANALGESICS
MEPERIDINE HYDROCHLORIDE, U.S.P. (DEMEROL)
Actions

- Produces analgesia and euphoria but is less likely than the opiates to produce sleep.

Indications

- Relieves moderate to severe pain.
- Often used preoperatively, especially when combined with a sedative.

Adverse Effects, Contraindications

- Dizziness, nausea and vomiting, sweating, and flushing are common.
- Mental confusion, disorientation, and hypotension occur.
- *Respiratory depression* and *convulsions* may be fatal.

- Tolerance and dependence similar to that which results from morphine develops.
- Patients with *liver dysfunction, increased intracranial pressure,* or *chronic obstructive pulmonary disease* should not receive meperidine.
- Patients taking such drugs as other narcotic analgesics, sedatives, tranquilizers, alcohol, *monoamine oxidase* (MAO) inhibitors, or *tricyclic antidepressants* along with meperidine could have severe reactions (*e.g.,* respiratory depression, hypotension, and profound sedation or coma).

Dosage, Administration

- Usual adult dosage range is 50 to 100 mg, p.o. or IM, every 3 to 4 hours.

Nursing Tips

- When patients are also receiving other central nervous system (CNS) depressants, the dosage of meperidine should be reduced.
- Dosage should be reduced for elderly patients.
- Postoperative patients who are ambulating (especially for the first few times) may experience postural hypotension and should be protected against injury from falls.

OXYCODONE HYDROCHLORIDE (PERCODAN)
Actions

- Analgesic

Indications

- Relieves moderate to severe pain.

Adverse Effects, Contraindications

- Similar to other narcotic analgesics.
- Tolerance and dependency develop to a greater extent than with codeine.

Dosage, Administration

- Usual dosage range is 5 to 10 mg, p.o., of oxycodone.
- In the United States, oxycodone is available in combination with aspirin. One tablet is usually taken q. 6 hr.

Nursing Tips

- Be sure to question patients receiving oxycodone about aspirin allergy.

PENTAZOCINE, N.F. (TALWIN)
Actions

- Analgesic.

Indications

- Relieves moderate to severe pain.
- The oral form is often used to treat chronic pain because of its low potential for producing dependency.

Adverse Effects, Contraindications

- Nausea, vomiting, dizziness, and drowsiness are common.
- Constipation, euphoria, disorientation, and confusion are rare.
- Overdose can produce respiratory depression.
- Use cautiously for patients whose respirations are depressed (*e.g.*, chronic obstructive pulmonary disease).
- Tolerance and dependency develop, especially with the parenteral forms.

Dosage, Administration

- Usual oral adult dosage is 50 mg q. 3 to 4 hr (should not exceed 600 mg daily).
- Usual IM adult dosage is 30 mg q. 3 to 4 hr (should not exceed 360 mg daily).

Nursing Tips

- Subcutaneous injections should be avoided because of possible tissue damage.
- Overdose is counteracted by naloxone (Narcan). *(See PH, Narcotic antagonist)*

PROPOXYPHENE HYDROCHLORIDE, U.S.P. (DARVON)
Actions

- Analgesic.

Indications

- Relieves mild to moderate pain.

Adverse Effects, Contraindications

- Drowsiness, dizziness, and headache may occur.
- Nausea, vomiting, and constipation are possible.
- Both physical and psychic dependence develop if abused.
- Overdose produces *convulsions, coma, circulatory collapse,* and *respiratory failure.*

Dosage, Administration

- Usual adult dosage ranges from 32 to 65 mg, p.o., 3 to 4 times each day.
- For Darvon-N the dose ranges from 50 to 100 mg, p.o.
- Propoxyphene is often combined with aspirin; with acetaminophen; or with aspirin, phenacetin, and caffeine to increase its effectiveness.

Nursing Tips

- This drug is widely prescribed and frequently abused, and its effectiveness is being questioned.
- When people take propoxyphene with other CNS depressants (*e.g.*, alcohol, sedatives, or tranquilizers), death can result.

NARCOTIC ANTAGONIST: NALOXONE HYDROCHLORIDE, U.S.P. (NARCAN)

Actions

- Displaces the narcotic drugs from the nerve cell receptors.

Indications

- Reverses respiratory depression and hypotension resulting from overdose with opiates and other synthetic narcotics.
- Naloxone is considered capable of diagnosing opiate overdose because it is so effective in reversing the effects.

Adverse Effects, Contraindications

- Severe withdrawal occurs in patients who are physically dependent on narcotics.

Dosage, Administration

- For treating narcotic overdose, 1 ml (0.4 mg) is administered IV, IM, or SC. May be repeated every 2 to 3 minutes until respiratory function improves.
- Narcotic addicts and patients with postoperative respiratory depression may receive smaller doses.
- Newborn dosage is usually 0.01 mg/kg IV, IM, or SC. Again, dosage may be repeated every 2 to 3 minutes.

Nursing Tips

- Observe patients carefully for signs of narcotic withdrawal (*e.g.*, nausea, vomiting, sweating, and hypertension).

- Maintain an open airway and have resuscitation equipment and personnel available.

ENDOCRINE SYSTEM
ADRENOCORTICOSTEROIDS

Actions

- Important pharmacologic effects of steroid drug action are anti-inflammatory, antiallergic, antipyretic and antistress.

Indications

- Replacement therapy for adrenocortical insufficiency.
- Rheumatoid arthritis and osteoarthritis.
- Collagen diseases (*e.g.,* lupus erythematosus).
- Severe or incapacitating allergic problems.
- Chronic obstructive pulmonary disease.
- Skin disorders (*e.g.,* psoriasis, erythema multiforme).
- Reduces cerebral edema.
- Severe acute and chronic inflammatory processes of the eye.
- Blood dyscrasias (*e.g.,* hemolytic anemia).
- Neoplastic diseases (*e.g.,* lymphocytic leukemia).
- Gastrointestinal diseases (*e.g.,* exacerbations of ulcerative colitis).
- Nephrotic syndrome.

Adverse Effects, Contraindications

- Cushing's-type symptoms (*e.g.,* moon face, buffalo hump, hirsutism, edema). (*See SS, Endocrine*)
- Delayed wound healing.
- Peptic ulcer.
- Amenorrhea.
- Reduced resistance to infections.
- Thrombophlebitis (with possible embolism).
- Headache.
- Mood changes (*e.g.,* euphoria, depression, insomnia).
- Osteoporosis.
- Increased blood sugar.
- Suppression of growth in children.
- Caution *must* be used when administering steroids to patients with infections (including a history of tuberculosis); osteoporosis; diabetes; hypertension; peptic ulcer; acute heart and kidney disease; emotional problems; and thrombophlebitis; and to women in the first trimester of pregnancy.

Dosage, Administration

- Dexamethasone, U.S.P. (Decadron): 500 mcg to 6 mg daily, or 750 mcg, two to four times daily.
- Hydrocortisone sodium succinate, U.S.P. (Solu-Cortef): Doses vary greatly depending on the problem and its severity. Range is from 50 to 300 mg daily, IV or IM.
- Methylprednisolone sodium succinate, N.F. (Solu-Medrol): 10 to 40 mg daily, IV or IM.
- Prednisone, U.S.P. (Meticorten): *(See PH, Respiratory)* Again, dosage will vary greatly. Range is from 5 to 80 mg, p.o., q.d.
- Whenever possible, steroids that act at local sites (*e.g.*, joints, eyes, lungs) are used to help reduce systemic toxicity.
- The physician will always attempt to determine the *smallest dosage* that will relieve the symptoms, and then reduce that dosage (*e.g.*, during remission).
- Using massive dosages for short periods is acceptable treatment in emergency situations (*e.g.*, anaphylactic shock or adrenal crisis).
- Another measure used to reduce systemic toxicity is an intermittent dosage schedule. For example, the total daily dose may be taken with the morning meal, or the total dose for 2 days may be taken q.o.d. with the morning meal.
- Steroids are best given between 7 and 8 AM. This is when the body's own production of glucocorticoids is highest (between 6 and 9 AM). Fewer side effects will occur because there will be less suppression of the hypothalamus, pituitary, and adrenals.

Nursing Tips

- Help patients to understand that steroids cannot cure or prevent progress of their diseases. They are used to minimize symptoms. Also, it may not be possible to take large enough doses to completely eliminate the symptoms because the chance of toxicity may be too great.
- Patients on long-term therapy should receive ophthalmic exams to check for glaucoma and cataracts. Blood sugar should be checked, especially if the person is already diabetic. Insulin, oral hypoglycemics, or diet may need adjustment. X-rays to determine bone thinning and demineralization are indicated because osteoporosis may develop. Patients may need antacid therapy to prevent peptic ulcer or its recurrence.
- Long-term therapy causes atrophy of the adrenal glands.
- Patients on long-term therapy may not be able to cope with stress for many months after the drugs are discontinued.
- Patients on steroid therapy should always carry an ID card to that

effect. They may require IV infusion of steriods following an accident or other trauma.
- Do not omit doses, and wean patient from the drug gradually.
- Administer with antacids, meals, or milk to minimize gastric distress.
- Patients must be aware that steroids mask symptoms of infection.

ANTITHYROID DRUGS
IODIDES
Actions
- Rapidly reduce size and vascularity of the thyroid gland by interfering with formation, release, or action of thyroid hormones.

Indications
- Used preoperatively in patients who require thyroidectomy.
- May also be used to treat thyroid crisis and to control symptoms of thyrotoxicosis until the radioisotope takes effect. *(See SS, Endocrine)*

Adverse Effects, Contraindications
- Sore gums, excessive salivation, nausea and vomiting, sinusitis with frontal headache, and acne.
- Hypothyroidism is not common but can occur.

Dosage, Administration
- Iodine solution, strong, U.S.P. (Lugol's solution): Usual daily dose is 5 to 10 gtt.
- Potassium iodide solution, U.S.P. (SSKI): Usual daily dose is 0.1 to 1 ml.
- Mix iodine solutions in one-third to one-half of a glass of milk or juice to prevent gastric irritation.
- To prevent discoloration of the teeth, give through a straw.

Nursing Tips
- Failure to take proper dose can result in the return of more severe symptoms.
- These drugs are used only on a temporary basis to assist other treatments or to prepare for thyroidectomy.
- Sodium iodide I-131 is a radioactive isotope. Dosage depends on purpose of treatment: diagnostic or therapeutic. Consult the radiology or nuclear medicine departments to find out any necessary precautions.

THIOAMIDES
Actions
- Block synthesis of thyroid hormones.

Indications
- Used to treat hyperthyroidism and thyrotoxicosis, and used pre-operatively in patients undergoing thyroidectomy. These are the most commonly used antithyroid drugs.

Adverse Effects, Contraindications
- May experience skin rashes, nausea, headache, and dizziness.
- If jaundice develops, drugs must be discontinued.
- Hypothyroidism can occur.

Dosage, Administration
- Methimazole, U.S.P. (Tapazole): Usual dosage is to 5 to 20 mg, p.o., q.d.
- Prophylthiouracil, U.S.P. (Propacil): Usual dosage is 50 to 500 mg, p.o., q.d.

CALCIUM GLUCONATE, U.S.P.

Actions
- Assists in maintaining normal neuromuscular activity.
- Assists in regulating the rhythm of the heart.
- Essential factor in the body's blood-clotting mechanism.

Indications
- Treats hypocalcemic tetany no matter what the underlying cause (*e.g.*, deprivation of calcium and vitamin D, hypoparathyroidism, and advanced renal insufficiency, or following thyroidectomy if the parathyroid glands are removed).
- Improves cardiac contractility, and may be used during resuscitation efforts following cardiac arrest.

Adverse Effects, Contraindications
- Calcium overdose may cause hypercalcemia—which results in anorexia, nausea, vomiting, weakness, depression, polyuria, and polydipsia.
- Use cautiously for patients receiving digitalis preparations because calcium potentiates the action of digitalis and may precipitate arrhythmias.

Dosage, Administration

- For severe hypocalcemic tetany, calcium gluconate injection, U.S.P. is administered intravenously at a slow rate. Usually a 10%-solution is used, and from 5 to 30 ml are given.
- For mild hypocalcemic tetany, a usual adult dosage is 5 g orally, three times daily, 1 to $1\frac{1}{2}$ hr after meals.
- The intramuscular route should not be used because abscesses may form.

Nursing Tips

- Serum calcium levels must be monitored carefully to prevent hypercalcemia.
- Patients receiving IV calcium should have their EKG monitored.

CORTICOTROPIN INJECTION, U.S.P. (ACTHAR, ACTH)

Actions

- Stimulates the adrenal glands to secrete their hormones (*e.g.,* the corticosteroids). *(See PH, Adrenocorticosteroids; actions)*

Indications

(See PH, Adrenocorticosteroids; indications)
- The steroids are usually considered safer than corticotropin in the treatment of these diseases.
- Corticotropin is also used to aid in the diagnosis of adrenal insufficiency. *(See SS Endocrine)*

Adverse Effects, Contraindications

(See PH, Adrenocorticosteroids: adverse effects)
- Allergic reactions may occur because of the foreign protein in the injectable solution.

Dosage, Administration

- Dosage differs according to the condition being treated. Usual range is 25 to 40 units, IM or SC, t.i.d.
- Intravenously, 10 to 25 units are mixed in 500 ml of D_5W.

Nursing Tips

- This drug must be given parenterally because if administered orally it would be destroyed by enzymes in the gastrointestinal tract.
- Skin tests may be done to determine if a patient is allergic to this drug.

INSULIN

Actions

- Assists in regulating carbohydrate metabolism by affecting the process by which glucose is stored, released, and utilized.
- Also affects the conversion of lipids into fat and of amino acids into protein.
- Administration of insulin assists in the control of hyperglycemia (elevated blood sugar), glycosuria (glucose in the urine), and ketosis (excess ketones in the blood), as well as the diabetic complications that can develop.

Indications

- Used in the treatment of all cases of juvenile-onset diabetes. *(See SS, Endocrine)*
- Also used in maturity-onset diabetes for those people who do not respond to oral hypoglycemics and changes in diet.
- Indicated in the treatment of diabetic ketoacidosis.
- Hyperglycemic patients who are subjected to stressful situations (*e.g.,* surgery, infection, or pregnancy) may also receive insulin.

Adverse Effects, Contraindications

- The most common adverse effect is a *hypoglycemic reaction. (See SS Endocrine)*
- If insulin injection sites are not rotated, changes in subcutaneous fat content will occur (lipodystrophy and hypertrophy), causing adverse cosmetic effects and interfering with insulin's absorption.
- Resistance to insulin and allergy do develop in some cases.

Dosage, Administration

- Dosages are adjusted on the basis of blood and urine glucose levels.
- The patient's needs may change if illness is present or if exercise is increased or decreased.
- Various preparations of insulin are available. They do not differ in action, only in their onset and duration of action (see Table 4-2).

Nursing Tips

- Insulin is given subcutaneously at a 90° or 45° angle. A very thin patient may require the 45° angle. Diabetics who are learning to give their own insulin will probably find the 90° angle easier.
- Insulin is available in two strengths: U-40 and U-100. U-100 is the one you will see most frequently. The ADA is encouraging phy-

TABLE 4-2. **Insulin Preparations**

	Time of administration	Time of onset	Peak action	Duration of action	Hypoglycemia most likely
Insulin injection, U.S.P. (Regular Insulin)	15–20 min a.c.	within 1 hr	2–4 hr	6–8 hr	2–4 hr after injection
Isophane insulin suspension, U.S.P. (NPH Insulin)	about 30 min a.c. breakfast	2–4 hr	8–12 hr	24–28 hr	3 PM to dinner
Insulin zinc suspension, U.S.P. (Lente Insulin)	about 30 min a.c. breakfast	2–4 hr	8–12 hr	24–28 hr	3 PM to dinner

sicians to place all their diabetic patients on U-100 because measurement is less confusing. "U-100" indicates there are 100 units of insulin per milliliter.

- Always match the strength of insulin with the correct syringe (*e.g.,* U-100 insulin with U-100 syringe).
- Insulin does not need to be refrigerated, but extremes of temperature should be avoided.
- If you observe signs of hypoglycemia in your patient, treat it *immediately.* An untreated insulin reaction can progress very quickly to coma or convulsions. Mixing two or three packs of sugar in orange juice is a quick, effective, early treatment.
- Preparations such as NPH and Lente are suspensions and need to be mixed before they are drawn up. The vial should be rotated gently between the hands and inverted end to end several times. Never shake vigorously.
- If a patient is n.p.o. for surgery or a diagnostic test, the time of his insulin may need to be adjusted to avoid a hypoglycemic reaction. Consult with his physician.
- Whenever possible, a patient should continue to give his own insulin while hospitalized. This is a good time for you to observe his technique and help him with any difficulties.
- The patient will recognize the importance of site rotation only if *you* emphasize it and help him develop a systematic approach. Insulin injections should be at least 1 $\frac{1}{2}$ inches from each other, and a site should not be reused for 6 to 8 weeks. Areas to use include the subcutaneous tissue of the deltoids, the anterior and lateral thighs, and the abdomen and buttocks (see Fig. 4-3). Use one area for a week before proceeding to the next body area. Covering the daily site with a spot Band-aid assists in locating a new site for the next day.

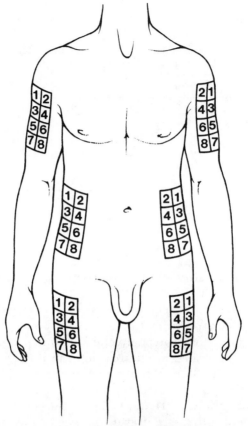

FIG. 4-3. *Rotation sites for the administration of insulin.*

ORAL HYPOGLYCEMICS

Actions

- Stimulates the beta cells of the pancreas to secrete insulin and therefore lowers blood sugar levels.

Indications

- Used to treat maturity-onset diabetes when diet and weight reduction alone do not reduce the blood sugar levels.
- Also used when insulin cannot be employed (*e.g.*, if patient is allergic or unwilling to take the injections).

Adverse Effects, Contraindications

- Hypoglycemia, gastrointestinal disturbances (*e.g.*, anorexia, nausea, and vomiting), and headache.

- Not effective for juvenile or brittle diabetes or for patients in coma or those with ketoacidosis.

Nursing Tips

- The following drugs can potentiate the action of the oral hypoglycemics: coumarin-type anticoagulants, alcohol, phenylbutazone-type anti-inflammatory agents, salicylates, and the sulfonamides.
- Use of thiazide diuretics may necessitate an increase in the dosage of oral hypoglycemics.
- Both the safety and effectiveness of these drugs are being investigated, especially their ability to prevent diabetic complications and reduce cardiovascular mortality. Great reduction in usage has occurred since the study done by the University Group Diabetes Program (UGDP). They reported that diabetic patients receiving oral hypoglycemics had a death rate from cardiovascular disease that was much higher than those being treated with diet alone, insulin, or placebos.
- The following are examples of oral hypoglycemics: acetohexamide, N.F. (Dymelor); chlorpropamide, U.S.P. (Diabinese); tolazamide, U.S.P. (Tolinase); tolbutamide, U.S.P. (Orinase)

THYROID-REPLACEMENT THERAPY

Actions

(See SS, Endocrine, thyroid: description)

Indications

- Used as replacement therapy in various forms of hypothyroidism (*e.g.*, myxedema, cretinism, and nontoxic goiter). *(See SS Endocrine)*

Adverse Effects, Contraindications

- Overdose results in signs and symptoms of hyperthyroidism. *(See SS Endocrine, thyroid, hyperthyroidism)*
- Use cautiously in patients with a history of angina pectoris, congestive heart failure, hypertension, or recent myocardial infarction.
- Adrenal deficiencies must be corrected before thyroid therapy is started.

Dosage, Administration

- Preparations differ mainly in potency, duration of action, and composition (*e.g.*, synthetic T_3, synthetic T_3 & T_4, thyroid extract, thyroglobulin extract, and synthetic T_4).
- Liotrix, (Thyrolar): initially, one tablet with 25 to 30 mcg levothyroxine (T_4) and 6.25 to 7.5 mcg liothyronine (T_3). Maintenance: 50 to 180 mcg (T_4) and 6.25 to 45 mcg (T_3), p.o. daily.

- Sodium levothyroxine (T_4), U.S.P. (Synthroid, Levothroid): initially, 25 to 100 mcg, p.o., q.d. Maintenance, 150 to 300 mcg, p.o., q.d.
- Thyroid, U.S.P. (Desiccated thyroid): initially, 15 to 60 mg, p.o., q.d. Maintenance, 60 to 180 mg, p.o., q.d.

Nursing Tips

- Average dosage levels are lower than previously. The patient's clinical response is used as a guide.
- Thyroid-replacement therapy is frequently life-long, and patients may need assistance and support in understanding this.
- Thyroid drugs potentiate anticoagulants. Insulin or oral hypoglycemics may require dosage adjustment.

VASOPRESSIN INJECTION, U.S.P. (PITRESSIN)

Actions

- This purified preparation, also known as the antidiuretic hormone (ADH) keeps the body from becoming excessively dehydrated. It stimulates the kidneys to conserve water by increasing reabsorption of water by the renal tubules.

Indications

- Used in the treatment of diabetes insipidus.
- Because of its vasoconstricting effect it is used to treat esophageal bleeding (*e.g.,* secondary to cirrhosis). *(See SS Gastrointestinal)*

Adverse Effects, Contraindications

- Overdose may result in sodium and fluid retention.
- Cramps and diarrhea may occur because of smooth muscle contraction. This constriction may also lead to hypertension when it effects the blood vessels.
- Coronary blood vessel constriction can precipitate attacks of angina or cause an acute coronary attack.

Dosage, Administration

- Usual range is 5 to 10 units IM or SC, two or three times daily.
- When Pitressin is administered intranasally by spray or on pledgets, the dosage and interval between treatments must be determined for each patient.
- Vasopressin tannate, U.S.P. (Pitressin Tannate): Long-acting form: 1.25 to 5 units IM, every 1 to 3 days.

Nursing Tips

- Observe patients for signs of drowsiness and mental confusion that could indicate water intoxication.

GASTROINTESTINAL SYSTEM
ANTACIDS

Actions
- Neutralize secreted stomach acid.
- Relieve peptic pain and assist in the healing of gastric and duodenal ulcers.

Indications
- Treat peptic ulcer and relieve other types of gastric distress (*e.g.*, heartburn) caused by hyperacidity. *(See SS, Gastrointestinal)*

Adverse Effects, Contraindications
- The aluminum antacids (*e.g.*, Amphojel) frequently cause constipation; occasionally, they cuase nausea and vomiting.
- The magnesium antacids (*e.g.*, milk of magnesia) frequently cause diarrhea.
- Electrolyte imbalance, especially if kidney function is compromised, can lead to an accumulation of the aluminum and magnesium in the central nervous system. Kidney stones and edema may also occur.
- Extended intake of high doses of the aluminum antacids may remove phosphate from the bones and lead to a softening of the bones (osteomalacia).

Dosage, Administration
- Aluminum hydroxide gel, U.S.P. (Amphojel): 5 to 40 ml, p.o., several times daily. Dosage of tablets is 300 to 600 mg several times daily. The liquid may be given by continuous intragastric drip in severe cases of peptic disease.
  1. May also be used to treat patients with phosphate-type kidney stones.
- Magnesia and alumina oral suspension, U.S.P. (Maalox): 5 to 30 ml, p.o., several times daily. Dosage of tablets is 200 to 400 mg several times daily. Continuous intragastric drip may be used in severe cases of peptic disease.
- Magaldrate, U.S.P. (Riopan): 400 to 800 mg, p.o., several times daily.
  1. Contains less sodium than many other antacids and may be preferred for patients with compromised function of the heart and kidneys.

Nursing Tips
- Patients with a history of heart and kidney disease should be closely monitored. Because of the sodium content of some antacids, fluid

retention is a possibility, especially if frequent, large doses are used. Kidney stone formation from excess calcium and phosphate is also possible.

- Although most antacids are considered relatively insoluble, some systemic absorption of ions (*e.g.,* magnesium, aluminum, calcium, and sodium) can occur. Observe patients for lethargy, fatigue, weight gain, muscle weakness, and coma.
- Antacids interfere with the absorption of tetracycline-type antibiotics, oral iron salts, warfarin, and the sulfonamides.
- Patients should be assisted in self-care as soon as possible because their therapy must continue when they go home. Antacid tablets must be thoroughly chewed. Liquid suspensions must be shaken each time and followed by a small amount of water or milk. Greatest amounts of gastric acid are usually secreted 1 to $1\frac{1}{2}$ hours after meals and at night. Therefore, taking the antacids about 1 hour after meals and at night can protect the patient when he is most vulnerable.
- Problems with constipation and diarrhea can be reduced by alternating the magnesium and aluminum products or by using a combination product (*e.g.,* Mylanta).
- Antacids relieve *symptoms.* They do not always assist in the correction of the underlying problem.

ANTIDIARRHEALS

Overview

- Diarrhea is usually a self-limiting symptom and treatment may not be necessary. Because diarrhea is a defense mechanism that helps rid the body of irritants, bacteria, viruses, and so forth, slowing the intestinal motility may actually prolong the underlying problem.
- Severe or prolonged diarrhea can quickly lead to dehydration and electrolyte imbalance, especially in children and the elderly.
- The cause for chronic diarrhea should always be determined. Colon and rectal cancer must be ruled out, and appropriate treatment must be determined.

DIPHENOXYLATE HYDROCHLORIDE WITH ATROPINE SULFATE, N.F. (LOMOTIL)

Actions

- The antiperistaltic action slows intestinal motility and reduces the number of stools.

Indications

- Used for both acute and chronic diarrhea resulting from functional, inflammatory, and other types of disorders.
- May assist in keeping dosages of corticosteroids *(see PH, Adrenocorticosteroids)* low in the treatment of chronic inflammatory bowel problems *(e.g.,* Crohn's disease and ulcerative colitis).

Adverse Effects, Contraindications

- A derivative of meperidine (Demerol), lomotil could produce dependency in large doses. Occasionally, drowsiness and constipation may result from ordinary doses.
- Use cautiously in patients with liver problems.
- The atropine *(see PH, Autonomic nervous system)* in the drug could result in abdominal distention and cause serious problems for patients with ulcerative colitis.
- This drug should not be used to treat diarrhea caused by the antibiotics lincomycin and clindamycin.
- Overdoses can result in lethargy, coma, and respiratory depression and may necessitate the use of naloxone. *(See PH, Central nervous system)*

Dosage, Administration

- Initially the adult dosage is usually 5 mg, p.o., q.i.d. and may be reduced to 5 mg, q.d.

Nursing Tips

(See PH, Antidiarrheals, overview)

KAOLIN MIXTURE WITH PECTIN, N.F. (KAOPECTATE)
Actions

- Kaolin functions as an absorbent. It binds and removes irritants, bacteria, and toxins from the intestinal tract.
- Pectin is a demulcent and soothes the irritated bowel lining.

Indications

- Used to control acute diarrhea.

Adverse Effects, Contraindications

- This drug is relatively safe when used in the recommended dosage range.
- Not recommended for use in chronic diarrhea.

Dosage, Administration

- Usual adult dosage range is 30 ml, p.o., several times daily or after each loose stool.

Nursing Tips

(See PH, Antidiarrheals, overview)

PAREGORIC, U.S.P. (CAMPHORATED TINCTURE OF OPIUM)
Actions

- Lessens hyperperistaltic activity, thereby delaying passage of the intestinal contents.

Indications

- Used to control acute diarrhea.

Adverse Effects, Contraindications

- Because this is an opium preparation, dependency could result if dosages are abused.
- Because small dosages are usually employed, side-effects are infrequent and minimal, but they can occur. *(See PH, Central nervous system, opiates: adverse effects)*

Dosage, Administration

- Usual adult dosage is 5 to 10 ml, p.o., several times daily. May also be added to nonprescription products, such as kaolin and pectin.

Nursing Tips

(See PH, Antidiarrheals, overview)

ANTIEMETICS

Overview

- Severe vomiting can lead to dehydration and electrolyte imbalance, especially in children and the elderly.
- Nausea and vomiting can be symptoms of a huge variety of problems. It is important to determine the cause of the nausea and vomiting and to eliminate it if possible.

DIMENHYDRINATE, U.S.P. (DRAMAMINE)
Actions

- Prevents nausea and vomiting by blocking nerve impulses from the inner ear to the vomiting center in the brain.

Indications

- Prevents motion sickness and problems due to inner ear dysfunction (*e.g.*, Meniere's syndrome).
- Also may be used to alleviate postoperative nausea and vomiting.

Adverse Effects, Contraindications

- Drowsiness occurs in some patients.

Dosage, Administration

- Usual adult dosage is 50 mg, p.o., q. 4 to 6 hr. The drug may also be administered rectally or parenterally.

Nursing Tips

(See PH, Antiemetics, overview)
- Because of the drowsiness that can occur, patients should be cautioned against driving or operating machinery.

PHENOTHIAZINES
Actions

- Control nausea and vomiting by reducing the responsiveness of the chemoreceptor trigger zone (CTZ) in the medulla to emetic stimuli.
- For a more complete listing of actions referring to care of psychiatric patients, see *PH, Psychotropics, major tranquilizers.*

Indications

- Controls postoperative vomiting.
- Effective for vomiting secondary to severe infections.
- Use cautiously for severe vomiting due to pregnancy (hyperemesis gravidarum).
- Effective for cancer patients receiving radiation therapy and chemotherapy.
- Also may be used to treat psychiatric problems. *(See PH, Psychotropics)*

Adverse Effects, Contraindications

- Used cautiously in children and pregnant women.
- Because small doses are used in the treatment of nausea and vomiting, most adverse effects of the phenothiazines are not experienced. However, side-effects can occur, and the following are examples *(see also PH, Psychotropics):*
  1. Extrapyramidal stimulation (*e.g.*, sudden contraction of muscle groups in spasms, extreme restlessness, muscular rigidity).

2. Atropinelike effects (*e.g.*, dry mouth, blurred vision, constipation, postural hypotension).
3. Quinidinelike effects (*e.g.*, slowed conduction, ventricular arrythmias).
4. Hepatitis with obstructive jaundice.
5. Agranulocytosis and other blood dyscrasias.
6. Endocrine imbalances (*e.g.*, delayed ovulation and menstruation).
7. Skin reactions ranging from mild to severe and photosensitivity.

Dosage, Administration

- Prochlorperazine maleate, U.S.P. (Compazine): For treatment of nausea and vomiting, the drug may be administered orally, parenterally, or rectally. Adult dosage range is 5 to 10 mg, q. 4 hr as needed (maximum is usually 30 mg per day). *(See PH, Psychotropics)*
- Promethazine hydrochloride, U.S.P. (Phenergan): Usually, adult dosage is 25 to 50 mg, q. 4 hr as needed IM.

Nursing Tips

(See PH, Antiemetics, overview)
- Promethazine HCl has a synergistic (additive) effect when combined with narcotics. The combination potentiates the analgesic effect of the narcotic.

TRIMETHOBENZAMIDE HYDROCHLORIDE, N.F. (TIGAN)
Actions

- Relieves nausea and vomiting by blocking nerve impulses from the inner ear to receptors in the brain.

Indications

- Used to treat nausea and vomiting caused by radiation sickness, infection, and operative procedures.

Adverse Effects, Contraindications

- May occasionally cause drowsiness, dizziness, and diarrhea, but the incidence of adverse effects is low.

Dosage, Administration

- Usual oral adult dosage is 100 to 250 mg, q. 4 to 6 hr as needed. Usual IM adult dose is 200 mg, q. 4 to 6 hr as needed. Tigan is also available in suppositories.

Nursing Tips

(See PH, Antiemetics, overview)
- Because of the drowsiness that can occur, patients should be cautioned against driving or operating machinery.

ANTISECRETORY: CIMETIDINE (TAGAMET)

Actions
- Blocks the action of histamine at the histamine H_2 receptors of the parietal cells of the stomach. Therefore, the secretion of gastric acid is reduced.

Indications
- Used to relieve peptic pain both during the day and at night.
- Very effective for healing duodenal ulcers.
- Also used to treat stomach and esophageal ulcers. Can help control or prevent bleeding secondary to the ulcers.
- Patients with Zollinger-Ellison syndrome (gastrin-secreting pancreatic tumors) have responded to this drug.
- May be used prophylactically to prevent stress ulcers (*e.g.,* in burn patients).
- Because gastric acid inactivates pancreatic enzymes, cimetidine increases the effectiveness of these enzymes, and patients receiving replacement therapy may benefit.

Adverse Effects, Contraindications
- Occasional mild diarrhea, dizziness, rash, mental confusion, and muscle pains have occurred.
- Toxicity can produce coma and seizures.
- Rarely, agranulocytosis occurs.
- This drug is relatively new, and more side-effects may be reported as use increases. *Rebound ulcer perforation* may be a problem, and gradual dosage reduction at the end of therapy is suggested.
- Patients with impaired liver and kidney function may need reduced dosages to prevent confusion from high serum levels of the drug.
- Drug safety during pregnancy and nursing has not been established.
- *High intravenous bolus doses* may induce bradycardia and hypotension.

Dosage, Administration
- Usual adult dosage is 300 mg, p.o., q.i.d. with meals and at bedtime for 4 to 6 weeks.
- Intravenous doses have been given to help control gastrointestinal bleeding.

Nursing Tips
- Monitor blood pressure and pulse carefully, especially during IV administration of the drug.

- Monitor the patient's white blood count, and observe for sore throat or infection.
- To lessen risk of sudden hypotension from IV administration, dilute a 2-ml vial in 100 ml of 0.9% NaCl or 5% DW and run in over 15 to 20 min.
- *Antacids* may interfere with cimetidine absorption and should be administered at different times (*e.g.,* cimetidine *with* meals and the antacids 1 to 1 ½ hours *after meals*).
- Serum *Valium* levels may be increased by the concurrent use of cimetidine. Observe patients for drowsiness and dizziness.
- *Warfarin* and cimetidine interact, so prothrombin times must be watched carefully.

PSYCHOTROPICS
MAJOR TRANQUILIZERS: ANTIPSYCHOTIC AGENTS
PHENOTHIAZINES
Actions

- Sedate and calm patients who are anxious or severely agitated. (tranquilizing effect)
- Reduce psychotic patients' hallucinations and delusions, and assist in improving disturbed behavior (antipsychotic effect).
- Control nausea and vomiting (antiemetic effect).
- Block both cholinergic and adrenergic effects of the autonomic nervous system.

Indications

- Relieve symptoms of psychosis in schizophrenia, in the manic phase of the manic-depressive psychosis, and in confused, senile patients.
- Treat toxic psychoses caused by alcohol, amphetamines, and LSD.
- Effective to relieve alcohol withdrawal syndrome.
- Control postoperative vomiting and assist in preventing vomiting induced by antineoplastic drugs.
- Produce preoperative sedation.

Adverse Effects, Contraindications

- Drowsiness is common but may disappear after the first few weeks. Lethargy, fatigue, and weakness also occur.
- Extrapyramidal motor system reactions include the following:
  1. acute and persistent dyskinesias (*e.g.,* abnormal movements of extremities and facial disturbances such as lateral jaw movements, sucking and smacking of the lips, and in-and-out tongue movement)

2. pseudoparkinsonism (*e.g.*, tremor, rigidity, drooling, masklike facial expression, and restlessness)
3. akinesia (*e.g.*, fatigue and weakness of arms and legs)
4. akathisia (*e.g.*, motor restlessness)

- Postural hypotension occurs, and the hypotension may progress to a shocklike state. Heart palpitations and cardiac arrest are possible.
- Atropinelike side-effects include dry mouth, blurred vision, constipation, paralytic ileus, urinary retention, and decreased sweating.
- Nasal stuffiness and inhibition of ejaculation result from adrenergic blockage.
- Amenorrhea, false-positive pregnancy tests, gynecomastia and lactation, and a reduction in libido have all occurred.
- Patients may experience weight gain, edema, and increased appetite.
- Phenothiazines can produce hyperglycemia and glycosuria.
- Blood dyscrasias can include leukopenia, agranulocytosis, hemolytic anemia, thrombocytic purpura, and pancytopenia, but occurrences are rare.
- Skin rashes and eruptions, photosensitivity, and jaundice have occurred.
- Long-term therapy may result in skin pigmentation and ocular changes (deposits in the lens and cornea may form opacities).
- Use cautiously for patients with cardiovascular disease, liver disease, chronic obstructive lung disease, blood dyscrasias, peptic ulcer, glaucoma, or epilepsy.
- Not recommended for use during pregnancy.

Dosage, Administration

- Chlorpromazine hydrochloride, U.S.P. (Thorazine): Dosage ranges from 10 mg to 1 g daily. Oral administration is most common.
- When using the intramuscular (IM) route, inject slowly, deep into the upper outer quadrant of the buttocks. Patients should remain lying down for $\frac{1}{2}$ hour after injection because of the possible hypotensive effects.
- The IV route is reserved for surgery and severe hiccups.
- Chlorpromazine is the prototype of antipsychotic drugs.
- Fluphenazine decanoate, U.S.P. (Prolixin Decanoate): Dosage ranges from 12.5 to 50 mg, every 2 or 3 weeks.
- Fluphenazine may be given either IM or SC. A dry syringe and needle of at least 21 gauge should be used. (Solution may become cloudy if wet needles or syringes are used.)

- Trifluoperazine hydrochloride, N.F. (Stelazine): Dosage ranges from 2 to 20 mg daily. Trifluoperazine is administered orally or IM.
- Thioridazine hydrochloride, U.S.P. (Mellaril): Dosage ranges from 20 to 800 mg daily, orally.
- Extrapyramidal side-effects are common with thioridazine.

Nursing Tips

- Dosage of the phenothiazines is adjusted on an individual basis. The goal is to administer the smallest effective dose.
- These medications should be withdrawn gradually to avoid nausea, vomiting, dizziness, and tremulousness.
- The drugs in this family are closely related chemically. Cross-sensitivity within the family is likely.
- Blood counts and liver function should be monitored, especially for patients on long-term therapy.
- Patients receiving long-term therapy should also have periodic eye exams to detect opacities and other drug-induced damage to the eyes.
- Observe patients for clinical signs of agranulocytosis, such as sore throat and infection. Patients most commonly develop the problem between the fourth and tenth weeks of therapy.
- The dosages of barbiturates and narcotic analgesics should be cut one-quarter to one-half when phenothiazines are added.
- Patients should not use alcohol when taking the phenothiazines because of the additive central nervous system (CNS) depression.
- The use of atropine with the phenothiazines will potentiate the cholinergic blockade. *(See PH, Autonomic nervous system, anticholinergics)*
- A single daily dose, taken at bedtime, is usually well-tolerated. Dizziness and faintness are less noticeable when the patient is lying down and the drowsiness is desirable.

HALOPERIDOL, U.S.P. (HALDOL)
Actions

- Antagonizes the neurotransmitter action of dopamine.

Indications

- Treats psychotic disorders.
- Controls the tics and vocal utterances of Gilles de la Tourette's syndrome in children and adults.
- Reduces behavior problems in children with combative, explosive hyperexcitability.

Adverse Effects, Contraindications

- Extrapyramidal reactions are frequent. They include parkinson-like symptoms and akathisia. Persistent tardive dyskinesias also may occur. *(For extrapyramidal symptoms, see PH, Psychotropics, phenothiazines: adverse effects)*
- Insomnia, restlessness, anxiety, drowsiness, depression, confusion, grand mal seizures, and exacerbation of psychotic symptoms have been reported.
- Tachycardia and hypotension may occur.
- Leukopenia and anemia are usually mild and transient.
- Jaundice and impaired liver function can occur.
- Breast engorgement and lactation, menstrual irregularities, impotence, and increased libido have resulted.
- Hyperglycemia and glycosuria have been produced.
- Gastrointestinal effects include anorexia, constipation, diarrhea, nausea, and vomiting.
- Autonomic reactions such as dry mouth, blurred vision, urinary retention, and diaphoresis occur.
- Laryngospasm and bronchospasm are possible.
- Patients with CNS depression or Parkinson's disease should not receive haloperidol.
- Use cautiously for patients with cardiovascular disease or glaucoma, those using anticonvulsants or anticoagulants, and those who have allergies to other drugs.

Dosage, Administration

- Usual dosage range is 1 to 15 mg daily, orally or IM.
- Patients with moderate symptoms and elderly patients receive 0.5 to 2.0 mg, two or three times daily. The doses should be evenly spaced to maintain therapeutic blood levels.

Nursing Tips

- Haloperidol may potentiate the actions of other CNS depressants, such as barbituates, narcotic analgesics, and alcohol.
- Patients should be cautioned against driving or operating machinery.
- A few patients treated with haloperidol plus lithium have developed an encephalopathic syndrome followed by irreversible brain damage. Observe patients for neurological toxicity.

MINOR TRANQUILIZERS: ANTIANXIETY AGENTS
CHLORDIAZEPOXIDE HYDROCHLORIDE, U.S.P. (LIBRIUM)
Actions

- Possesses antianxiety properties.

Indications

- Relieves anxiety and tension in various disease states.
- Treats withdrawal symptoms of acute alcoholism.
- Manages preoperative apprehension and anxiety.

Adverse Effects, Contraindications

- Drowsiness, ataxia, and confusion occur.
- Rarely, patients have experienced skin eruptions, edema, nausea, and constipation.
- Blood dyscrasias such as agranulocytosis occur occasionally.
- Physical and psychological dependence are possible.
- Use cautiously for patients with impaired liver and kidney function.
- Paradoxical reactions (*e.g.*, excitation) have been reported.

Dosage, Administration

- Usual adult dosage for mild to moderate anxiety is 5 to 10 mg orally, three or four times daily.
- Severe anxiety is treated with 20 to 25 mg orally, three or four times daily.
- Alcoholic patients receive 50 to 100 mg in repeated doses, IM or IV. Maximum is 300 mg per 24 hours.
- Elderly or debilitated patients receive 10 mg or less, orally, per day. Dosage is gradually increased as tolerance develops.

Nursing Tips

- Blood counts and liver function should be monitored in patients receiving long-term therapy.
- Patients should be cautioned against driving or operating machinery because of the drowsiness that can occur.
- Chlordiazepoxide may potentiate the actions of other CNS depressants, such as barbiturates, narcotic analgesics, and alcohol.
- Patients with suicidal tendencies may require protective measures.

DIAZEPAM, U.S.P. (VALIUM)

Actions

- Possesses antianxiety, anticonvulsant, and skeletal muscle relaxant properties.

Indications

- Relieves anxiety and tension in transient situational disturbances, functional or organic disorders, and psychoneurotic states.
- In acute alcohol withdrawal, diazepam relieves acute agitation, tremors, and delirium tremens.

- Large parenteral doses reduce muscle spasticity in cerebral palsy and athetosis, and control recurring convulsions in status epilepticus, tetanus, and other seizure states.
- Produces sedation preoperatively and prior to cardioversion, gastroscopy, and esophagoscopy.
- Relieves skeletal muscle spasticity and spasm.

Adverse Effects, Contraindications

- Frequent side-effects include drowsiness, fatigue, and ataxia.
- Physical and especially psychological dependence can develop.
- Use cautiously in patients with impaired liver and kidney function.
- Paradoxical reactions (*e.g.*, excitation, hallucinations, and rage) sometimes occur and necessitate discontinuing the drug.
- Do not give to patients with acute narrow-angle glaucoma.

Dosage, Administration

- Usual adult dosage for anxiety and muscle spasm is 2 to 10 mg orally, two to four times daily.
- Alcoholic withdrawal may require 10 mg orally, three or four times daily.
- Elderly or debilitated patients usually receive 2 mg orally, one or two times daily.
- For control of convulsions and acute agitation, repeated doses of 5 to 10 mg are given IM or IV every 3 to 4 hours.
- Do not mix or dilute diazepam with other solutions or drugs.
- For IV administration take at least 1 minute for each 5 mg (1 ml) given. Maximum single dose is 30 mg.
- If direct IV injection is not possible, give slowly through infusion tubing as close as possible to vein insertion.

Nursing Tips

- Caution patients against driving or operating machinery because of the drowsiness that can occur.
- Diazepam may potentiate the actions of other CNS depressants, such as barbiturates, narcotic analgesics, and alcohol.
- Blood counts and liver function should be monitored in patients receiving long-term therapy.
- Patients with suicidal tendencies may require protective measures.

HYDROXYZINE HYDROCHLORIDE, N.F. (ATARAX); HYDROXYZINE PAMOATE, N.F. (VISTARIL)

Actions

- Antianxiety agents that also possess antihistaminic, antiemetic, and antispasmodic effects.

Indications

- Relieve anxiety and tension associated with psychoneurosis and some organic diseases.
- Used to manage some cases of pruritus due to allergies.
- Used to sedate patients preoperatively and following general anesthesia.

Adverse Effects, Contraindications

- Side-effects are usually mild and transitory.
- Dry mouth and drowsiness occur.
- Tremor and convulsions may result from higher-than-recommended doses.

Dosage, Administration

- Usual adult dosage range is 25 to 150 mg orally per day.
- Parenteral solutions are administered IM because the IV and SC routes are too irritating.

Nursing Tips

- Caution patients against driving or operating machinery because of the drowsiness that can occur.
- Hydroxyzine may potentiate the actions of other CNS depressants, such as barbiturates, narcotic analgesics, and alcohol.

DRUGS FOR AFFECTIVE DISORDERS
LITHIUM CARBONATE, U.S.P. (LITHANE, LITHONATE)
Actions

- Alters sodium transport in muscle and nerve cells, and affects the metabolism of catecholamines.
- Specific mechanism for treating mania is unknown.

Indications

- Treats manic episodes of manic-depressive illness.
- Prevents or reduces the intensity of further episodes.

Adverse Effects, Contraindications

- Use *cautiously* in patients with cardiovascular or kidney disease, low serum sodium, and dehydration, and in those receiving diuretics. In these instances, the risk of lithium toxicity is very high.
- Initial therapy may produce mild nausea, thirst, and fine hand tremors. These side-effects usually subside, but occasionally they continue throughout therapy.

- Early signs of lithium toxicity include diarrhea, vomiting, drowsiness, muscular weakness, and lack of coordination. These can occur at serum lithium levels below 2 mEq per liter.
- Ataxia, giddiness, tinnitus, blurred vision, and a large amount of dilute urine occur at higher levels.
- Severe toxicity produces the following:
  1. tremor, twitching, hyperreflexia, and clonic spasms
  2. restlessness, confusion, convulsive seizures, stupor, and coma
  3. cardiac arrhythmias, hypotension, circulatory collapse

Dosage, Administration

- Acute episodes of mania are usually treated with 600 mg, t.i.d., orally. Serum lithium levels range from 1 to 1.5 mEq per liter.
- Maintenance dosages usually are 300 mg, t.i.d. or q.i.d., orally. Serum levels should range between 0.6 and 1.2 mEq per liter.

Nursing Tips

- Lithium toxicity can occur at doses close to therapeutic levels. Serum lithium levels must be closely monitored.
- The blood should be drawn 8 to 12 hours after the previous dose.
- The patient's ability to tolerate lithium appears to be greater during acute episodes and to decline during long-term therapy.
- It is very important to maintain a normal diet, including salt, and to drink adequate fluids (at least 2500 to 3000 ml during initial therapy).
- It may be necessary to temporarily reduce lithium dosage if the patient develops infection with elevated temperature, diarrhea, or sweating.
- A few patients treated with lithium plus haloperidol have developed an encephalopathic syndrome followed by irreversible brain damage. Observe patients for neurological toxicity.
- Encourage patients to notify their physicians immediately if they experience symptoms of toxicity *(see adverse effects)*. The drug should be discontinued, and serum levels should be checked.

ISOCARBOXAZID, N.F. (MARPLAN): MAO INHIBITOR
Actions

- Inhibits the enzyme monoamine oxidase (MAO).
- Produces antidepressant activity.

Indications

- Treats depressed patients who do not respond to tricyclic antidepressants or electroconvulsive therapy.

Adverse Effects, Contraindications

- Postural hypotension is a frequent side-effect. Patients may experience weakness, dizziness, and faintness.
- Other autonomic side-effects include hypertension, mouth dryness, blurred vision, constipation, difficulty in urination, impotence, and sweating.
- Effects on the CNS include euphoria, hyperactivity and hyperreflexia, confusion, hallucinations, delirium, tremors, and convulsions.
- Patients may also experience skin rashes and photosensitivity, and edema and weight gain.
- Do not give to patients with severely impaired liver or kidney function, congestive heart failure, or pheochromocytoma.

Dosage, Administration

- Usual starting dosage is 30 mg orally, daily.
- Because of the cumulative effects that occur, maintenance dosages are usually 10 to 20 mg orally, daily.

Nursing Tips

- The numerous potential drug interactions are a major deterrent to the use of MAO inhibitors.
- MAO inhibitors such as isocarboxazid potentiate the activity of sympathomimetic substances and can produce a hypertensive crisis.
  1. Drugs in this category are amphetamines, methyldopa, levodopa, dopamine, tryptophan, epinephrine and norepinephrine. Over-the-counter preparations to treat colds and hay fever and reducing preparations also contain sympathomimetics.
  2. Foods high in tryptophan include cheese, beer, wine, pickled herring, chicken livers, and yeast extract.
- Excessive caffeine intake can also precipitate a hypertensive crisis.
- The use of MAO inhibitors with CNS depressants and general anesthesia can lead to circulatory collapse and death. MAO inhibitors should be discontinued at least 10 days before elective surgery.
- The use of MAO inhibitors with other psychotropics decreases the margin of safety.
- Isocarboxazid should not be given with other MAO inhibitors (*e.g.*, pargyline hydrochloride—Eutonyl; phenelzine sulfate—Nardil; and tranylcypromine—Parnate), or the dibenzepines (*e.g.*, amitriptyline hydrochloride—Elavil; desipramine hydrochloride—Norpramin; and imipramine hydrochloride—Tofranil). The combi-

nation can result in hypertensive crisis, fever, convulsions, coma, and circulatory collapse. A 14-day interval should occur between discontinuing one of these drugs and starting therapy with another.

- The hypertensive crisis seen with MAO inhibitors is frequently treated with 5 mg of phentolamine, administered intravenously at a slow rate.
- Patients receiving MAO inhibitors should have their liver function monitored.

TRICYCLIC ANTIDEPRESSANTS
Actions

- Potentiate action of norepinephrine by blocking neuronal reuptake.
- Increase release of norepinephrine by blocking alpha adrenergic receptor sites controlling norepinephrine release.

Indications

- Relieve symptoms of depression.
- Treat enuresis and neurogenic bladder.

Adverse Effects, Contraindications

- Autonomic side-effects include dry mouth, blurred vision, constipation, difficulty in urinating, postural hypotension, localized sweating, impotence, nausea, and vomiting.
- Early CNS effects are drowsiness and fatigue. Patients may also experience restlessness, agitation, mania, confusion, hallucinations, tremors, and convulsions.
- Numbness, tingling of extremities, and ringing in the ears can occur.
- Hypersensitive patients may develop skin rashes, photosensitivity, jaundice, and agranulocytosis.
- Cardiovascular problems include hypertension, tachycardia, myocardial infarction, arrhythmias, precipitation of congestive heart failure, and stroke.
- Patients with glaucoma or an enlarged prostate should not receive tricyclics.
- Use cautiously for patients with a history of liver, kidney, or cardiovascular disease.

Dosage, Administration

- Amitriptyline hydrochloride, U.S.P. (Elavil): Oral dosage ranges from 25 to 300 mg per day, but most patients respond to 75 mg per day (25 mg t.i.d.).

- For maintenance therapy 40 mg per day may be sufficient and is taken in a single dose, preferably at bedtime.
- Imipramine hydrochloride, U.S.P. (Tofranil): Usual adult oral dosage is 150 mg per day but may range from 25 to 300 mg.
- Imipramine is also used to treat childhood enuresis in children 6-years-old and older. Initially, 25 mg is given orally 1 hour before bedtime. Dosage may be increased but should not exceed 2.5 mg/kg/day.

Nursing Tips

- Tricyclic antidepressants should not be given with MAO inhibitors. The combination can result in hypertensive crisis, fever, convulsions, coma, and circulatory collapse. A 14-day interval should occur between discontinuing one of these drugs and beginning therapy with another.
- Patients should be cautioned against driving and operating machinery because these drugs cause drowsiness and impair alertness.
- Tricyclics can enhance the CNS-depressant effects of alcohol.
- The risk of suicide may increase as the patient's depression is relieved.

RESPIRATORY SYSTEM
ADRENOCORTICOSTEROIDS

See *PH, Endocrine system* for actions, adverse effects, and nursing tips.

Indications

- Used for chronic asthma when bronchodilators and other antiasthmatic drugs cannot stabilize the patient.
- Also used in short term IV therapy, in very high doses, for status asthmaticus.

Dosage, Administration

- Beclomethasone dipropionate (Vanceril Inhaler; Beclovent): Delivered by inhalation, usually two inhalations (100 mcg) three or four times q.d. The low doses produce local therapeutic effects and the medication absorbed is rapidly eliminated. Systemic toxicity is greatly reduced or eliminated. May take 1 to 2 weeks to become effective, and then may be possible to gradually reduce oral steroids.
- Prednisone, U.S.P. (Deltasone): *(See PH, Endocrine)* May be started on 60 mg, p.o., q.d. and tapered to about one-third of the dose after 1 to 2 weeks. Later it may be reduced further, to 10 mg or

less. With low maintenance doses chance of habituation is reduced and discontinuing the drug is easier. To further reduce the suppressant effect on the pituitary and adrenal glands, an intermittent dosage schedule may be used (*e.g.*, the full daily dose is given with the morning meal or the full dosage for 2 days is given q.o.d. with the morning meal).

Nursing Tips

- Weaning a patient from steroids can be very difficult because the asthmatic symptoms may become worse.

BRONCHODILATORS
AMINOPHYLLINE, U.S.P. (THEOPHYLLINE ETHYLENEDIAMINE)
Actions

- Relaxes smooth muscle of the bronchi and bronchioles and of the pulmonary blood vessels.
- Stimulates cardiac muscle and may increase cardiac output.
- Produces diuresis.
- Dilates coronary blood vessels.

Indications

- Treats intermittent and recurring bronchial constriction (*e.g.*, from chronic obstructive pulmonary disease, or COPD), asthma, and acute respiratory distress in children.
- Also used for the treatment of pulmonary edema. *(See SS, Cardiovascular)*

Adverse Effects, Contraindications

- Gastrointestinal (GI) irritation is common and may cause nausea and vomiting. Intestinal bleeding may occur.
- Restlessness, irritability, and insomnia may result from central nervous system (CNS) stimulation.
- Serious, and at times fatal, cardiac arrhythmias and convulsions occur.
- Rapid IV administration can precipitate severe hypotension and circulatory collapse. An IV pump and microdrip tubing should be used.

Dosage, Administration

- Average adult dosage p.o. is 130 to 250 mg, t.i.d. or q.i.d. Rectally, 300 mg may be given up to t.i.d.
- The initial infusion rate for IV aminophylline is ordered in mg/kg/hr and is based on lean body weight. Check package inserts for

rates. After the first 12 to 24 hr, dosage should be based on serum levels. Therapeutic range is 10 to 20 mcg/ml.

Nursing Tips

- Monitor BP, pulse, and respirations very carefully, especially during IV administration.
- Patients metabolize aminophylline at very different rates. Therefore, a therapeutic dose for one person could produce toxic symptoms in another.
- Aminophylline levels should be checked every other day. The recommended initial IV infusion rates have recently been reduced. New guidelines are in the package insert but may not be in standard drug references.
- Gastrointestinal absorption can be unpredictable, so aminophylline should be given on an empty stomach. The nausea and vomiting that can occur come from stimulation of the central emetic mechanism in the brain rather than from local GI irritation.
- Long-term use of rectal suppositories can produce local irritation and is not recommended. Long-acting forms of oral aminophylline are available for nighttime use.
- There are many over-the-counter bronchodilators available. Patients must be carefully counseled about the side-effects of these drugs. Tolerance develops easily, and patients may therefore overdose themselves. Severe hypertension, pulmonary edema, and cardiac arrhythmias can occur. These drugs also contain additives that can dry secretions (antihistamines) and cause sedation.

EPINEPHRINE, U.S.P. (ADRENALIN)

(See PH, Autonomic nervous system)

ISOPROTERENOL HYDROCHLORIDE, U.S.P. (ISUPREL HYDROCHLORIDE)

(See PH, Autonomic nervous system)

TERBUTALINE SULFATE (BRETHINE)

Actions

- Relaxes smooth muscle of the bronchi and bronchioles and the peripheral vasculature.
- At normal doses, causes much less cardiovascular stimulation than isoproterenol.

Indications

- Used mainly in the treatment of bronchial asthma and bronchospasm.

Adverse Effects, Contraindications

- Increases in heart rate, nervousness, tremor, and dizziness are common.
- Headache, nausea and vomiting, anxiety, and restlessness also occur.
- Use cautiously in patients with diabetes, hypertension, hyperthyroidism, or cardiac disorders with arrhythmias.

Dosage, Administration

- Adult SC dose is 0.25 mg. Adult oral dosage range is from 2.5 to 5 mg, t.i.d., at 6-hr intervals. Maximum dosage is 15 mg, q.d.

Nursing Tips

- Should not be given with other sympathomimetic drugs *(see PH, Autonomic nervous system, catecholamines)*. The cardiovascular side-effects can be additive.

EXPECTORANTS

Actions

- Expectorants stimulate the secretion of the natural lubricant fluid of the lower respiratory tract. This liquifies thick mucus and assists in its expulsion. Coughing becomes productive.

Indications

- Used in treatment of COPD, asthma, bronchitis, colds, and pneumonia.

GUAIFENESIN, N.F. (GLYCERYL QUAIACOLATE)

(See PH, Expectorants: actions and indications)

Adverse Effects, Contraindications

- Few side-effects at ordinary doses.
- Higher doses may cause nausea and vomiting.

Dosage, Administration

- Average adult dosage is 100 to 200 mg orally, q. 3 to 4 hr.
- For greater effects, 200 to 400 mg may be given orally, q. 4 hr.

Nursing Tips

- Guaifenesin can interfere with laboratory tests done to determine the presence of excess chemicals in pheochromocytoma and carcinoid syndrome.

POTASSIUM IODIDE, U.S.P.

(See PH, Expectorants: actions and indications)

Adverse Effects, Contraindications

- Iodine sensitivity may produce skin eruptions similar to acne.
- Frontal sinus pain and a mumpslike swelling of the parotid gland may occur.
- Gastrointestinal irritation may result in nausea, vomiting, and diarrhea.
- Tuberculosis patients should not receive potassium iodide.

Dosage, Administration

- 300 mg, p.o., diluted in a liquid vehicle or in a saturated solution containing 1 g/ml; usually given q.i.d.
- Mix iodine solutions in one-third to one-half of a glass of milk or juice to prevent gastric irritation.
- To prevent discoloration of the teeth, give through a straw.

Nursing Tips

- Patients should be well-hydrated in order to increase the effectiveness of the drug and to reduce GI irritation.

TERPIN HYDRATE, N.F.

Actions and Indications

(See PH, Expectorants: actions and indications)
- Often used as a vehicle for other drugs (*e.g.,* codeine).

Adverse Effects, Contraindications

- May cause gastric irritation (from the alcohol content).
- Side-effects may occur from the drugs mixed with terpin hydrate.

Dosage, Administration

- Usual adult dosage is 5 ml q. 4 to 6 hr.

MUCOLYTIC AGENTS

ACETYLCYSTEINE, N.S. (MUCOMYST)

Actions

- Reduces the thickness and adhesiveness of pulmonary secretions. Its chemical action breaks up the mucus.

Indications

- Used for COPD, cystic fibrosis, and pneumonia, and used to assist in tracheostomy care.

- Effective as an antidote to acetaminophen toxicity if used within 24 hr of the poisoning.

Adverse Effects, Contraindications

- Asthmatic patients may experience bronchospasm.
- Acetylcysteine has a wide margin of safety, but it may cause stomatitis, nausea, or rhinorrhea.

Dosage, Administration

- Usually given by nebulization for about 15 min, t.i.d. or q.i.d. It takes 5 to 10 min for maximum effects to occur.
- When used as an antidote to acetaminophen toxicity, Acetylcysteine is given orally. Initial dose is 140 mg/kg, followed by 70 mg/kg every 4 hours for 17 doses (total of 1,330 mg/kg). If the patient is unconscious, acetylcysteine is given through a nasogastric tube.

Nursing Tips

- Remember other methods for liquifying secretions (e.g. forcing fluids, using a vaporizer).
- Postural drainage and coughing and deep breathing following the treatment are usually helpful.

NEBULIZATION THERAPY

Overview

Many of the medications used to treat chronic obstructive pulmonary disease (COPD) and other respiratory problems *(see SS, Respiratory)* are delivered through nebulization therapy. In nebulization therapy, the medication is suspended in air in the form of small droplets. Ultrasonic nebulization, which makes use of even smaller drops, is frequently employed because the smaller the drops, the more likely they will reach the aveoli. The following types of apparatus are used: hand-held nebulizers, oral inhalers, pump-driven nebulizers, and intermittent positive pressure breathing machines (IPPBs). The following types of drugs are used: bronchodilators, mucolytic agents, antibiotics, and steroids.

Nursing Tips

- When using the oral nebulizers the patient should hold his breath for several seconds before exhaling slowly through pursed lips.
- It is important for patients to avoid overuse of the apparatus and medications because tolerance develops and rebound bronchospasm and adverse cardiac effects can occur.

URINARY SYSTEM
DIURETICS
Nursing Tips

- Diuretics can remove sodium, potassium, hydrogen, chloride, and bicarbonate; therefore all types of electrolyte and acid–base imbalances can occur.
- Monitor serum electrolytes.
- Observe patients for signs of muscle cramps, weakness, fatigue, anorexia, thirst, mental confusion, and vomiting.
- An accurate intake and output must be recorded either by the nurse or the patient. This does not require a physician's order and is a nursing responsibility.
- The patient should be weighed daily, at the same time and on the same scale, while wearing the same type of clothing. Usually, weights are done before breakfast.
- Examine patient for signs of edema. *(See SS, Cardiovascular)*
- Diuretics should be administered early in the day so that the patient's sleep is uninterrupted. Once-a-day diuretics can be administered at 8AM or 10AM; twice-a-day diuretics can be given at 8AM and 2PM.
- To avoid injury to your patients, carefully determine what assistance they will need. The urinal, bedpan, and call light should be within reach. If a patient is independently ambulatory, be sure that extra furniture will not be in his way if he must make a hurried trip to the bathroom.
- Many diuretics result in a loss of potassium, so patients may require a potassium supplement. However, some patients can replace the loss by eating potassium-rich foods (*e.g.,* bananas, tomatoes, citrus fruits and juices, and whole milk).
- Because of the potassium loss that occurs with most diuretic therapy, patients receiving digitalis are more likely to develop toxicity.
- Patients receiving lithium should not use diuretics because of the danger of lithium intoxication.
- Diuretics can potentiate the action of antihypertensives. Reduction in dosage may be necessary.

CARBONIC ANHYDRASE INHIBITORS

Actions

- Inhibit the enzyme carbonic anhydrase.
- In the eye, the secretion of aqueous humor is reduced, resulting in a decrease in intraocular pressure.
- In the kidneys, bicarbonate is lost, which results in the excretion of sodium, potassium, and water.

Indications

- Reduce intraocular pressure in chronic open-angle glaucoma and, preoperatively, in acute closed-angle glaucoma.
- Used with anticonvulsant drugs. Provide additional control of grand mal and petit mal seizures.

Adverse Effects, Contraindications

- Paresthesias (tingling and numbness of the extremities, especially the fingers, toes, and lips).
- Drowsiness and confusion.
- Metabolic acidosis can result from the accumulation of hydrogen and chloride ions in relation to the excretion of bicarbonate ions.
- Hypersensitivity reactions are possible (*e.g.,* fever, rash, and blood dyscrasias).
- Crystalluria and renal calculi are possible.
- Patients with low sodium and potassium levels should not receive carbonic anhydrase inhibitors.
- Do not give to patients with anuria.
- Contraindicated for patients with kidney and liver disease.
- Use carbonic anhydrase inhibitors cautiously for patients with chronic obstructive pulmonary disease (COPD) because these drugs may aggravate acidosis.
- Pregnant women, especially in the first trimester, should avoid all diuretics.

Dosage, Administration

- Acetazolamide, U.S.P. (Diamox)
  1. For congestive heart failure (CHF): Usually a dose of 250 to 375 mg is given p.o., every other day (alternating with another diuretic).
  2. For chronic open-angle glaucoma: Usual dose is 250 mg to 1 g orally per day in divided doses.
  3. For acute closed-angle glaucoma: Preoperative treatment is usually 250 mg orally q. 4 hr. For rapid relief of intraocular pressure the IV route is used (Acetazolamide sodium, U.S.P., Diamox Parenteral).
  4. For epilepsy: Usual range is 375 mg to 1 g, p.o., daily in divided doses. Therapy may begin with 250 mg, p.o., daily and is increased as needed.
  5. For drug-induced edema: Usual range is 250 to 375 mg, p.o., once daily for 1 or 2 days, alternating with a day of rest.

Nursing Tips

(See PH, Diuretics nursing tips)

LOOP OR HIGH-CEILING DIURETICS

Actions

- Inhibit reabsorption of sodium and chloride in the ascending loop of Henle and possibly in both the proximal and distal tubules.
- Cause a greater degree of diuresis than most other diuretics.

Indications

- Relieve edema associated with congestive heart failure, renal disease, and cirrhosis of the liver.
- Intravenous forms are used in acute pulmonary edema.
- Reduce blood pressure when used alone or with other antihypertensives.

Adverse Effects, Contraindications

- Can produce serious fluid and electrolyte imbalances (*e.g.,* hypokalemia—low serum potassium).
- Sudden, massive diuresis can precipitate cardiovascular collapse or blood clot formation.
- Ototoxicity may occur, especially in patients with impaired kidney function, resulting in hearing loss, tinnitus, and vertigo.
- Mild diarrhea may occur. However, Ethacrynic acid can produce profuse, watery diarrhea, which necessitates discontinuing the drug.
- Elevations of blood sugar and serum uric acid may precipitate diabetes and gout.
- Do not give to patients with anuria.
- Use cautiously for patients with advanced cirrhosis of the liver. The electrolyte imbalances may lead to hepatic coma and death.

Dosage, Administration

- The smallest dose necessary to produce a gradual weight loss of 1 to 2 lb per day is recommended.
- Ethacrynic acid, U.S.P. Edecrin: Usual adult daily dose is 50 to 200 mg orally. Treatment is usually started with 50 mg orally after breakfast and is gradually increased by 25 mg or 50 mg as needed. The maximum is usually 200 mg twice daily.
- In emergencies, 50 to 100 mg of sodium ethacrynate may be administered IV.
- Furosemide, U.S.P. (Lasix): Usual adult daily dose is 40 to 80 mg orally. Dosage may be increased carefully (20 to 40 mg every 6 to 8 hr) to a maximum of 600 mg per day.
- In emergencies, 20 to 40 mg of furosemide may be given IM or

IV. Intravenous injection should be given slowly (over 1 to 2 minutes). A second dose may be administered 2 hr after the first.
- If high-dose parenteral therapy is necessary, furosemide may be mixed with isotonic saline, lactated Ringer's or 5% dextrose. The pH of the solutions should be above 5.5. The rate should not exceed 4 mg/min.

Nursing Tips

(See PH, Diuretics: nursing tips)
- Ethacrynic acid can displace warfarin from plasma proteins so it may be necessary to reduce the dosage of the warfarin. Monitor patient's prothrombin time (PT).
- Furosemide and cephaloridine should not be administered concurrently because the chance of nephrotoxicity is increased.
- Furosemide competes with salicylates for renal excretion. Therefore, the salicylates may reach toxic levels in the body.

OSMOTIC DIURETICS

Actions

- These nonelectrolytes are given in quantities sufficient to ensure that only a small amount can be reabsorbed by the renal tubules. The rest remains in the tubules and acts (by osmosis) to keep water from leaving the tubules. Thus the volume of urine produced is increased.
- When in the bloodstream, osmotic diuretics draw fluid from the extravascular spaces into the plasma.

Indications

- Prevent renal failure in situations in which glomerular filtration is severely reduced, for example, when patients have been severely injured and burned, have undergone heart surgery, or have had transfusion reactions.
- Reduce elevated intracranial and intraocular pressure. Therefore, these diuretics are useful during neurosurgery and in treating head injuries, and prior to surgery for acute closed-angle glaucoma or detached retina.

Adverse Effects, Contraindications

- Disorientation, confusion, and headache.
- Nausea and vomiting.
- Give cautiously to patients with severely impaired kidney, liver, or cardiac function.

- Dehydrated patients or those with active intracranial bleeding should not receive osmotic diuretics.
- Extravasation of the fluid into the surrounding tissue causes irritation and possible tissue necrosis.
- Convulsions and anaphylaxis have been reported with *mannitol.*
- Not indicated for use with chronic edema.
- Do not give to patients with anuria.

Dosage Administration

- Mannitol, U.S.P. (Osmitrol): Usual daily adult dose is 50 to 100 g, IV, in a 15%-20% solution.
- Urea, U.S.P. (Ureaphil): Usual daily dose is 40 to 120 g, IV, in a 4% or 30% solution.
  1. The 30% solution is used for reducing intracranial pressure. Infuse slowly (3 or 4 ml per minute).
  2. The 4% solution is used to treat oliguria. Infuse slowly (1500 to 3000 ml in 24 hr).

Nursing Tips

- Osmotic diuretics are usually indicated for use in short-term therapy.
  (See PH, Diuretics: nursing tips)

POTASSIUM-SPARING DIURETICS
SPIRONOLACTONE, U.S.P. (ALDACTONE)
Actions

- Blocks the action of aldosterone in the distal portion of the renal tubule.
- Increased amounts of sodium and water are excreted, and potassium is retained.

Indications

- Assists in management of primary hyperaldosteronism.
- Used adjunctively to relieve the edema of congestive heart failure and the nephrotic syndrome when other diuretics do not produce a satisfactory response.
- Relieves the edema and ascites of cirrhosis of the liver.
- Used in combination with other drugs to manage essential hypertension.
- Treats hypokalemia (low potassium) when other measures do not produce a satisfactory response. Used on a prophylactic basis for patients receiving digitalis.

Adverse Effects, Contraindications

- Potassium retention resulting in hyperkalemia. The high potassium levels can precipitate cardiac arrhythmias and arrest.
- Excessive loss of sodium (hyponatremia) can result in mouth dryness, thirst, lethargy, and drowsiness.
- Spironolactone is a steroid that can cause gynecomastia, deepening of the voice, hirsutism, irregular menses or amenorrhea, and impotence.
- Do not give to patients with anuria.

Dosage, Administration

- For edema: Usual adult dosage is 25 mg, q.i.d., orally. After 5 days, if response is inadequate, a diuretic that acts in the proximal renal tubule may be added.
- For essential hypertension: Usual adult dosage is 50 to 100 mg per day, orally, in divided doses. Frequently given with antihypertensives and other diuretics.
- For hypokalemia: Usual adult dosage is 25 to 100 mg per day, orally.
- For primary hyperaldosteronism: Usual adult dosage is 100 to 400 mg per day, orally, in preparation for surgery.

Nursing Tips

(See PH, Diuretics: nursing tips)

- When spironolactone is used all potassium supplements are usually discontinued, and a diet high in potassium is discouraged.
- Diabetics, the elderly, and patients with impaired kidney function are at greatest risk for developing hyperkalemia.
- Only one potassium-sparing diuretic should be used at a time because of the danger of hyperkalemia.

TRIAMTERENE, U.S.P. (DYRENIUM)

Actions

- Acts on the distal portion of the renal tubule to block sodium–potassium and sodium–hydrogen exchange mechanisms.

Indications

- Reduces the edema of congestive heart failure, the nephrotic syndrome, and cirrhosis of the liver.
- Relieves steroid-induced edema.
- Aids in preventing hypokalemia, thereby reducing the danger of toxicity in patients taking digitalis.

Adverse Effects, Contraindications

- Potassium retention resulting in hyperkalemia. The high potassium levels can precipitate cardiac arrhythmias and arrest.
- Excessive loss of sodium (hyponatremia) can result in mouth dryness, thirst, lethargy, and drowsiness.
- Diarrhea, nausea, and vomiting can occur.
- Weakness, headache, rash, and photosensitivity are possible.
- Blood dyscrasias have been reported.
- Do not give to patients with anuria.
- Use cautiously in patients with impaired liver and kidney function.

Dosage, Administration

- Usual adult daily dose is 100 to 200 mg orally (frequently given 100 mg twice daily after meals).

Nursing Tips

(See PH, Diuretics: nursing tips)
- When triamterene is used all potassium supplements are usually discontinued, and a diet high in potassium is discouraged.
- Diabetics, the elderly, and patients with impaired kidney function are at greatest risk for developing hyperkalemia.
- Only one potassium-sparing diuretic should be used at a time because of the danger of hyperkalemia.
- Monitor blood counts for evidence of blood dyscrasias.

THIAZIDES

Actions

- Block active tubular reabsorption of chloride and sodium in the ascending loop of Henle.
- Reduce elevated blood pressure.

Indications

- Reduce the edema of congestive heart failure, cirrhosis, and renal dysfunctions.
- Relieve drug-induced edema from steroid and estrogen therapy.
- Reduce hypertension. May be used alone in mild hypertension or concurrently with other antihypertensive drugs for more severe hypertension.
- Produce a more concentrated urine in some patients with diabetes insipidus.

Adverse Effects, Contraindications

- Hypokalemia (low serum potassium) is a common electrolyte imbalance resulting from thiazide therapy.

- Serum glucose levels may rise, resulting in the symptoms of diabetes mellitus.
- Blood levels of uric acid may rise, precipitating an attack of gout.
- Patients with severe liver or kidney disease should use the thiazides cautiously. Hepatic coma or kidney failure are possible.
- Do not give to patients with anuria.
- Anorexia, nausea, vomiting, diarrhea, or constipation can occur.

Dosage, Administration

- Chlorothiazide, U.S.P. (Diuril)
  1. For edema: Usual adult dosage is 0.5 to 1 g, p.o., daily. Some patients may achieve good results by taking the drug only 3 to 5 days per week. With an intermittent schedule electrolyte imbalance is less likely.
  2. For hypertension: Usual adult starting dosage is 0.5 to 1 g, p.o., daily. Rarely, up to 2 g per day in divided doses is used.
- Hydrochlorothiazide, U.S.P. (Hydrodiuril)
  1. For edema: Usual adult dosage is 50 to 200 mg, p.o., daily in divided doses. As with chlorothiazide, an intermittent schedule (3 to 5 days per week) may be sufficient.
  2. For hypertension: Usual initial adult dosage is 50 to 100 mg, p.o., daily. Rarely, up to 200 mg per day in divided doses is used.

Nursing Tips

(See PH, Diuretics: nursing tips)

BIBLIOGRAPHY

BOOKS

Bergersen B: Pharmacology in Nursing, 14th ed. St Louis, CV Mosby, 1979

Curren A: Math for Meds, 3rd ed. Seal Beach, CA, Wallcur, 1979

Gilman AG, Goodman L, Gilman A (eds): The Pharmacological Basis of Therapeutics, 6th ed. New York, MacMillan, 1980

Lamy P: Prescribing for the Elderly. Littleton, MA, PSG Publishing, 1980

Physicians' Desk Reference, 34th ed. Oradell, NJ, Medical Economics Company, 1980

Rodman M, Smith D: Pharmacology and Drug Therapy in Nursing, 2nd ed. Philadelphia, JB Lippincott, 1979

JOURNALS

Allen M: Drug therapy in the elderly. Am J Nurs 80(8): 1474–1475, August, 1980

Burkle W: What you should know about tagamet. Nursing 80 10(4):86–87, April 1980

Chamberlain S: Low-dose heparin therapy. Am J Nurs 80(6):1115–1117, June, 1980

Fuller E: The effect of antianginal drugs on myocardial oxygen consumption. Am J Nurs 80(2):250–254, February, 1980

Gever L: Acetaminophen overdose. Nursing 80 10(6):57, June, 1980

Gever L: New thinking about parenteral iron supplements. Nursing 80 10(8):60, August, 1980

Gever L: Reducing the side effects of steroid therapy. Nursing 80 10(9):59, September, 1980

Gresh C: Helpful tips you can give your patients with Parkinson's disease. Nursing 80 10(1):26–33, January, 1980

Hansen MS, Woods S: Nitroglycerin ointment—where and how to apply it. Am J Nurs 80(6):1122–1124, June, 1980

Hussar D: New Drugs. Nursing 80 10(5):24–32, May, 1980

Maxwell M: Scalp tourniquets for chemotherapy—induced alopecia. Am J Nurs 80(5):900–903, May, 1980

Meissner J, Gever L: Reducing the risks of digitalis toxicity. Nursing 80 10(9):32–38, September, 1980

Satterwhite B: What to do when adriamycin infiltrates. Nursing 80 10(2):37, February, 1980

Smith–Collins A: Dobutamine, a new inotropic agent. Nursing 80 10(3):62–66, March, 1980

Stanford J, Felner J, Arensberg D: Antiarrhythmic drug therapy. Am J Nurs 80(7):1288–1295, July, 1980

Webber–Jones J, Bryant M: Over-the-counter bronchodilators. Nursing 80 10(1):34–39, January, 1980

Welch D, Lewis K: Alopecia and chemotherapy. Am J Nurs 80(5):903–905, May, 1980

5

Systems and Specialties (SS)

Thyroid
Simple goiter
Hypothyroidism (myxedema)
Hyperthyroidism (Graves' disease)
Thyroidectomy and subtotal thyroidectomy
Thyroid storm (thyroid crisis)
Gastrointestinal system
Anorectal conditions
Adenomatous polyps
Esophageal varices
Gallbladder
Gastrointestinal bleeding (the GI bleeder)
Hernia
Abdominal hernia
Hiatal hernia
Inflammation of the intestinal tract
Appendicitis
Diverticulitis and diverticulosis
Meckel's diverticulum
Peritonitis
Regional enteritis (Crohn's disease)
Ulcerative colitis
Liver
Cirrhosis
Hepatic tumors
Liver abscess
Viral hepatitis
Obstruction of the intestinal tract
Pancreas
Acute pancreatitis
Chronic pancreatitis
Peptic ulcer
Pilonidal cysts
Surgery (gastrointestinal)
Gastric surgery
Intestinal surgery
Neurological system
Chronic organic brain syndrome
Increased intracranial pressure
Infections
Acute bacterial meningitis
Acute viral encephalitis
Multiple sclerosis

Introduction

ASSESSMENTS
NEUROLOGICAL

Reliable and consistent assessments of consciousness levels are required, especially when brain damage is present. This can be obtained through the use of the Glasgow Coma Scale (GCS), which was developed at the University of Glasgow (Fig. 5-1). It is widely used as a method of grading changes in motor, verbal, and eye responses of patients with recent brain damage. Additionally, pupil size and reaction, along with vital signs, are recorded when "neuro checks" are indicated.

SYSTEMS
Assessment

For systems assessment, write heading on left of page and chart assessment information to the right after each heading in narrative form.*

- Central Nervous System (CNS)
  1. Level of consciousness; orientation to time, place, and person.
  2. Pupil reaction; movement and degree of strength or weakness of extremities.
  3. Appropriateness of speech and behavior; sensitivity to pain.
- Skin
  1. Color.
  2. Skin temperature and general condition (dryness, turgor, lesions).
  3. Condition of IV insertion site.
- Cardiovascular System (CVS)
  1. Signs of Congestive Heart Failure (CHF)

*Developed by Carolyn Smith Marker, R.N.

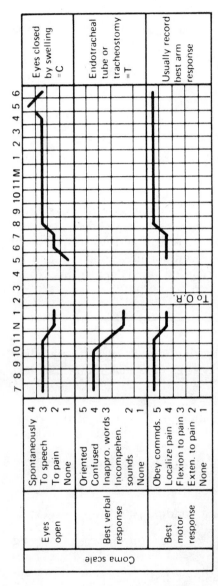

FIG. 5-1. *The Glasgow Coma Scale (GCS). The scale includes three parts—assessment of eye opening, verbal response, and motor response. Each can be assessed hourly, given a numerical value, and plotted graphically. A patient's neurological status—unchanged, deteriorating, or improving—can then be monitored. In the GCS above, the patient remained stable until 10 AM, rapidly deteriorated between 10 AM and 1 PM, at which time he went to the operating room. Postoperatively, his GCS improved.* (Jones C: The Glasgow coma scale. Am J Nurs, Vol 79, No 9, 1979. Copyright © 1979, American Journal of Nursing Company. Reproduced with permission.)

   a. Auscultate chest for quality of breath sounds and congestion.
   b. Presence of dyspnea at rest or with exertion.
   c. Appearance of neck veins at 45 degrees (flat or distended).
   d. Presence of peripheral edema (hands, sacrum, lower extremities).
2. Heart tones (strong, regular, distant, muffled), murmurs, friction rub, and so forth.
3. Vital signs
   a. Quality of pulses; absence or presence of peripheral pulses.
   b. Quality of blood pressure (BP) as well as numerical value
   c. Apical/radial pulse (document presence of deficit).
- Pulmonary
1. Respiratory rate and quality (labored, shallow, and so forth).
2. Chest auscultation (quality of breath sounds, retained secretions).
3. Description of quality and quantity of secretions.
4. Mode of oxygenation (tracheostomy, mask, nasal prongs).
5. Type and frequency of chest physiotherapy.
6. Chest dressings or tubes (quality/quantity of drainage and suction).
- Gastrointestinal (GI)
1. Palpate and auscultate abdomen (for bowel sounds, distention, tenderness, softness).
2. Describe appetite, or if the patient is not to eat, write n.p.o.
3. Nasogastric tubes (quality and quantity of drainage, type of tube, amount of suction).
4. Abdominal dressings (dry, saturated, changed, reinforced).
5. Wound (describe appearance).
- Genitourinary (GU)
1. Foley: voiding/not voiding.
2. Quality/quantity of drainage and specific gravity if necessary.

Subjective Data

Document subjective data from patient interview/discussion. (State how your patient says he feels; *e.g.,* SOB, tired, weak.)

Evaluation

Document effectiveness of your nursing approaches in meeting present nursing-care goals. Notes should contain evaluative statements and should describe patient appearance (assessment), verbalization, or any action that indicates achievement of or direction toward stated nursing-care goal. It should be understood that goals of care are incorporated into the nursing-care plan.

PREOPERATIVE CARE

The following are the highlights of general preoperative care. Care for a specific situation is included in the section in Systems and Specialties that deals with that situation (*e.g.*, gastrointestinal surgery, thyroidectomy).

ON ADMISSION

- Confirm that the information on the patient's identification bracelet is correct.
- Obtain nursing history. Question patient as to his most recent use of aspirin. Some surgeons will not operate on a patient who has taken aspirin during the previous two weeks.
- Collect specimens and arrange for laboratory tests as needed.
- Orient patient to his environment, making sure that the call bell is within his reach.
- Assessment of vital signs is essential to provide baseline data.
- Provide emotional support.

PREOPERATIVE TEACHING

The goal of preoperative teaching is to prepare the patient for his postoperative situation. Inclusion of family members in the instruction is especially helpful if they will be at the patient's bedside when he returns from surgery. Both the patient and his family should have a realistic idea about what his condition is likely to be and what therapies may be in progress (*e.g.*, oxygen administration, nasogastric suction, chest tubes, casts, traction). In addition

- They need to understand why he will be turned frequently and encouraged to move his arms and legs.
- Foreknowledge that frequent monitoring of the patient's blood pressure postoperatively is one of the usual ways of following a patient's progress may allay unnecessary fears.
- They should know that the patient's postoperative pain will be controlled and that he should ask for medication when the pain begins.
- The patient will need "how to" instruction and an opportunity to practice deep breathing techniques. (*See NR, Deep breathing techniques*)

GENERAL PREOPERATIVE ORDERS

- An *enema* is usually ordered. Results and how procedure was tolerated should be noted.
- *Skin preparation of the operative site* and the area around it will usually be ordered (see Fig. 5-2).

1. The skin will be washed with soap and water or a bacterial skin cleanser.
2. The shave should be carefully done with a sharp razor. The skin must not be broken.
3. Follow with a scrub or shower, using povidone-iodine solution (Betadine or Isodine) or other antibacterial solution, if ordered. In some cases, the area is patted dry with a sterile towel and covered with another one. Check for hospital procedure or specific orders.

- A sedative is usually ordered for the evening before surgery. The patient should be encouraged to take it. Side rails should be up.
- The patient receives nothing by mouth (n.p.o.) for at least 8 hours prior to surgery, and his cooperation should be enlisted. If the patient is scheduled for morning surgery, his chart and room will be marked "n.p.o. after midnight" or with the appropriate directions. *Caution:* Check with the physician as to whether any medications are to be given in spite of the n.p.o. instruction (*e.g.,* some cardiac medications and antithyroid medications are often given right up to the time of surgery).
- Check to be sure that "consent for surgery" forms have been signed and that appropriate laboratory reports for laboratory work as ordered, or as required by hospital policy, are in the chart. Variations from normal should be called to the attention of the surgeon. If blood has been ordered, slips indicating that blood has been typed and crossmatched, and that it is available, should be in the chart.

IMMEDIATE PREOPERATIVE CARE

- Vital signs should be taken before preoperative medications are given. Any variation from normal should be reported.
- A shower is usually encouraged if the patient's condition, the procedure regarding preparation of the operative site, and time permit.
- Antiembolism stockings are usually ordered.
- The patient is asked to void.
- The patient is asked to remove jewelry, hair pins, contact lenses, dentures, and removable bridges, though some hospitals allow full dentures to be left in. Check hospital policy. Follow hospital policy regarding care of valuables.
- An intravenous infusion may be started in the patient's room with a needle of large enough gauge (#19) for administration of blood.
- A preoperative intramuscular injection is usually scheduled to be given 1 hour before anesthesia is scheduled. It usually contains a

(*Text continues on p. 276*)

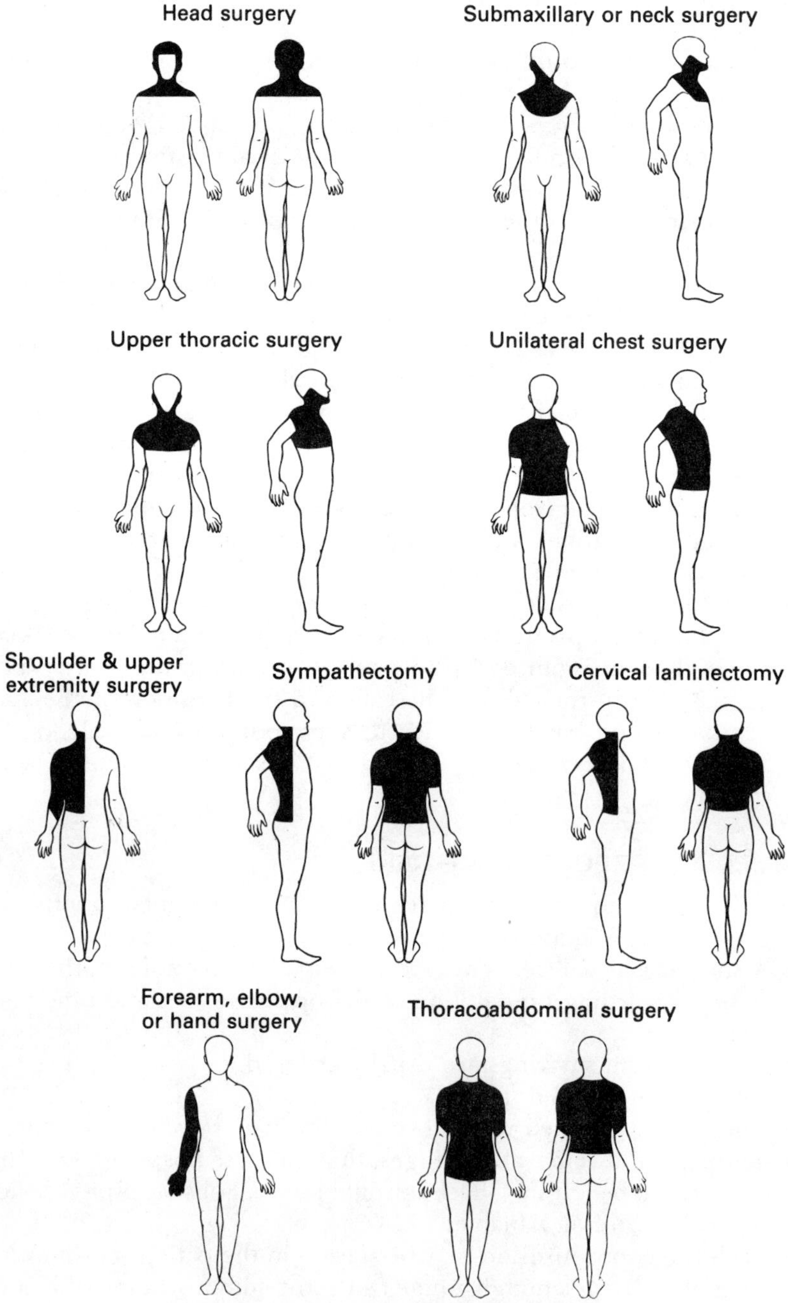

FIG. 5-2. *Preoperative preparation chart.*

Abdominal surgery

Lumbar laminectomy

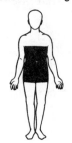

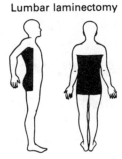

Unilateral surgery of
posterior lumbar region

Renal & upper ureteral surgery

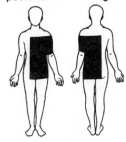

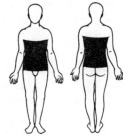

Gynecological & genito-
urinary surgery

Anorectal surgery

Unilateral
hip surgery

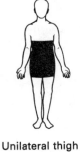

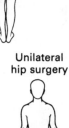

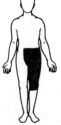

Unilateral thigh
& leg surgery

Lower leg &
foot surgery

Ankle, foot,
or toe surgery

Inguinal area
surgery

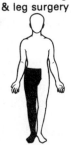

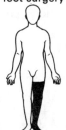

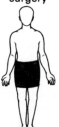

FIG. 5-2. *Continued.*

narcotic and an anticholinergic. Advise the patient that his mouth will feel dry, that he will feel drowsy, and that he must stay in bed. Side rails should be up.

POSTOPERATIVE CARE

IMMEDIATE CARE (when patient returns from surgery)

Positioning:

- The unconscious patient should always be positioned on his side to prevent aspiration of vomitus or obstruction of his airway by his tongue.
- Head should be to the side. The airway should remain in place until the patient coughs it out.
- Side rails should be up.

Extra warmth: enough for comfort, but not enough to cause the patient to perspire profusely.

- The patient may require an extra thermal blanket. Remember that to be effective the thermal blanket should be covered with a bath blanket or some covering with a closer weave.
- Bath blankets next to the patient provide extra warmth.

Monitor for signs of shock and hemorrhage:

- Preoperative assessment of vital signs is essential to provide a baseline.
- Vital signs are monitored carefully, usually q. 15 min, 8 times, and then q. 30 min, 4 times, or until stable.

SHOCK

What to Look for

- Baseline vital signs: watch trends.
- Falling blood pressure (BP): systolic reading dropping over 20 mm Hg, or drops in BP shown consistently when taken q. 15 min.
- Narrow pulse pressure (the difference between systolic and diastolic blood pressures).
- Rapid, weak pulse; rapid breathing.
- Cold, moist, pale skin.
- Failure of a compressed nail bed to fill within a fraction of a second after compression. In shock, capillary filling may take several seconds.
- Patient's level of consciousness. How does he feel?
- Fluid intake and output during surgery; estimated blood loss.

Laboratory

- Arterial blood gases (ABGs).
- Serum lactate (the higher the elevation above normal, the greater the oxygen need).
- Hematocrit.

Treatment

- Elevate the legs about 20°, leaving the rest of the body flat. *Caution:* In cases of possible increased intracranial pressure, keep the patient's position flat.
- If no IV is running, start one, so that line is available. *(See NR, Intravenous therapy)*
- Blood volume will be restored according to need, with blood, electrolyte solutions, or volume expanders.
- Cover patient with light blanket to keep him warm, though not warm enough to perspire.
- Oxygen therapy may be required. *(See NR, Oxygen administration)*
- Cardiovascular medications, as ordered.
- Indwelling catheter with urinometer, for accurate measurement of urinary output. Output under 30 ml/hr should be called to the attention of the physician. *(See NR, Urinary bladder catheterization)*

HEMORRHAGE

What to Look for

- Apprehensiveness, restlessness, and thirst (salivary glands, especially in shock from hemorrhage, are very sensitive to even slight decreases in circulating blood volume).
- Tachycardia (rapid heart rate), deep rapid respirations, falling blood pressure (BP), and orthostatic hypotension. *(See NR, Postural hypotension)*
- Cool, moist, pale skin.
- Symptoms of shock. *(See above, "shock: what to look for")*
- Look for visible evidence of bleeding. Check under the patient with your hand. Blood or drainage may seep out of the dressing and pool underneath the patient and may be unseen on superficial inspection.
- Check the dressing. Mark the perimeters of any fresh spot on top of the dressing with a pen, and include the time. If the perimeter of the spot extends, you will have objective evidence that bleeding continues.

Treatment

- Start IV to replace blood volume with appropriate component.
- Treat shock if present.

PAIN CONTROL

Pain control is vital for the patient's comfort and postoperative recovery. *(See MNS, Pain management)*

PREVENTION OF VASCULAR COMPLICATIONS

(See SS, Cardiovascular system, Thrombophlebitis)

- Reposition the postoperative patient every 2 hours. Teach him to use the side rail to help himself (if appropriate).
- Range of motion exercises—first passive and then active. *(See NR, Range of Motion Exercises)*
- Early ambulation, on surgeon's order.
- Assessment for phlebothrombosis (clot formation in a vein)
  1. *Homan's sign:* pain in the calf upon dorsiflexion of the foot with the leg extended.
  2. Pain in the calf at gentle pressure.
- Elastic support stockings are usually applied preoperatively, are changed daily, and are worn postoperatively until danger of thrombosis is minimal.

PREVENTION OF RESPIRATORY COMPLICATIONS

- Identify patients who are at higher risk: those with existing respiratory problems (*e.g.* chronic obstructive pulmonary disease (COPD) or upper respiratory infections); those with high abdominal incisions or chest incisions; those with congestive heart failure; those who are overweight, malnourished, anemic, or elderly; and those who have had a prolonged time in surgery, particularly if an endotracheal tube or oxygen have been used.
- Watch for signs of atelectasis: elevated temperature, respirations that are labored or shallow and rigid, cyanosis (a late symptom), confusion (caused by anoxia), agitation (caused by hypoxia), and diminished breath sounds on the affected side.
- Watch for signs of pneumonia: elevated temperature, rusty-colored sputum, cough, chest pain, decreased chest movement on the affected side, and absence of chest sounds on the affected side. *(See SS, Pneumonia)*
- Assist patient to ventilate completely (5 to 10 deep breaths every hour) by teaching him to splint his incision and to use one of the deep breathing techniques *(see NR, Deep breathing techniques)*. En-

courage patient responsibility for this and for frequent position changes, if possible. Involve the family.

- Oxygen therapy is sometimes ordered. *(See NR, Oxygen administration)*

MANAGEMENT OF NAUSEA AND VOMITING

- Important not only for the patient's comfort, but also to prevent strain on the incision.
- Position patient on his side while he is recovering from anesthesia to prevent aspiration of vomitus.
- Describe symptoms and amount and character of vomitus.
- Administer antiemetic medications, as ordered. *(See PH, Gastrointestinal system)*
- Nasogastric tube to suction may be ordered. *(See NR, Gastrointestinal intubation)*
- Monitor for electrolyte imbalances. If they occur, correct with IV therapy as ordered. *(See LAB and NR, Intravenous therapy, electrolyte imbalances)*

MANAGEMENT OF ABDOMINAL DISTENTION

- Auscultate (listen with a stethoscope) for bowel sounds. Nothing by mouth until peristalsis has returned, signaled by passing of flatus (gas), or stool or the return of bowel sounds. *(See SS, Paralytic ileus)*
- Nasogastric tube to low intermittent suction. Be sure tube is patent.
- Turn the patient q. 2 hr. Have him move.
- Rectal tubes or enemas may be ordered.

PREVENTION OF ELECTROLYTE IMBALANCES

(See LAB)
- Monitor for electrolyte imbalances, especially when nasogastric suction is in use, drainage is profuse, vomiting persists, or diarrhea is present.
- Measure intake and output accurately. Monitor weight.
- Imbalances are corrected with supplements ordered by the physician and usually administered in IV therapy. *(See NR, Intravenous therapy, electrolyte imbalances)*

MANAGEMENT OF VOIDING PROBLEMS

- Most patients will urinate within the first 12 hours following surgery. Check doctor's orders or hospital policy to find out when physician should be notified if this has not occurred.
- Try nursing measures to promote voiding (*e.g.*, allowing male pa-

tient to stand at the bedside—if permitted; running water within earshot of the patient; and providing privacy and a warm bedpan or urinal).

- Palpate for a distended bladder, especially if patient is voiding small amounts of urine frequently. The patient may be experiencing retention with overflow.
- Catheterization should be avoided if possible, but may be ordered if problem persists. *(See NR, Urinary bladder catheterization)*

PROMOTION OF WOUND HEALING

- Identify patients who are at high risk for wound complications. Factors that increase risk are anemia, being overweight or underweight, smoking, low serum albumin level, diabetes, radiation therapy at proposed operative site, certain cancers, and certain medications (*e.g.*, aspirin and the steroids).
- The surgeon may prefer to do the first dressing change. Thereafter if dressing changes are ordered, use scrupulous sterile technique. Remove soiled dressing down to the primary dressing or wound, and apply a sterile one. Never simply cover a wet dressing with a dry one.
- Inspect the wound during dressing changes for closure, drainage, and signs of infection (*e.g.*, redness or pus formation). Document appearance of the wound.
- If there is copious drainage from the wound or a drain, protect the skin by keeping it dry. Apply a collecting bag, when appropriate. *(See NR, Ostomies, fistulas, and draining wounds)*
  1. Montgomery straps facilitate ease of dressing changes in any situation where a wound with copious drainage requires a large dressing (see Fig. 5-3). Since the straps eliminate frequent tape changes, they also protect the skin. Ties should be tied shoelace style for greater security.
- Dry wounds are now often being left open to the air (without a dressing). Inspect and palpate the wound frequently. Look for the following:
  1. Warmth along the wound should disappear after approximately 72 hours postoperatively. Palpate with the back of the hand.
  2. Thereafter, warmth in one area of the incision may indicate impending infection.
  3. Healing ridge is normal and healthy, developing after 5 to 7 days postoperatively. If it is not easy to palpate, complications (*e.g.*, hernia or wound dehiscence) may be anticipated.
- Surgical drains, tubes, and catheters may be used when there is an

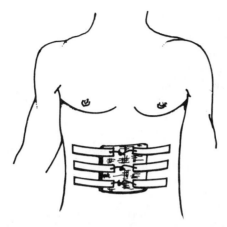

FIG. 5-3. *Montgomery straps are used for dressings that must be changed frequently.* (Wolff L, Weitzel MH, Fuerst EV: Fundamentals of Nursing, 6th ed, p 543. Philadelphia, JB Lippincott, 1980)

abscess cavity; insecure closure of the GI tract; anticipated leakage, as in gallbladder or pancreatic surgery; trauma; or radical surgery. The nurse should

1. Understand why drain is in place.
2. Know what is expected if tube is draining properly.
3. Be sure that tube is adequately secured.
4. Observe and record the nature and volume of the drainage.

- Wound complications include infection, dehiscence, and eviscera-tion. *(See SS, Wound dehiscence and evisceration)*

POSTOPERATIVE COMPLICATIONS
PARALYTIC ILEUS
Description

Paralytic (adynamic) ileus describes the condition in which intes-tinal peristalsis is absent or decreased. Some measure of ileus is com-mon the first 2 or 3 days following abdominal surgery and usually disappears spontaneously. It is also associated frequently with peri-tonitis, trauma, vertebral compression fracture, electrolyte deficien-cies (especially hypokalemia), and mechanical obstruction.

Common Diagnostic Tests

- X-ray: flat plate of abdomen shows loops of small bowel distended with gas.

What to Look for

- Abdominal distention and tenderness.
- Persistent gas pains.
- Vomiting after eating.
- Absence of bowel sounds.
- Failure to pass feces or gas.

Prevention

- Nasointestinal tube to suction postoperatively, until peristalsis has returned. Most physicians withhold food and fluids until that time.

Treatment

- Nasointestinal tube to suction. *(See NR, Gastrointestinal intubation)*
- Intravenous fluids. *(See NR, Intravenous therapy)*
- Medications that stimulate intestinal activity are occasionally used, *e.g.*, dexpanthenol (Ilopan), vasopressin (Pitressin), bethanechol (Urecholine), and neostigmine (Prostigmin). *Caution:* If there is a possibility of mechanical obstruction, medications are used cautiously, since they could cause perforation.
- Rectal tube for 30 minutes t.i.d. may be ordered.

Nursing Tips

- Watch for return of normal function, signaled by the return of bowel sounds heard with a stethoscope and the passage of flatus. The patient should be instructed to tell the nurse when "gas" is first passed.
- Manage the nasointestinal tube to suction. Record the amount and describe the drainage. *(See NR, Gastrointestinal intubation)*

SEPTIC SHOCK

Description

Septic shock is a complication of a complication, the result of a potentially avoidable nosocomial (hospital acquired) infection. It is believed to be due to the effects of cell damage caused by endotoxins produced by gram-negative bacteria, especially *Escherichia coli, Proteus,* and *Pseudomonas.* (Gram-positive bacteria rarely cause shock.) Patients at risk include those who are debilitated, those over 60 years of age, and those who have undergone urinary, gastrointestinal, or biliary tract instrumentation. The urinary tract is the portal of entry in over 50% of these infections.

Common Diagnostic Tests

- Blood culture and sensitivity: to identify offending organism. *(See LAB, Cultures)*

- Complete blood count (CBC), arterial blood gases (ABGs), electrolyte screen, and central venous pressure (CVP).

What to Look for

- Baseline clinical data is vital: trends are important.
- Early signs include
  1. Chills and fever; warm, dry, flushed skin.
  2. Increasing pulse and respiratory rates (pulse may be full and often bounding).
  3. Urine output may be normal or increased.
  4. Blood pressure normal or slightly elevated, with widening pulse pressure. (Pulse pressure is the difference between systolic and diastolic pressure).
  5. Deteriorating mental status (confusion, restlessness, apprehension, lethargy).
- Untreated septic shock progresses rapidly.
- Late signs include
  1. Elevated pulse and respiratory rates.
  2. Cool, clammy, mottled, cyanotic skin.
  3. Oliguria (markedly decreased urine output).
  4. Decreased blood pressure.

Treatment

- Identification and treatment of infections before they reach the shock stage.
- When shock exists:
  1. Oxygen therapy. *(See NR, Oxygen administration)*
  2. Mechanical ventilation may be started.
  3. Intravenous fluids immediately. *(See NR, Intravenous therapy)*
  4. Specific antibiotics to treat infection. *(See PH, Antimicrobials)*

Nursing Tips

- Hand washing, good catheter care *(see NR, Urinary bladder drainage)*, and the use of aseptic technique when providing wound care are vital measures in the prevention of infection.
- Observe all patients carefully for signs of infection. Be aware of those who are at high risk for septic shock, especially those with long-term indwelling catheters.

WOUND DEHISCENCE AND EVISCERATION
Description

Separation of the edges of a wound is called *dehiscence*. This complication is especially serious in abdominal wounds. It is more likely to occur in a lengthy vertical incision or following hasty, emergency surgery. In *evisceration,* intestinal contents protrude. Malignancy, prolonged paralytic ileus, malnutrition, and advanced age are predisposing factors.

What to Look for

- The patient may feel something pop, as sutures give way and the wound opens.
- This may be followed by the escape of large amounts of serous fluid.
- Evisceration usually occurs suddenly, in the debilitated or obese patient after a sudden cough or strain.

Nursing Tips

- Cover the wound and the evisceration with a sterile towel moistened with sterile normal saline. Do not try to return the intestines to their place.
- Keep the patient flat in bed with knees slightly flexed.
- Notify the physician immediately. The operating room will also be notified.
- Stay with the patient.
- Treat for shock. *(See SS, Postoperative care)*

Cardiovascular System

ARTERIAL OCCLUSIVE DISEASE OF THE LOWER EXTREMITIES

Description

Arterial occlusive disease is the result of a decreased arterial blood flow to the lower extremities, generally caused by a gradual narrowing of the arteries. It manifests itself by pain, skin breakdown, and slow healing often accompanied by infection and gangrene. This disease is often seen in diabetics. An acute arterial occlusion may occur as the result of an embolism that has traveled to the site or a thrombus that has formed at the site.

Common Diagnostic Tests

- Doppler measurements of the lower extremities. *(See NR, Ultrasound)*
- Arteriograms (angiograms).
- Tests to rule out or confirm diabetes. *(See LAB)*

What to Look for

- Intermittent claudication—a muscle pain commonly in the calf of the leg or in the foot, which occurs during exercise and is relieved by rest.
- Rest pain—occurs in advanced cases in which the pain may awaken a sleeping person.
- Pedal pulses are absent or weak; hair loss on the leg and foot.
- Cyanosis and coolness of the legs and feet, frequently starting with just the toes.
- Taut and shiny skin and toenails that are thick and distorted are signs of poor circulation.
- Leg ulcers, resulting from vascular insufficiency.

- Sudden severe pain in the leg(s) and loss of sensation and function with cold and pale skin, which indicates an arterial occlusion. *RE-QUIRES IMMEDIATE MEDICAL ATTENTION.*

Treatment

- Anticoagulants (*e.g.*, heparin, warfarin). *(See PH, Cardiovascular system)*
- Pain management. *(See PH, Central nervous system)*
- Regulation of diabetes, including diabetic teaching. *(See SS, Diabetes)*
- Leg ulcers are treated in a variety of ways, but the basic procedure is to first medicate for pain before beginning treatment. A wound culture is taken *(see LAB)* and often oral or topical antibiotics are prescribed *(see PH, Antimicrobials).* The ulcer is washed with sterile saline, patted dry, and sterile saline-soaked gauze or one of a variety of ointments is applied. When simple debridement is necessary, it can often be done with hydrogen peroxide; in severe cases surgical intervention may be required. Skin grafts may be necessary for those ulcers that do not heal. *(See MNS, Decubitus ulcer prevention and treatment)*
- Surgical replacement or bypass of a severely occluded area of an artery using either a synthetic or a venous graft. An endarterectomy (incision and removal of an obstruction in an artery) may also be done.

Nursing Tips

- The treatment of arterial occlusive disease of the lower extremities is aimed at preventing skin breakdown, infection, and leg ulcers.
- In daily assessment, emphasize the necessity of keeping the feet clean and dry; of wearing shoes that are well fitted; of getting prompt medical attention for any cut or sore before it becomes infected; of never wearing garters; of not crossing the knees or standing or sitting too long; and of not smoking, which causes venous constriction and vulnerability to burns because of decreased sensation to heat and cold.
- When the pedal, popliteal, and femoral pulses are located, mark each spot with a magic marker, so they will be easy to locate for future palpation.
- Breakdown of the skin of the heel is common in the bedridden patient, especially with diabetics, so do not allow the heels to rest directly on the mattress.
- Inspect the skin between the toes; this is often the first place that cracks in the skin occur.

- When an obstruction occurs in a major blood vessel and ischemia jeopardizes the survival of a limb, vascular surgery is necessary.
- Thrombosis and hemorrhage are the most common complications that occur during the postoperative period. Check the circulation in the feet every 2 hours. Check for circulatory status with a Doppler ultrasound pulse detector if available. Skin temperature and color and nail bed color are conditions that can also be used to check circulatory status. Any changes or fresh bleeding must be reported to the surgeon *immediately.*
- Avoid flexing the knees to prevent pooling of blood and the formation of thrombi in the lower leg.
- When the patient begins to ambulate, encourage walking and deter sitting except for the use of the toilet. This is especially important after arterial grafts have been done to prevent pressure on the graft.
- Following arterial grafts, be especially aware of any evidence of infection externally on the suture line or internally as evidenced by an elevation in temperature. An infection will destroy the graft.

CARDIAC PACEMAKERS

Description

A pacemaker is an electronic device that delivers electrical stimulation to the heart for individuals with low cardiac output due to impaired cardiac electrical impulses. It consists of a pulse generator attached to a catheter with an electrode tip. The catheter is threaded through a large vein into the superior vena cava and from there into the heart where the electrode tip rests on the apex of the right ventricle. Occasionally a thoracotomy is performed, and the electrode is attached directly to the left ventricle. The pulse generator is usually implanted in a pocket of skin in the right upper chest. It is powered by lithium batteries that last 7 to 10 years.

Demand pacemakers are the most commonly used. These are set at a rate consistent with the patient's need for cardiac output. They sense the heart's rate and only fire (called capture) when the heart rate falls below the set rate of the pacemaker.

Nursing Tips

- Patients with new pacemaker insertions are cared for in units having cardiac monitoring equipment. However, they often enter regular hospital units when being treated for unrelated illnesses.
- Know the rate set in the patient's pacemaker. Paste it in large numbers on the front of the chart, so that everyone knows the patient has a pacemaker and the rate.

- Know that hiccups, fainting, and dizziness are signs of pacemaker displacement, generally of the catheter element or the electrode element.
- Pacemakers do not cure heart disease. The need for cardiac medications still exists. A person with a pacemaker needs to take his pulse for 1 full minute daily and report any changes. A decrease of as little as two beats per minute may be significant. Remember, even if a pacemaker patient goes into shock the cardiac rate may not change.
- An identification bracelet should be worn to signify that the person has a pacemaker.
- Review with the patient what he knows and be prepared to fill in the gaps. Note that specific cautions should be observed by avoiding interference from items such as microwave ovens, large motors or generators, and electrical substations. Such interference generally is not encountered unless the patient is within close proximity to the radiation device. Standard home appliances, such as hair dryers and shavers, do not bother modern pacemakers.

CEREBROVASCULAR ACCIDENT

Description

A cerebrovascular accident (CVA), or stroke, occurs when the blood supply to a part of the brain tissue is cut off and the nerve cells in that part of the brain can then no longer function.

A CVA may be described as extracranial or intracranial in origin. Extracranial CVAs are occlusive and are most commonly the result of a thrombus forming on plaque at the bifurcation of the carotid artery. Occasionally an embolus, carried in the blood stream from a damaged heart, will lodge in a cerebral vessel. This is called a cerebral embolism. Intracranial CVAs may be hemorrhagic and are the result of a damaged artery. This type of CVA is most likely to occur in patients with a combination of hypertension and diabetes. The most common CVA is intracranial, resulting from thrombus formation with the lumen of cerebral vessels that have become progressively occluded with plaque.

A stroke in evolution refers to continuing neurological changes over a period of 24 to 48 hours. When the patient ceases to show further progression in neurological impairment, a completed stroke has taken place.

A transient ischemic attack (TIA) is caused by momentary impairment of cerebral blood flow. It may last from 5 to 30 minutes, accompanied by numbness of extremities, fainting or a brief dizzy spell. About 40% of patients experiencing TIAs suffer a full CVA within 2 years if untreated.

Common Diagnostic Tests

- Neurological examination. *(See SS, Assessment)*
- Cerebral arteriogram.
- Brain scan. *(See NR, Scans)*
- CAT scan. *(See NR, Scans)*

What To Look For

- Stroke victims who show some stability or improvement within 24 hours have a good prognosis.
- The most visible sign of a stroke is paralysis of one side of the body. Watch to be sure that the patient can swallow and that the eye on the affected side has a blink reflex. When one cheek puffs out with each expiration, it indicates paralysis of that side of the face.
- Patients with occlusive disease rarely lose consciousness. They only display neurological changes. *(See SS, Neurological System, Increased intracranial pressure)*
- When a hemorrhage is the cause of a CVA, the patient will often have lost consciousness.
- Right-sided hemiplegia (paralysis) indicates injury to the left side of the brain. Symptoms of this type of injury are aphasia, or trouble in speaking and understanding; use of inappropriate words; inability to see on far right; and slowness and caution in movement.
- Left-sided hemiplegia indicates injury to the right side of the brain. Symptoms of this type of injury are spatial and perceptual difficulty, such as trouble in steering a wheelchair and inability to keep place while reading or eating; impulsive movements; and inability to see on far left.
- These symptoms may be very mild and gradually disappear, or they may be severe and lasting, depending on the location and pervasiveness of the CVA.

Treatment

- Anticoagulants (*e.g.,* heparin, warfarin). *(See PH, Cardiovascular system)*
- IV for vein access. *(See NR, Intravenous therapy)*
- Nasogastric tube for feeding. *(See NR, Gastrointestinal intubation)*

Nursing Tips

- Place the patient, when both in and out of bed, so that his unimpaired side is toward the movement in the room. Left hemiplegics have left field cuts, meaning that they have difficulty seeing objects left of center in the field of vision. The opposite is true of right hemiplegics.

- If a patient needs to be fed, never leave him unattended with a tray of hot food. An uncoordinated hand movement can result in burns.
- An unconscious or otherwise disabled patient must be turned from side to side every 2 hours and maintained in a semi-prone position.
- Check unconscious patients for contact lenses and remove them. *(See SS, Eye-patient care)*
- When the eyelids do not close, they must be taped closed. Check with the physician for lubricating drops.
- Airway obstruction caused by the tongue falling backward leads to atelectasis and pneumonia and can result from leaving a helpless patient on his back.
- In dealing with an aphasic patient, remember that speechlessness does not mean deafness or a loss of understanding. Don't shout. Test the patient by asking him to perform a simple task such as winking his eye or by asking him a nonsense question such as "Am I green?" A speech therapist should start therapy as soon as possible and also should be able to help with swallowing difficulties. The nurse must be sure that there is a system of communication. A magic slate is useful, or alphabet cards are good for the patient who is unable to write. Be sure the nurse-call system is one the patient is able to use.
- There are often some memory and personality changes in CVA patients. These may be manifested by difficulty in remembering new information or by carryover learning from one situation to another. Some patients may laugh or cry inappropriately. It is possible to interrupt this behavior by abruptly changing the subject or snapping the fingers, if it is due to emotional instability rather than depression or euphoria. The family needs to be aware of this potential memory and personality change.
- Mouth care is absolutely essential after each feeding. It is especially important to check for food left in the mouth.
- Soft foods are often easier to swallow than liquids. Milk and milk products thicken saliva and mucous secretions, making swallowing more difficult.
- Nighttime darkness is disturbing, and increased restlessness and confusion often occur. Keeping on the lights, radio, or TV is helpful. *(See MNS, Disoriented patients)*
- Physiotherapy should be started at the bedside with range of motion (ROM) exercises as early as possible. The physiotherapist can come to evaluate the patient 24 hours after a completed stroke. Remind the physician to order this.
- The voiding reflex is diminished when a Foley catheter is used for a long time. Also, the incidence of urinary tract infection (UTI)

increases. Within a week after a completed stroke, a toileting schedule of every 1 to 2 hours should begin for relearning bladder control.

CONGESTIVE HEART FAILURE

Description

Congestive Heart Failure (CHF) is a condition in which circulatory congestion exists as a result of the inability of the heart to pump an adequate supply of blood. This manifests itself as left-sided heart failure (LSF) or as right-sided heart failure (RSF) and can range from mild to life-threatening. Failure of either side is generally followed by some degree of failure in the other side. LSF results in lung congestion, which may lead to pulmonary edema, an immediate life-threatening situation. RSF affects primarily the systemic system, with resulting liver congestion and peripheral edema. When CHF is caused solely by lung disease, it is called cor pulmonale. This is common in patients with chronic obstructive pulmonary disease.

Common Diagnostic Tests
- Chest x-ray.
- Arterial blood gases (ABGs). *(See LAB)*

What to Look for
- Restlessness and confusion—symptoms of cerebral anoxia—are early symptoms of CHF.
- LSF can produce rales, cough (productive or nonproductive), and dyspnea. Paroxysmal nocturnal dyspnea (PND) and orthopnea are specific signs of LSF.
- Pulmonary edema is a common complication of LSF that may develop over a period of several hours or within minutes. *It must be treated as an extreme emergency.* Pallor, tachycardia, hypotension or hypertension, increased rales, and cough with blood-tinged sputum are typical of pulmonary edema.
- Pitting edema of the extremities and sacral area generally indicates RSF. As the failure increases the edema may progress bilaterally up the legs and extend into all body tissues. Generalized body edema is called anasarca. In a bedridden patient, leg edema may be absent, and sacral edema may be the only sign of RSF. Presence of jugular vein distention (JVD), most evident when the patient is at a 45° angle, is an indication of increased venous pressure resulting from RSF. Hepatic congestion results in abdominal pain and fluid accumulation (ascites).

Treatment

- Oxygen therapy. *(See NR, Oxygen administration)*
- Rest and restful conditions constitute at least 50% of any treatment. Hot and humid conditions aggravate the problem.
- Diet must contain low sodium, and often includes a fluid restriction.
- Medication typically includes diuretics *(e.g., furosemide, Lasix) (see PH, Urinary system)*; digitalis preparations *(see PH, Cardiovascular system);* and a potassium supplement *(e.g.,* Kaon) *(see PH, Cardiovascular system).*
- The patient should have a clear understanding of diet, activity, and medication for effective lifelong management of the condition.
- Emergency treatment for pulmonary edema includes IV for vein access *(see NR, Intravenous therapy)*; morphine sulfate *(see PH, Central nervous system);* furosemide (Lasix) *(see PH, Urinary system);* aminophyllin medications *(e.g.,* Theophylline ethylenediamine) *(see PH, Respiratory system);* rotating tourniquets *(see NR, Rotating tourniquets);* indwelling urinary catheter *(see NR, Urinary bladder catheterization);* and ABGs *(see LAB).* As soon as possible a pulmonary artery catheter *(e.g.,* Swan-Ganz) is inserted through a large peripheral vein into the pulmonary artery to determine left ventricular function.

Nursing Tips

- The nurse's skilled observations throughout a shift can provide an early detection of increasing CHF, especially lung congestion. Assess the lungs of all cardiac patients at the beginning of each shift to establish baselines. Any patient who suddenly develops a cough should be watched carefully.
- Jugular vein distention should be assessed; if present, it should be reported and monitored frequently.
- Diuretics should be given early in the day. There is often a large fluid loss in a short period of time, causing weakness and affecting electrolyte balances. Weigh daily after voiding and before breakfast and on the same scale. The amount of fluid retention indicates the effectiveness of treatment. Patients who are usually independent may need assistance getting out of bed. Postural hypotension is an early sign of hypovolemia.
- It is extremely important that a shift to above or below the normal serum potassium level be reported to the physician at any hour of the day or night *(see LAB).* Severe cardiac arrythmias may develop from potassium imbalance. A low potassium level may cause digitalis toxicity.

- Measure ascites daily, using a tape measure at the level of the umbilicus, and mark where the tape is placed with a magic marker.
- IVs should be monitored very closely to prevent a sudden rate increase that would cause a fluid overload. The tubing should be out of reach of a confused patient. It is good practice to hang a 100 ml bottle with a microdrip or pediatric drip to ensure that if anything does increase the rate the patient will receive only an acceptable amount of fluid.
- Cerebral anoxia often occurs; restlessness and confusion are early symptoms *(see MNS, Disoriented patients)*. Be sure the patient is receiving oxygen. The brain is very susceptible to hypoxia. Keep the lights on in the room—and often the radio or TV—to allay the patient's fear of being left alone.
- Sedatives may increase the level of restlessness because they are detoxified in the liver, and its function may be compromised by CHF.

CORONARY ARTERY DISEASE

ANGINA PECTORIS

Description

Angina pectoris describes transient insufficient coronary blood flow caused by an obstruction or constriction of the coronary arteries. It does not result in cell death within the heart muscle. *Stable angina* refers to pain that occurs after physical or emotional exertion that increases the metabolic demand for oxygen (the oxygen requirement of the myocardium is three times that of any other body tissue). Stable angina tends to follow a consistent pattern of cause, intensity, and duration, and is relieved by rest and vasodilators within 15 minutes.

As the disease progresses—as a result of further decrease in coronary blood flow—pain occurs with less provocation and lasts longer. This is called *coronary insufficiency* or *preinfarction angina*. It is unrelieved by vasodilators, and may waken the patient at night.

Intractable angina is chronic chest pain or discomfort that is incapacitating and does not respond to medical treatment.

Common Diagnostic Tests

- EKG, which should be done during any angina attack to rule out myocardial infarction. *(See NR, Electrocardiogram leads and how to place them)*
- Coronary arteriography determines the patency of coronary arteries through injection of a contrast substance directly into them by way of a catheter threaded through the arterial system.

What to Look for

- Chest pains may be intense, as characterized by the fist drawn to the chest; symptoms may be described as a mild discomfort, indigestion, tightness, or a "funny feeling," rather than as pain.
- Extreme fear may be expressed or apparent during subjective observation.
- Elevated blood pressure (BP) at the onset of pain, as the body attempts to increase the blood flow to the coronary arteries, with a fall in BP after the administration of a vasodilator, *e.g.*, nitroglycerine (NTG).
- A fall in BP at the onset of pain may indicate severe insufficiency or an impending infarction. *This should be reported immediately to the physician.*

Treatment

- Raise the head of the bed.
- Vasodilator *(e.g.,* NTG) taken immediately for pain. *(See PH, Cardiovascular system)*
- Oxygen, to relieve ischemia. If a specific flow rate has not been ordered, 2 liters is safe as an emergency administration. *(See NR, Oxygen administration)*
- Prepare for an EKG. *(See NR, Electrocardiogram leads and how to place them)*
- Typical medications are NTG, Nitrol Paste, and isosorbide dinitrate (Isordil). Propranolol hydrochloride (Inderal) is not usually given during an acute attack, but it is an effective preventive drug. *(See PH, Cardiovascular system)*

Nursing Tips

- Give the vasodilator medication immediately at the onset of pain. If the patient is allowed to keep the medication at his bedside, be sure that he understands that the nurse must be notified immediately when it is taken. NTG may be repeated at five-minute intervals three times. If no relief, notify the physician. EKG should be taken with any episode of chest pain. Explain this so the patient doesn't become apprehensive about the number being done.
- Fear and apprehension are often severe during an angina attack, especially if the patient is awakened at night. Stay with the patient during the attack. Obtain a sedation order. Be especially aware at night of the patient's complaining of "indigestion," or of getting out of bed and moving about the room while denying pain. The nurse may be the only person to witness an attack. Document all you observe. Later, ask the patient to describe the site, duration,

and intensity of the pain or "feeling" and whether there were precipitating factors. Document this carefully. When a patient understands what activities may bring on an attack, he will be able to take NTG prophylactically.

- Be prepared to explain any diagnostic tests. If surgery is contemplated, help the patient find out as much as he wants to know.

MYOCARDIAL INFARCTION

Description

A myocardial infarction (MI) is a localized area of cell death in the heart muscle. It results from a lack of blood supply to the area caused by a partial or complete occlusion of a coronary artery.

Common Diagnostic Tests

- Enzymes: test for increased SGOT, CPK, and LDH myocardial specific isoenzymes, which are released into the blood from damaged heart tissue *(see LAB)*. The most important and specific test is for CPK with its isoenzymes that will elevate in a few hours.
- Leukocyte count: usually elevates within a few hours and soon returns to normal.
- EKG: frequently, changes are not immediately evident, but most often they do occur within 3 days. *(See NR, Electrocardiogram leads and how to place them)*

What to Look for

- Pain: usually severe, but may be described as heaviness or a burning sensation anywhere above the waistline, including the jaws, and may extend down the arms to the back and to the fingers of either hand. It is unchanged on inspiration or expiration, and is not relieved by change of position.
- Severe apprehension: patients will often ask "am I going to die?"
- Diaphoresis: very common as cold sweat along with skin pallor.
- Nausea and vomiting.
- Chest congestion: heard as rales; indicative of heart failure.

Treatment

Patients are usually admitted to an ICU. In the event this cannot be done, the following are the immediate needs:

- Oxygen: start with what is immediately available, usually a nasal cannula. Although the flow rate needs to be ordered by a physician, 2 liters is safe in an emergency while awaiting specific orders. *(See NR, Oxygen administration)*
- Pain management: usually with IV morphine sulfate. *(See PH, Central nervous system)*

- Intravenous line: for immediate access for medications. Start with 5% dextrose in water at a very slow rate (10 to 20 ml/min) with microdrip or a pediatric drip and preferably on a pump. Remember the high incidence of congestive heart failure (CHF) with these patients.
- Medications: antiarrythmics, *e.g.,* lidocaine hydrochloride, procainamide hydrochloride (Pronestyl), and quinidine; anticoagulants, *e.g.,* heparin; and diuretics, *e.g.,* furosemide (Lasix), and digitalis preparation. *(See PH, Cardiovascular system and Urinary system)*
- Daily weight and intake and output (I and O) are used to determine how well the heart is performing in relation to kidney function. These also determine the effectiveness of diuretics if they are being administered.

Nursing Tips

- Life-threatening arrhythmias often develop in the first few hours of infarction, so establish vital sign baselines immediately, *e.g.,* blood pressure (BP), apical/radial pulse (ARP), and respirations (RESP). Take BP the first time in both arms, documenting any difference and the arm (right arm, RA; left arm, LA). Continue taking in one arm every 15 minutes for 1 hour or until stable. Be sure to use the same arm each time. Take ARP for 1 full minute, each time documenting irregularity, pulse deficit (difference between apical and radial rate), and quality (bounding or weak). Count respirations, and note dyspnea and quality (shallow or labored).
- Pain relief is imperative. Continued uncontrollable pain is a poor prognostic sign.
- Anxiety level in MI patients is very high. The constant attendance of calm and competent personnel is imperative. Talk as you work, explaining what you are doing. If the family is present include them in your explanations. It is important that visitors do not upset the patient. Position the patient for his comfort. Clear the area around the bed for ease of movement for personnel and equipment.
- Observation of the patient is extremely important. Restlessness or confusion, resulting from cerebral anoxia, can be an early symptom of a failing heart.
- Know how to assess the lungs. If there is any question ask for assistance. Report presence of rales to physician immediately. Sixty per cent of MI patients develop left-sided heart failure.
- Patients with MI should never use a bedpan or strain at producing a stool. Provide a bedside commode, and be sure that stool softeners are ordered.

- Pulmonary embolism is a possible complication of bed rest *(See SS, Pulmonary embolism)*. Check with the physician regarding orders for elastic stockings and range of motion (ROM) exercises.
- Denial of having an MI is very common, especially when the pain disappears and there is no dyspnea.
- Cardiac teaching needs to start as early as possible, by using the material provided in each hospital or by contacting the American Heart Association.

HYPERTENSION

Description

Hypertension is a persistent elevation of arterial blood pressure, characterized primarily by an increased diastolic pressure. This indicates increased resistance of the peripheral arterial vessels during the resting phase of the heart's pumping action. It is usually defined by blood pressure (BP) levels above 150mm Hg systolic and 90mm Hg diastolic. Primary hypertension (also called essential hypertension) evolves over a period of years with no known cause. Over 90% of the cases fall in this category. Secondary hypertension is the result of a specific disease such as renal failure and endocrine dysfunction. Malignant hypertension is a sudden severe increase in BP that quickly causes damage to vital organs. It is generally fatal if not treated immediately.

Common Diagnostic Tests

- Urinalysis and renal function tests. *(See LAB)*
- Endocrine function tests (for pheochromocytoma and Cushing's syndrome). *(See SS, Endocrine)*

What to Look for

- BP that remains elevated when measured in the sitting, lying, and standing positions; taken at 15-minute intervals.
- History of headaches, vertigo, nosebleeds, blurring of vision, and spots before the eyes.

Treatment

- Patients with a diastolic pressure above 90 are generally started on antihypertensive medication, *e.g.,* reserpine (Serpasil) and methyldopa (Aldomet) *(see PH, Cardiovascular system)*, and are regularly checked by their physician.
- Immediate hospitalization is usually ordered for a diastolic BP over 130. This is a life-threatening situation.

Nursing Tips

- Take BP with the cuff and limb at the level of the heart. Be sure that the manometer indicator is at zero before starting to pump up cuff pressure. The cuff needs to fit snugly around the limb. A false high reading will be obtained if it is too narrow. A false low reading will result if too wide a cuff is used. There are oversize and pediatric cuffs available. Note on the chart which arm was used for the BP measurement.
- Potassium levels need to be checked frequently. *(See LAB)*
- When the hypertension is severe and potent antihypertensives are given, monitor the BP every hour for the first 24 hours.
- A frequent side effect of the hypertensive medications is postural hypotension. Under this condition, the drop in the systolic pressure when standing is more than 20mm Hg. Patients with this condition should be cautioned to stand up slowly.
- The nurse is in a unique position to help the patients prepare themselves for a lifetime condition which, although not curable, is controllable. Sustained hypertension is the most important factor predisposing to strokes, myocardial infarctions, and renal disease.
- Weight control, elimination of smoking, and a restricted sodium diet go along with medication as integral parts of the treatment in the lifelong control of hypertension.
- It is estimated that as many as 80% of hypertensive patients quit taking their medications within 5 years. It must be emphasized that, although there may be no symptoms, patients must continue to take medications to prevent complication of stroke, heart disease, and renal failure.

THROMBOPHLEBITIS

Description

Thrombophlebitis is an inflammation of the veins in conjunction with a blood clot (thrombus). Usually the deep veins are involved. Any alteration of or injury to a vein that restricts blood flow (venous stasis) tends to result in blood clots and thrombophlebitis. This is often a complication of prolonged bed rest. Phlebothrombosis refers to thrombosis not accompanied by symptoms of inflammation.

What to Look for

- Swelling, redness, and warmth and tenderness of a leg area commonly occur when superficial veins are involved.
- Sometimes the thrombus in such surface veins can be felt as a hard spot.

- A positive Homan's sign (pain in the calf on dorsiflexion of the foot with the leg extended) may be the only external evidence of thrombophlebitis in deep veins. Frequently this is accompanied by a temperature elevation.

Treatment

- Bed rest, elevation of the leg on pillows, and warm, moist packs to the leg are commonly prescribed.
- Anticoagulants (*e.g.,* heparin and warfarin). *(See PH, Cardiovascular system)*
- Analgesics as necessary for pain. *(See PH, Central nervous system)*
- The insertion of a filter device in the vena cava is done occasionally in patients with frequently recurring thrombophlebitis or where anticoagulant therapy is contraindicated or ineffective. The filter is made of fine mesh, which prevents emboli from traveling to the lung.

Nursing Tips

- Read the pharmacy section on anticoagulants *(see PH, Cardiovascular system)*. There are many drugs that should not be taken while on anticoagulants. Be prepared to discuss this with the patient. Patients should consult their physician about any medication, including over-the-counter ones.
- Patients are often allowed to use a commode rather than a bedpan. Watch carefully while moving patient from and to bed (and immediately afterward) for any signs of an embolism. Caution them not to strain.
- A special effort should be made to prevent thrombophlebitis in any hospitalized patient. Those on bed rest must have ROM exercises. Sitting in chairs for long periods should be avoided. Venous stasis occurs rapidly in anyone with impaired circulation.
- Check with the physician regarding the patient's use of elastic stockings both when in the hospital and when discharged.
- Patients are often discharged on a prophylactic anticoagulant regime. Emphasize the importance of blood tests and prothrombin levels, as ordered by the physician. Emphasize to the patient that any unusual bleeding should be reported.
- An identifying bracelet should be worn noting that this person is on an anticoagulant.
- Any evidence of a pulmonary embolism must be reported to the physician at once. *(See SS, Pulmonary embolism)*

VARICOSE VEINS

Description

Varicose veins are abnormally dilated veins that have an impaired valve function. They usually occur in the lower extremities, with the long saphenous vein most often affected. Varicose veins occur as hemorrhoids and also as esophageal varices, which result from complications of liver diseases. *(See SS, Esophageal varices)*

What to Look for

- Disfigurement in the lower extremities, with large discolored veins, usually accompanied by edema, fibrosis, and pigmentation of the skin that may become pruritic. This is called stasis dermatitis. There is an increased susceptibility of this tissue to infection and trauma.
- Varicose ulcers often develop because of venous stasis and the poor condition of the skin.

Treatment

- Support stockings, prescribed by a physician's measurements and made to order.
- Surgical: stripping or removal of the saphenous vein, provided the deep veins are able to supply collateral circulation. This is done under a general anesthetic.
- Injection of a caustic solution into a vein, which causes sclerosis of the vein. This is done usually with smaller veins or for patients unable to undergo surgery.

Nursing Tips

- These patients are often allowed to walk the day of surgery. They need pain medication and thus assistance in walking. Sometimes bed rest is ordered for the first 24 hours.
- Check the dressings frequently for excessive bleeding for the first 24 hours.
- Check pedal pulses every 2 hours for the first 24 hours.
- Since it is a weakness of vessel walls that predisposes to varicose veins, the patient should know the problem may recur in the collateral veins.
- If elastic stockings are to be worn, arrangements should be made to have them fitted as soon as possible after surgery.
- Have the patient avoid excess weight, crossing of the legs, prolonged standing or sitting with legs not elevated, and constriction by garters or a tight girdle.

- Varicose ulcers are often very painful. Medicate for pain before beginning their care; use sterile technique. *(See SS, Arterial occlusive disease of the lower extremities)*
- A care plan with step-by-step directions should be prepared and followed by everyone caring for the ulcer; this demonstrates to the patient the necessity for continuity of care. If a family member or a visiting nurse will be continuing care at home, have them come to observe and participate in the procedure in the hospital.
- When skin grafts are necessary, infection prevention measures become even more important during the healing period.

Endocrine System

Overview

The endocrine glands contain highly specialized cells that secrete hormones that act as chemical messengers, creating an intricate chain of interactions between body systems. Hormones are released directly into the blood stream, and when delivered to target organs they elicit specific responses. In some cases, as with the thyroid, there is a more general effect on the entire body. In other cases the effect is exceedingly specific; such is the case with the follicle stimulating hormone, which influences the ovarian cycle. The adrenal medulla, the posterior pituitary, and to a lesser extent, the pancreas are connected to the autonomic nervous system, secreting their hormones in response to electrical stimuli originating in the higher centers of the brain. By controlling and integrating the body's functions, the endocrine glands help the body interact with its environment.

In general, dysfunction of the endocrine system involves underproduction or overproduction of hormones, or failure to secrete them according to the normal checks and balances of the body. Causes include congenital and genetic defects, surgery, atrophy, and neoplastic and nonneoplastic overactivity. Since the organs of the endocrine system are interdependent, dysfunction in one area can cause reciprocal dysfunction in another. Treatment involves correction of over- or underproduction.

Nursing Tips

- Nursing care involves
  1. *Absolute accuracy in collecting specimens* for sophisticated laboratory tests (check agency laboratory manual for specific instructions).
  2. *Administration of hormones* to patients with deficiencies.
  3. *Patient teaching and emotional support* for patients who may face lifelong alterations in their bodies, activities, and life-style, and possibly a lifelong program of therapy.

ADRENAL CORTEX

Description

The adrenal cortex produces hormones (corticosteroids) that control the body's adaptation to stress and are essential to life. The gland acts principally, though not entirely, under the influence of the anterior lobe of the pituitary gland and its hormone messenger, the adrenocorticotropic hormone (ACTH).

Overview

Functions

- Glucocorticoids increase the catabolism of protein and fat, elevate the blood sugar, inhibit protein synthesis, influence emotions, and suppress inflammation.
- Mineralocorticoids retain sodium in the body and decrease the amount of body potassium.
- All corticoids are important for defense against stress or injury to body tissues.
- Adrenal androgens (weak male hormones found in both men and women) govern certain secondary sex characteristics.

Adrenocortical insufficiency: may be caused by inadequate stimulation of the hypothalmus or pituitary, surgical removal of the adrenals, the inability of the adrenal cortex to function following abrupt withdrawal of steroid therapy, idiopathic atrophy, malignancy, possible autoimmune factors, or an infection such as tuberculosis.

Hypersecretion by the adrenal cortex: may be caused by cortisol-secreting adrenal tumors or by hyperplasia of the adrenal cortex resulting from hypersecretion of ACTH by the pituitary or from ectopic hypersecretion of ACTH by malignancies in other areas, especially bronchogenic oat-cell carcinomas. Excessively high therapeutic dosages of steroids will produce the same effects as adrenocortical hypersecretion.

ADDISON'S DISEASE (PRIMARY ADRENOCORTICAL INSUFFICIENCY)

Common Diagnostic Tests

- Feedback test: The fundamental basis for the diagnosis involves establishing the inability of the adrenal gland to respond to stimulation with ACTH (ACTH stimulation test).
- Low levels of adrenocortical hormones in plasma and urine as reflected in plasma cortisol levels and in 24-hour urine tests for steroids (17-hydroxycorticosteroids, and 17-ketosteroids).
- Plasma ACTH levels: elevated in primary adrenal deficiency (also highly elevated in ectopic ACTH-producing tumors and in pituitary adenomas).

- Low serum sodium (less than 130 mEq/liter), low fasting blood sugar (less than 50 mg/100 ml), high serum potassium (greater than 5 mEq/liter), elevated BUN, decreased CO_2 combining power (less than 28 mEq/liter, and relative lymphocytosis *(see LAB)*. These findings, though, often are not present in a given case.

What to Look for

- Muscular weakness, fatigue, emaciation, anorexia, nausea and vomiting, generalized and specific dark pigmentation of the skin, hypotension, emotional disturbances, and diminished resistance to even minor stress.
- *Addisonian crisis:* critical drop in corticosteroids leading to severe hypotension, hyperkalemia, and vascular collapse. It may be caused by stress, infection, surgery, severe perspiration and salt loss, or the inadequate replacement or sudden withdrawal of steroids.

Treatment

- General: administration of replacement steroids. *(See PH, Adrenocorticosteroids, Endocrine system)*
- Addisonian crisis: reverse shock, restore circulation, replace steroids, treat hypoglycemia, and treat infection, if present. In crisis, fluid therapy provides more immediate benefit than does steroid replacement.

Nursing Tips

- Administer steroids, and instruct patient concerning them. *(See PH, Endocrine system)*
- Monitor fluid and electrolyte balances carefully.
- Educate patient as to the danger of infection; it could put him into Addisonian crisis. Increased steroid doses are often required during the stress of infection or other illness or injury. Infections should be treated promptly.
- Patient should wear an identifying tag or bracelet that indicates that he has adrenal insufficiency and that requests that his physician be notified in case of an accident.

CUSHING'S SYNDROME (HYPERSECRETION OF THE ADRENAL CORTEX)
Common Diagnostic Tests

- Plasma cortisol and urinary hydroxysteroids are usually elevated. Loss of diurnal variation of cortisol is present, with late afternoon cortisol levels equal to morning levels.
- Cortisone suppression test: generally dexamethasone (Decadron), which normally suppresses pituitary secretion of ACTH, is admin-

istered. In Cushing's syndrome, serum cortisone levels and urinary 17-hydroxycorticosteroids fail to drop.

- ACTH stimulation tests by administration of metyrapone (Metopirone).
- Androgen hypersecretion with elevated urinary 17-ketosteroids may be present.
- Abnormal glucose tolerance with hyperglycemia, hypernatremia (high blood sodium), hypokalemia (low blood potassium), low eosinophils, and low lymphocytes may be demonstrated.
- Other tests include intravenous pyelogram *(see NR, x-ray preparations)*, adrenal arteriography, ultrasound, skull x-rays, and computerized tomography of head and adrenal areas. *(See NR, Scans and Ultrasound)*

What to Look for

- Edema, hypertension, and abnormal fat production and distribution, *e.g.*, "moon face," protruding abdomen, and fat pads on the back of the shoulders (buffalo hump).
- Muscle weakness, osteoporosis, pathological fractures, increased capillary fragility and bruising, emotional instability or frank psychosis, steroid-induced diabetes, and increased susceptibility to infection. Thinning of scalp hair, the presence of facial hair, and acne are sometimes seen in female patients.

Treatment

- Removal of the cause (if possible). Excision of a tumor, chemotherapy, irradiation of the pituitary, or an adrenalectomy may be indicated.
- Reduce dosage of externally administered corticoids, if indicated.

Nursing Tips

- Give emotional support. Provide mental and physical rest. Depression and suicide are not rare in Cushing's disease.
- Diet should be low in sodium and high in protein and potassium, with calories dependent on weight and nutritional status.
- Test urine for sugar and acetone. *(See LAB)*
- Prevent or control infections.
- Give attention to safety factors because of potential for easy bruising and pathological fractures.

ADRENAL MEDULLA

Description

The adrenal medulla is under the control of the sympathetic nervous system and functions in conjunction with it. It is *not* essential to life. The effects of epinephrine and norepinephrine, hormones released by the adrenal medulla, are identical to those of the sympathetic nervous system.

Epinephrine elevates blood pressure converts glycogen to glucose when needed, increases heart rate, and dilates bronchioles.

Norepinephrine constricts peripheral blood vessels, causing increased blood pressure.

Underactivity or loss of the gland is rarely a problem.

PHEOCHROMOCYTOMA

Description

Overactivity of the adrenal medulla is usually caused by a catecholamine-producing tumor called pheochromocytoma. Usually benign, pheochromocytoma may also be found outside the adrenal medulla (*e.g.* in the urinary bladder).

Common Diagnostic Tests

- Assay of urinary catecholamines: elevation above normal.
- Assay of urinary vanillylmandelic acid (VMA), the principal metabolite of catecholamines: elevation above normal.
- Assay of catecholamines in blood: elevation above normal for epinephrine (0.48 to 0.51 µg/liter).
- X-ray, intravenous pyelogram (IVP), CAT scan. (*See NR, x-ray preparations and NR, Scans*)
- Blood sugar often elevated, and glycosuria often present. (*See LAB*)

What to Look for

- *Hypertension* (may be persistent, fluctuating, intermittent, or paroxysmal), pounding headache, sweating, apprehension, palpitations, nausea and vomiting, and hyperglycemia and glycosuria usually appear during attacks.
- Symptoms may develop spontaneously or may be precipitated by emotional stress, physical exertion, or position change.

Treatment

- Surgical removal, after preliminary control of hypertension.

Nursing Tips
Preoperative Care

- Promote rest and relief from emotional tension.
- Omit stimulants in diet.
- Monitor vital signs, especially blood pressure, frequently.
- Treat prior to surgery, on physician's order, with phenoxybenzamine (Dibenzyline) to block vasoconstricting effects of epinephrine or norepinephrine. Phentolamine (Regitine) may be used for the

rapid treatment of hypertensive episodes. *Caution:* Check blood pressure q. 30 min following administration of Regitine.

Postoperative Care

- Monitor blood pressure carefully. Watch for decrease as a result of catecholamine level drop or hemorrhage.
- Measure and record hourly urinary output. Report to physician if less than 30 ml/hr.
- Give intravenous fluids, as ordered.
- Give catecholamine support, as ordered.

ADRENALECTOMY

Description

Adrenalectomy may be performed in cases of Cushing's syndrome, primary aldosteronism, and adrenal tumors, and for carcinoma of the breast.

Nursing Tips

- Maintain appropriate replacement of hydrocortisone by IV drip intraoperatively and postoperatively.
- Monitor for shock, hypoglycemia, and infection.
- Administer corticosteroid therapy and instruct patient regarding it *(see PH, Endocrine system, adrenocorticosteroids)*. Patient will be on therapy for the rest of his life.

DIABETES MELLITUS

Description

Diabetes mellitus is a chronic disorder of carbohydrate, protein, and fat metabolism, due to inadequate production or utilization of insulin. Insulin is normally produced by the beta cells of the islands of Langerhans in the pancreas. It is currently thought that insulin acts primarily at cell membrane insulin receptor sites to facilitate transport of glucose into cells.

"Insulin dependent" diabetes (also called "brittle," "unstable," or "juvenile onset" diabetes) has an onset and is usually diagnosed prior to the age of fifteen years. The beta cells fail to produce insulin, probably most often as a result of viral damage.

"Insulin independent," or "maturity onset," diabetes is probably due most often to genetic factors. There is some production of insulin by the beta cells, and blood may contain supernormal amounts of insulin, but the body cannot use it efficiently. The patient may be able to control his diabetes through his diet or through diet and oral hypoglycemics.

Alterations in blood vessels and nerves frequently complicate long-standing diabetes.

Common Diagnostic Tests

- Fasting blood sugar (FBS) elevated above normal 65 to 110 mg/100 ml. *(See LAB)*
- Glucose tolerance tests: oral glucose tolerance test (OGTT) and intravenous glucose tolerance test (IVGT).
- Urine tests: for sugar and acetone. *(See LAB)*

What to Look for

- Hyperglycemia (elevated blood sugar or glucose)
- Glycosuria (presence of sugar in the urine)
- Polyuria (excessive urine production)
- Polydipsia (excessive thirst)
- Polyphagia (increased food intake)
- Weight loss
- Signs of diabetic complications, *e.g.,* diabetic acidosis *(see SS, Diabetic acidosis)*, low resistance to infections, increased incidence of toxemia of pregnancy and fetal wastage, cardiovascular disorders, eye disorders (retinopathy), nephropathy, and neuropathy

Treatment

- *Control requires a balance between food intake, activity, and medications* (if indicated).
- *Diet:* A balanced diet will be prescribed by the physician to meet the individual needs of the patient. The single most important dietary principle is the attainment of ideal body weight.
  1. *American Diabetic Association (ADA) diets* are based on six groups, or exchange lists, of food. Each list consists of foods that in the amounts described are nearly equal in calories, carbohydrates, proteins, and fats. The "exchanges," or groups, are milk, vegetables, fruit, bread, meat, and fat. Foods in the same list are interchangeable. Substitutions may be made within groups, but not between groups.
  2. The two food groups requiring significant restrictions are free sugars (sweets) and animal fats.
- *Exercise or activity:* Activity decreases the body's need for insulin. A regular exercise program (three or more times per week) is best.
- *Medication:*
  1. Insulin by injection (short-acting and long-acting) *(see PH, Endocrine system)*. Insulin pumps provide a more continuous supply of insulin.
  2. Oral hypoglycemic agents (presently seldom used; *e.g.,* Orinase, Tolinase). *(See PH, Endocrine system)*

DIABETIC ACIDOSIS

Description

Hyperglycemia, or a very high blood sugar, causes glycosuria, which results in water and electrolyte loss. In the absence of insulin, the body burns fat and protein, producing ketones and other acid residues.

- Blood sugar over 80 mg to 120 mg/100 ml blood.

What to Look for

- Symptoms may have a rapid onset, but they frequently come on gradually over a period of days or weeks.
- *Thirst;* dry mouth; dry, flushed skin
- Excessive urination
- Nausea and vomiting, abdominal pain
- Sweet odor to breath, "fruity" odor of acetone
- Deep rapid breathing, air hunger (Kussmaul respiration)
- Coma

Treatment

- Give short-acting (Regular) insulin, intravenously or subcutaneously.
- Correct electrolyte and water imbalance (*Caution:* myocardial infarction and strokes often complicate diabetic acidosis in older patients).
- Treat for shock, if present.
- Monitor blood sugar, CO_2, potassium, and serum acetone.
- Indwelling catheter to check urine every hour for sugar and acetone.

HYPOGLYCEMIC REACTION: INSULIN SHOCK

Description

Insulin reaction can occur if too much insulin is given, if food intake is less than usual, or if physical activity is greater than usual. Blood sugar falls below normal (55 mg/100 ml or less).

What to Look for

Symptoms frequently have rapid onset, may be minutes to hours.

- *Hunger*
- Weakness, nervousness, tremor
- Sweating
- Blurred vision
- Changes in behavior: irritability, confusion
- Headaches
- Unconsciousness

Treatment

- Give sugar (*e.g.,* sugar, orange juice, ginger ale, cola, honey, sugar candy, or cake frosting in a tube). A packet or two of sugar mixed in orange juice provides a quick way of supplying sugar. Record time and amount given.
- Fifty percent glucose IV. Viscosity makes it difficult to administer. Give over period of 2 to 5 minutes. While administering, aspirate blood frequently to counteract sclerosing effect of glucose.
- Glucagon stimulates the liver to release glucose from stored glycogen; it is sometimes ordered for very unstable diabetics. *Caution:* If there is doubt as to whether the patient's blood glucose is too high or too low, *always give glucose first.* If the patient is hypoglycemic, the response usually will be almost immediate.

Nursing Tips for the General Care of Diabetics

- General hygienic care; meticulous skin, foot, and mouth care. *Caution:* if neuropathy is present, patient may be more susceptible to burns from heating pads and so forth and to other injuries, especially to the feet.
- Administration of medication: insulin and, infrequently, oral hypoglycemic agents. *(See PH, Endocrine system)*
- Collection of specimens and testing of urine. *(See LAB)*
- Fasting blood sugar (FBS). If ordered, be sure blood is drawn before giving morning insulin or breakfast.
- Monitor for signs of hyperglycemia, hypoglycemia, and electrolyte imbalance.
- Fractional urines should be tested on all known hospitalized diabetic patients, because stress of surgery or infection can change body metabolism.
- Patient should wear an identifying bracelet to show that he is an insulin dependent diabetic.
- In cases where diabetics are receiving large amounts of intravenous glucose, blood sugars should be frequently monitored.
- Education of the patient and his cooperation in treatment are the keys to his staying well. Excellent informational materials are available through the American Diabetic Association, Inc., 600 Fifth Avenue, New York, 10020, or through local chapters.

PARATHYROID GLANDS

Description

The parathyroids are small bodies located on the lateral or posterior aspect of the thyroid gland. They produce the parathyroid hormone, parathormone (PTH), which acts on the bone, intestine, and kidney to maintain normal serum calcium levels. Parathormone maintains an inverse relationship between serum calcium and serum phosphate levels, thereby fostering normal excitability of nerves and muscles.

HYPERPARATHYROIDISM

Description

Hyperparathyroidism is overactivity of one or more of the parathyroid glands, caused most often by a single adenoma, by hyperplasia of all the glands, and occasionally by carcinoma of a single gland (primary hyperparathyroidism); or by compensatory oversecretion of PTH (secondary hyperparathyroidism); or by ectopic secretion of parathormone by tumors elsewhere. Symptoms arise from the elevated blood calcium, the increased resorption of calcium from bone, and the increased excretion of calcium in urine.

Common Diagnostic Tests

Diagnosis depends on demonstrating that hypercalcemia is *not* due to another of a great many causes of hypercalcemia.

- Measurement of parathyroid hormone in the blood by immunoassay.
- Elevated serum calcium, depressed serum phosphate levels, hypercalciuria (elevated calcium in the urine). *(See LAB)*
- Skeletal changes detected by x-ray, showing diffuse demineralization of bones, subperiosteal resorption, bone cysts, or vertebral compression fracture.
- Phosphate reabsorption test: indicates amount of phosphate reabsorbed by kidneys, reflecting the serum level of parathyroid hormone.

What to Look for

- Evidence of *hypercalcemia* (elevated blood calcium), *e.g.*, apathy, fatigue, thirst, muscular weakness, nausea, vomiting, constipation, cardiac arrhythmias, emotional irritability, neurosis or psychosis, and increased excitement of nerves and muscles.
- Evidence of *demineralization of bones*, possibly with pathological fractures; backache; joint pain.
- Evidence of *kidney damage*, (such as nephrocalcinosis, the precipitation of calcium phosphate in the renal tubules), or kidney stones.

Treatment

- Surgical removal of hyperfunctioning gland or glands.

Nursing Tips

Preoperative Care

- Force fluids. Give cranberry juice, low calcium diet.
- Avoid vitamin D preparations. Prevent constipation.
- Strain all urine if stones are suspected.
- Promote mobility of the patient (to minimize calcium resorption from bone), while protecting him from injury and falls.
- If the patient has heart disease, administer digitalis preparations cautiously. Interaction of calcium and digitalis can be hazardous. Watch for signs of digitalis toxicity. *(See PH, Cardiovascular system)*
- Severe hypercalcemia is an emergency that requires large volumes of fluid and vigorous therapy with Lasix.

Postoperative Care

- Same as for thyroidectomy. *(See SS, Thyroid)*
- Watch closely for signs of tetany, hyperirritability of nerves with spasms of hands and feet, generalized tremor, and incoordinated contractions. *(See SS, Hypoparathyroidism)*
- Monitor serum calcium and phosphorus frequently.

HYPOPARATHYROIDISM

Description

Hypoparathyroidism occurs when too much parathyroid tissue has been removed surgically, or as a result of idiopathic atrophy. Chief symptoms result from low serum calcium levels, which cause irritability of the neuromuscular system leading to tetany. Serum phosphate is increased.

Hypoparathyroidism occasionally occurs spontaneously, but it is seen most often following neck surgery with inadvertent loss of the parathyroids.

Common Diagnostic Tests

- Immunoassay measurement shows decreased parathyroid hormone.
- Serum calcium decreased; serum phosphate elevated. *(See LAB)*
- Skull x-ray shows basal ganglia calcification, but only in those with idiopathic hypoparathyroidism.
- Positive *Chvostek's sign:* spasms of facial muscles that occur when muscles or branches of facial nerves are tapped.
- Positive *Trousseau's sign:* carpal spasm induced by occluding the circulation in an arm with a blood-pressure cuff.

What to Look for

- *Tetany* (generalized tremor and incoordinated contractions).
- *Latent tetany,* which may cause numbness, tingling, and stiffness of hands and feet.
- *Overt tetany,* which may cause bronchospasm, laryngeal spasm, carpal spasm (flexion of the elbows and wrists and extension of the carpophalangeal joints), dysphagia, cardiac arrhythmias, and convulsions.
- Grand mal (major motor) seizures may occur.

Treatment and Nursing Tips

- Goal is to elevate serum calcium to approximately 9 to 10 mg/100 ml and to render patient free of symptoms.
- Mild hypoparathyroidism may prove to be transitory. Most patients get over the transitory hypocalcemic phase without therapy or with small amounts of calcium orally.
- In the acute phase, be prepared to administer calcium gluconate IV, if ordered. If convulsive tendencies continue, give sedatives as ordered. *Keep tracheostomy set, as well as calcium gluconate ready for IV administration at bedside following parathyroid and thyroid surgery. Caution:* Calcium gluconate and digitalis potentiate each other, so the cardiac patient requires constant monitoring. *(See PH, Endocrine system and Cardiovascular system)*
- Provide quiet environment.
- Long-term care when permanent hypoparathyroidism is diagnosed:
  1. Vitamin D and calcium lactate are used.
  2. Aluminum carbonate or aluminum hydroxide gel (Gelusil, Amphogel) p.c. may be used to keep phosphate levels down. *(See PH, Gastrointestinal system)*
  3. Diet should be high in calcium and low in phosphorus. Although milk products are high in calcium, they are also very high in phosphorus and are therefore restricted.
  4. Instruct patient about need for lifelong, follow-up medical supervision. Frequent calcium determinations are required. Hypercalcemia due to excessive vitamin D dosage is sometimes seen.

PITUITARY GLAND: DIABETES INSIPIDUS

Description

Diabetes insipidus (DI) is a disorder that results from a deficiency of the antidiuretic hormone (ADH), vasopressin. ADH is normally secreted by the posterior lobe of the pituitary gland. The deficiency may be caused by damage to the posterior pituitary itself from tumors (benign or malignant), trauma, or infectious processes, or the disorder may be due to idiopathic deterioration of part of the hypothalamus.

Common Diagnostic Tests

- Serum and urine osmolality tests (values decreased).
- Urine dilute and of low specific gravity, usually 1.001 to 1.005, with a maximum of 1.014 on a concentration test. *(See LAB)*
- No glycosuria.
- X-ray films of the skull.
- Fluid deprivation test. Normally urine will become more concentrated, but in DI it will not go above 1.014.
- Vasopressin injection test, to see if urinary output will decrease and specific gravity will rise after injection of vasopressin (ADH).

What to Look for

- Polyuria and polydipsia (patient may drink and excrete up to 5 to 40 liters of fluid per day). Urine is dilute.
- Signs of dehydration and hypovolemic shock, if patient is unable to drink fluids almost continuously.

Treatment

- Give vasopressin tannate (Pitressin tannate) in oil, deep IM or by topical application to nasal mucosa (lypressin or desmopressin). *(See PH, Endocrine system)*
- Chlorpropamide (Diabinese) may be used to potentiate vasopressin. Warn patient about possible hypoglycemic reactions. *(See PH, Endocrine systems)*
- Supplementary potassium is ordered to prevent depletion. *(See PH, Cardiovascular system)*
- Search for and try to correct any underlying intracranial pathology.
- Transphenoidal hypophysectomy.

Nursing Tips

- *Accurate measurement of intake and output is essential.*
- Check urine for specific gravity; monitor patient's weight closely.
- Follow special instructions in administration of vasopressin, and prepare patient for lifelong therapy.
- Keep patient well hydrated. Replace the amount of fluid lost in urine, because patient is very susceptible to dehydration, hypovo-

lemic shock, and collapse. (An otherwise healthy person with DI allowed to drink and eat as he pleases will maintain proper water balance without any therapy.)

- Excellent skin care is required.
- Emotional support is required to help patient deal with his frustrating symptoms of urgent need to allay thirst and to void. Additional support will be required when patient is studied for possible cranial pathology.
- Patient should wear a bracelet describing his condition and treatment.

THYROID

Description

The thyrotropin-releasing hormone (TRH), produced by the hypothalamus, stimulates the anterior pituitary gland to synthesize and release thyroid-stimulating hormone (TSH). TSH in turn stimulates the thyroid gland to synthesize and secrete its two principal hormones, *thyroxine (T_4)* and *triiodothyronine (T_3)*. These act to regulate body metabolism and energy production, to promote normal growth and cell reproduction, to influence fluid and electrolyte balance, and to control body use of fat, proteins, and carbohydrates. The manufacture of thyroid hormones requires protein and iodine. *Thyrocalcitonin* (calcitonin), a third hormone, is secreted by the parafollicular cells of the thyroid. Its functions are to help maintain blood calcium balance by inhibiting calcium release from bone and to promote calcium deposit in bone, thereby preventing hypercalcemia. Parathyroid hormone is antagonistic to calcitonin.

Most thyroid disorders are more common in women than in men. Common abnormalities include

- Enlargement of the thyroid gland (goiter), caused primarily by adenomatous hyperplasia, inflammation (thyroiditis), benign or malignant tumors, or iodine deficiency.
- Hypothyroidism (underactivity of the gland).
- Hyperthyroidism (overactivity of the gland).

Common Diagnostic Tests

Tests for thyroid function can help determine whether hyper- or hypo-function is present, whether it is primary or secondary to pituitary dysfunction, or whether some other malfunction is present. The tests are influenced greatly by the patient's sex hormone status, nutritional state, age, and exposure to drugs that alter the binding capacities of serum proteins, *e.g.*, oral contraceptives and phenytoin (Dilantin).

- Tests for evaluating thyroid function, none of which are influenced by exogenous iodides, are
  1. T_4 by radioimmunoassay (T_4-RIA).
  2. T_3 by radioimmunoassay (T_3-RIA).
  3. T_3 resin uptake.
  4. Free thyroxine index (FTI): the product of T_4 and T_3 resin uptake.
- Tests that involve homeostatic controls from the pituitary and the hypothalmus
  1. Serum thyroid-stimulating hormone (TSH).
  2. Thyroid-stimulating hormone (TSH) stimulation test.
  3. Thyrotropin-releasing hormone (TRH) stimulation test.
- Thyroid scan (radioiodine or technetium scintiscan) for evaluating the anatomic "geography" of the gland, including "hot" or "cold" nodules. *(See NR Scans, nuclear)*
- Radioiodine uptake: helpful in diagnosis of hyperthyroidism and essential for calculating dose for those to be treated with radioiodine. *(See NR, Scans, nuclear)*
- Sonogram: may help differentiate solid from cystic thyroid nodules. *(See NR, Ultrasound)*
- Other tests: thyroid-binding globulin (TBG), thyroid antibodies (in thyroiditis), serum calcitonin (increased in medullary carcinoma of the thyroid).

Nursing Tips

- A careful patient history regarding medication intake is essential for the correct evaluation of thyroid test results.
- Older tests, specifically protein-bound iodine (PBI), are greatly influenced by iodine-containing medications such as Lugol's solution, potassium iodide, x-ray contrast media, antiseptics, cough syrups, and nail strengtheners. Radioactive iodine uptake is also affected.
- Other medications that may alter results include estrogens, progesterone, androgen, antithyroid drugs, probenecid, dilantin, salicylates, large doses of corticosteroids or ACTH, and heparin.

SIMPLE GOITER
Description

The most common type of thyroid enlargement is most often due to adenomatous hyperplasia of unknown origin. It is often familial. In modern times it is rarely caused by inadequate iodine intake. It may be caused by ingestion of large amounts of goitrogenic substances (goiter-producing agents that inhibit thyroxine production), such as propylthiouracil, iodine in large doses, lithium, cabbage, and soybeans. Goiter often begins at puberty, often begins or worsens with pregnancy, and may come on at menopause.

What to Look for

- Enlarged thyroid gland—may cause difficulty in swallowing (dysphagia); respiratory difficulties (dyspnea); or voice changes.

Treatment and Nursing Tips

- Thyroid hormone: watch for symptoms of thyrotoxicosis *(e.g., rapid pulse, tremors, nervous symptoms, weight loss). (See PH, Endocrine system)*
- Subtotal thyroidectomy: may be necessary if thyroid hormone therapy fails to shrink goiter and symptoms or appearance require removal. *(See SS, Thyroidectomy and subtotal thyroidectomy)*

HYPOTHYROIDISM (MYXEDEMA)

Description

Primary hypothyroidism refers to hypofunction originating within the thyroid gland itself. It often has an autoimmune basis.

Secondary hypothyroidism involves disorders of the pituitary or hypothalmus that result in TSH deficiency.

Hypothyroidism may result from treatment of hyperthyroidism *(e.g.,* thyroidectomy or radioiodine therapy followed by too much destruction of thyroid tissue).

Myxedema refers to hypothyroidism of such a severe degree and duration that it causes extremely profound metabolic and anatomic changes in the patient.

Common Diagnostic Tests

- Free thyroxine index (FTI) and T_4 are decreased.
- Thyroid-stimulating hormone (TSH) level is elevated in primary hypothyroidism (but not in secondary hypothyroidism).

What to Look for

Symptoms and findings caused by low metabolic rate generally come on slowly. Every body system eventually becomes involved.

- Apathy, fatigue, mental slow down, weight gain, and constipation.
- Sensitivity to cold and diminished perspiration.
- Menstrual irregularities (usually menorrhagia).
- Decreased sex drive.
- Skin that becomes thickened, dry, flaky, and edematous; hair that thins and falls out; masklike expression of the face.
- Premature development of arteriosclerosis.

Treatment

- Correct deficiency by giving natural or synthetic thyroid hormones, *e.g.*, Thyroid, U.S.P. (desiccated), levothyroxine sodium (T_4), and Synthroid (T_4). *(See PH, Endocrine system)*
- Dose should be increased gradually to prevent undue strain on the heart if the patient has heart disease or is elderly, especially if the hypothyroidism is of long duration.

Nursing Tips

- Instruct patient as to life-long need for daily hormone therapy. (For important nursing implications regarding administration of thyroid hormones, see *PH, Endocrine system*)
- *Caution:* The myxedematous patient has decreased ability to handle barbiturates, anesthesia, narcotics, and sedatives.
- Provide a warm environment. Patient has intolerance to cold.
- Do not overtire the patient.
- Give good skin care, range of motion exercises, foods with roughage, stool softeners, and fluids (but not enough to cause patient to go into congestive heart failure or water intoxication).
- Be aware of possible complications: cardiovascular (angina, myocardial infarction, congestive heart failure), psychosis, myxedema coma (when all body systems come to almost a standstill), grand mal seizures, or death.

HYPERTHYROIDISM (GRAVES' DISEASE)

Description

Hyperthyroidism (Graves' disease) is caused by oversecretion of the two thyroid hormones. The phrase "exophthalmic goiter" describes two of the symptoms that are commonly seen: bulging of the eyeballs and enlargement of the thyroid gland. The condition is believed to have an autoimmune basis, and some evidence suggests an inherited factor. Hyperthyroidism may also be caused by a thyroid adenoma, very rarely by a pituitary adenoma, and not infrequently by overtreatment with thyroid hormone.

Common Diagnostic Tests

- Elevated T_4, T_3-RIA, T_3 resin uptake, and free thyroxine index (FTI). TSH normal or low normal.
- Thyroid scan to distinguish between diffuse goiter and a nodular goiter. Elevated radioiodine uptake.

What to Look for

- Nervousness, tremor, elevated pulse rate.
- Poor toleration of heat; flushed, hot skin; excessive perspiration.

- Exophthalmos (bulging eyes).
- Weight loss despite increased appetite.
- Enlargement of the thyroid gland is usually seen.

Treatment

- Antithyroid drugs, *e.g.,* propylthiouracil, methimazole, U.S.P. (Tapazole). *(See PH, Endocrine system)*
- Radioactive iodine therapy.
- Surgical removal of most of the thyroid tissue (subtotal thyroidectomy). Iodine to reduce vascularity of the thyroid preoperatively, *e.g.,* potassium iodide solution (SSKI). *(See PH, Endocrine system)*
- Propranolol (Inderal), for control of tachycardia and other symptomatic manifestations. *(See PH, Cardiovascular system)*

Nursing Tips

- *Patient must be brought to euthyroid (normal thyroid) state before surgery.*
- Administer medications, as ordered. Anithyroid drugs and propranolol (Inderal) must be given right up to the hours before surgery. *(See PH, Endocrine system, autonomic nervous system)*
- Provide a restful, cool environment. These patients are very intolerant of heat.
- Be accepting of behavior. These patients have poor control of their emotions and often fail to cooperate in their own care.
- Severe exopthalmos may require eye drops, dark glasses, eye exercises, and that eyelids be taped shut.
- Diet should be high in calories and fluids.
- Observe closely for arrhythmias, elevated blood pressure, and palpitations.

THYROIDECTOMY AND SUBTOTAL THYROIDECTOMY

Nursing Tips
Postoperative Care

- Care for the incision by maintaining semi-Fowler's position and support of the head, neck, and shoulders with sandbags and soft collar.
- Teach patient to support his own head and neck.
- Provide humidification. Oxygen therapy may be required. *(See NR, Oxygen administration)*
- *Watch for and be prepared for complications:*
    1. Hemorrhage (check dressing and vital signs frequently).
    2. Respiratory obstruction (have tracheostomy set at bedside).
    3. Laryngeal nerve damage (ask patient to speak every hour, but avoid unnecessary talking).

4. Tetany caused by inadvertent removal of parathyroid glands (have calcium gluconate available for IV administration).
5. Thyroid crisis or storm, seen with patients inadequately prepared for surgery (earliest manifestations are extreme tachycardia and hyperthermia). *(See SS, Thyroid storm)*

THYROID STORM (THYROID CRISIS)

Description

Thyroid storm (or thyroid crisis) is a life-threatening condition of thyrotoxicosis precipitated by stress, *(e.g.,* infection, injury, labor, or poor preparation for surgery).

What to Look for

- Severe tachycardia, hyperthermia (high fever), dehydration, delirium, and disturbances of all major systems.

Treatment

- Hypothermia (reduce fever).
  1. Nursing measures *(e.g.,* cold packs or hypothermia blanket). *(See NR, Hypothermia blanket)*
  2. Acetaminophen (Tylenol) preferred to salicylates. *(See PH, Analgesic antipyretics, anti-inflammatory agents, drugs for gout)*
- Iodine preparations *(e.g.,* Sodium Iodide IV initially, Lugol's solution p.o. after crisis has subsided). *(See PH, Endocrine system)*
- Intravenous fluids containing dextrose; may include antithyroid medication. *(See PH, Endocrine system)*
- Cardiac support, *e.g.,* propranolol (Inderal). *(See PH, Autonomic nervous system)*
- Corticosteroids (to treat shock or adrenal insufficiency). *(See PH, Endocrine system)*
- Oxygen therapy may be necessary. *(See NR, Oxygen administration)*
- Possible exchange transfusions or peritoneal dialysis.

Gastrointestinal System

ANORECTAL CONDITIONS

Description

Hemorrhoids are varicose veins of the anus; internal hemorrhoids lie above the anal sphincter and external ones lie below it. They may become inflamed or thrombosed, or they may bleed. The blood is bright red, and is usually on the outside of the stool, or appears on toilet tissue. Hemorrhoids and anal fissures are by far the most common cause of rectal bleeding, but other causes must be ruled out.

Anal fissure (fissure in ano) is an ulcerated, elongated laceration of the lower anal canal, usually caused by injury due to passage of large, hard stools. It is extremely painful upon defecation or rectal examination. Usually it will heal with conservative treatment.

Rectal fistulas (fistula in ano) are tracts that lead from the anorectal canal and open onto the skin near the anus. They are most commonly the result of neglect or poor treatment of anorectal abscesses, but are also complications of diseases of the large bowel, especially regional enteritis or Crohn's disease. They are accompanied by purulent, irritating discharge near the anus and by pain on defecation. They do not heal without treatment of the underlying disease and excision of the fistulous tract.

Common Diagnostic Tests

- Rectal examination by inspection and with a proctoscope (if it is not too painful for the patient).
- For fistula in ano
  1. Probe of the fistulous tract.
  2. Sigmoidoscopy to look for associated disease. *(See NR, Endoscopic procedures)*
  3. Barium x-rays, if regional enteritis or ulcerative colitis is suspected. *(See NR, x-ray preparations)*

Treatment

- Conservative treatment of hemorrhoids and anal fissure includes:
  1. Stool softeners to promote regular bowel movements without straining.
  2. Anesthetic ointments, applied topically.
  3. Witch hazel soaks *(e.g.,* Tucks).
  4. Sitz baths.
  5. External heat for thrombosed external hemorrhoids.
  6. Careful cleansing of the anal area after bowel movements.
- Surgical excision of hemorrhoids and anal fissure, if conservative measures are not successful.
- Wide excision of the fistulous tract and removal of the source of infection are required in rectal fistula. Temporary colostomy to provide for rest and healing of the area may be necessary for the patient with multiple fistulas.
- Some surgeons leave the excised areas open; others close them. Anorectal surgery is usually extremely painful the first day or two postoperative.

Nursing Tips

Postoperative care: The most common problems are hemorrhage, pain, and urinary retention.

- Hemorrhage: check the dressing or wound for signs of bleeding. Teach patient to check for bleeding. Monitor vital signs.
- Pain: analgesics for pain the first 24 to 48 hours postoperative, and immediately before or after the first bowel movement. *(See PH, Central nervous system)*
  1. Ice bags at first; later topical analgesics to the operative area may be helpful.
  2. Be with or near the patient when he has his first bowel movement. The pain may be severe enough for him to feel faint.
  3. Sitz baths, three or four times a day. Ice bag to head may prevent feelings of faintness.
- Urinary retention
  1. Restrict fluids drastically, preoperatively and postoperatively, as ordered.
  2. Check bladder for distention. Catheterize only if absolutely necessary. Some surgeons allow the patient to go 36 hours postoperatively without voiding, if fluids have been restricted and bladder is not distended.
  3. Getting patient out of bed to void is usually allowed.
  4. Try nursing measures to encourage patient to void *(e.g.,* pro-

viding a quiet, relaxed atmosphere, running water, blowing through a straw).
- Prevent constipation.
  1. Diet as tolerated; encourage roughage and fruits.
  2. Stool softeners, bulk laxatives.
  3. Encourage patient to develop good bowel habits to avoid constipation and to heed the desire to have a bowel movement—at a regular time of the day, if possible.

ADENOMATOUS POLYPS
Description

Most often found in the colon and stomach, adenomatous polyps are the most common benign tumor of the GI tract. They may be single or multiple, sessile (on a broad base) or pedunculated (on a stalk).
- Usually polyps are asymptomatic and are diagnosed by visualization on a proctosigmoidoscopic examination.
- Bleeding may be gross or occult; occasionally obstruction occurs if the polyp is large.
- Polyps of the colon are now frequently removed through the rectum by the use of the flexible colonoscope. *(See NR, Endoscopic procedures)*
- Familial polyposis, an inherited condition of multiple polyps, has an associated high incidence of cancer development. Colectomy is usually done to prevent malignancy.

ESOPHAGEAL VARICES

Description

Esophageal varices (varicose veins of the esophagus) are due generally to cirrhosis of the liver with intrahepatic portal venous obstruction and portal hypertension. Because of the hepatocellular dysfunction caused by the underlying cirrhosis, these patients are usually poor surgical risks. Extrahepatic compression of the portal circulation by adjacent tumors, cysts, aneurysms, and so forth are rare causes of esophageal varices. Because liver function is normal in this latter group of patients, the underlying problem can be treated surgically.

Ruptured esophageal varices may be caused by any increase in intra-abdominal pressure, such as coughing or vomiting, by erosion of the esophageal mucosa caused by esophagitis, by gastric acid reflux, by alcohol use, and by any drug that directly or indirectly injures the mucosal lining *(e.g.,* salicylates and corticoids). Bleeding esophageal varices constitute a life-threatening emergency because blood loss under such pressure is rapid and great.

Common Diagnostic Tests

- Esophagoscopy with flexible fiberoptic endoscope. *(See NR, Endoscopic procedures)*
- Barium swallow x-ray. *(See NR, x-ray preparations)*
- Portal venography.
- Hemoglobin, hematocrit, followed by type and crossmatch. *(See LAB)*
- Liver function tests, coagulation studies, electrolyte screen. *(See LAB and SS, Liver disorders)*

What to Look for

- Bleeding tends to be sudden and unexpected, in large volume, and bright red in color. *(See SS, Gastrointestinal bleeding)*
- History of alcoholism or evidence of cirrhosis. *(See SS, Liver disorders, cirrhosis)*

Treatment

For bleeding esophageal varices *(See SS, Gastrointestinal bleeding)*
- Blood replacement.
- Iced water lavage.
- Intravenous vasopressin injection, U.S.P. (Pitressin). *(See PH, Endocrine system)*
- Tamponade (direct pressure) applied by the balloons of the Sengstaken-Blakemore gastric tube. *(See NR, Sengstaken-Blakemore tube)*
- To prevent hepatic coma following massive bleeding, cathartics and enemas may be ordered to clear the GI tract of blood. Neomycin may be ordered to further reduce ammonia formation, the absorption of which can lead to coma and death. *(See PH, Antimicrobials)*

Surgical:
- Preferably, surgical procedures are done after the patient's condition has stabilized. The following procedures may be attempted: sclerosing of the varices, done endoscopically, and reduction of the portal hypertension through the use of one of several types of portal system shunts.

Nursing Tips

- Nurses, the patient, and his family must understand that vomited blood constitutes a medical emergency. Every member of the family should know or have at hand the telephone number of the rescue squad.
- Both the patient and family require emotional support. The patient faces a life-threatening situation and an uncomfortable, po-

tentially dangerous treatment if the Sengstaken-Blakemore tube is required.

- When in the hospital, these patients should have blood that has been typed and crossmatched on hold at all times. Check on its availability.
- Antacids may be ordered.
- To reduce the chance of hemorrhage, the patient should avoid use of aspirin and alcohol; he should also avoid constipation, coughing, and heavy lifting—anything that increases intrathoracic pressure.

GALLBLADDER

Description

The gallbladder stores bile produced in the liver for later delivery to the duodenum for the digestion of dietary fats. Disorders of the gallbladder and the bile ducts usually relate to inflammation, with or without the presence of stones. Terms that define the location of either the pathology or the surgical procedure involved in the biliary tract include the following: *chole* (pertaining to bile); *cyst* (bladder); *cholang* (bile ducts); *choledocho* (common duct); and *lith* (stone). *Cholelithiasis,* for example, refers to biliary stones. Symptoms are caused by inflammation of the gallbladder (cholecystitis) or the attempt of the body to "pass" a stone down the bile duct.

Common Diagnostic Tests

- Conventional tests have involved visualization of the biliary system by means of x-ray and a contrast dye. *Caution:* Before dye is administered, question patient about allergies to seafood, iodine, or dyes used in previous contrast studies. These dyes have an iodine base. Nausea, vomiting, hypotension, and rash may indicate allergy.
- Oral cholecystography: a radiopaque dye *(e.g.,* Telepaque or Oragrafin), which concentrates in the biliary system, is given orally. X-rays visualize the gallbladder and biliary ducts. *(See NR, x-ray preparations)*
- Intravenous cholangiography: dye is given slowly (over 20 min). Intravenous method may visualize the bile ducts better than oral cholecystography; useful in visualizing the biliary tree in the patient who has had a cholecystectomy. *(See NR, x-ray preparations)*
- Percutaneous transhepatic cholangiography: a needle is inserted into the liver and into an intrahepatic duct; bile is then drained out and dye is injected. This test is good for differentiating between obstructive and hepatocellular jaundice. Before procedure, patient should be questioned about bleeding history. After pro-

cedure watch for signs of bile leakage—fever, distention, and jaundice—and for signs of bleeding.
- Postoperative T-tube cholangiogram: dye is injected into common duct under fluoroscopy. *(See NR, x-ray preparations)*
- Endoscopic retrograde cholangiopancreatogram: direct visualization of the common bile duct and the pancreatic duct with a fiberoptic instrument after contrast medium has been injected into them. *(See NR, Endoscopic procedures)*
- Echogram or sonogram: noninvasive scan that may indicate presence of stones. *(See NR, Ultrasound, sonogram)*
- Laboratory work may show
  1. Moderately elevated WBC. *(See LAB)*
  2. Elevated serum bilirubin or urine bilirubin, or both, in obstruction of the common bile duct. *(See LAB)*
  3. Elevated prothrombin time if there is a defect in the coagulation mechanism. *(See LAB)*

What to Look for
- Pain in the right upper quadrant of the abdomen; may radiate to the right shoulder and back; may be dull and achy or, usually following ingestion of fatty foods, severe and colicky. There may be tenderness over the gallbladder area and abdominal rigidity.
- History of digestive disturbances, especially related to ingestion of fatty foods: nausea, vomiting, anorexia, belching, flatulence.
- Jaundice: due to edema or to a stone blocking the common bile duct. Watch for changes in the color of stool and urine. Stools may become clay-colored; urine may become dark orange.

Treatment
Medical
- Bed rest during the acute attack.
- IV fluids, especially when nausea and vomiting are present. *(See NR, Intravenous therapy)*
- Nasogastric tube with decompression. *(See NR, Gastrointestinal intubation)*
- Intake and output measured and recorded.
- Maintenance of electrolyte balance. *(See NR, Intravenous therapy, electrolyte imbalances)*
- Medications:
  1. Analgesics for the relief of severe pain, usually meperidine (Demerol). Morphine sulfate is avoided because it is believed to constrict the common duct sphincter. *(See PH, Central nervous system)*

2. Sedatives; antiemetics; antibiotics; phytonadione, U.S.P. (vitamin K). *(See PH, Central nervous system, Gastrointestinal system, Antimicrobials, and Cardiovascular system)*
- Diet, if tolerated: low fat, high protein, high carbohydrate.

Surgical

- *Cholecystectomy:* the operative procedure for 90% of patients with acute cholecystitis.
- Other procedures include: *choledocholithotomy* (incision of the common duct with removal of a stone) and *cholecystostomy* (drainage of the gallbladder). When there is evidence of gallstones, the gallbladder and ducts are explored. Usually a Penrose drain is left in the gallbladder area. A T-tube may be inserted into the duct with drainage to the outside in an effort to keep the duct open. *(For care of T-tube, see Nursing Tips)*
- Nonoperative manipulation and extraction or crushing of retained stones. This is done under fluoroscopy by inserting a catheter and basket through a sinus tract left by a T-tube that has been retained 6 weeks postoperatively.
- Endoscopic retrograde cholangiopancreatography (ERCP) may be done to retrieve stone if it is lodged in the lower common bile duct.

Nursing Tips

- Preoperative teaching should prepare patient for post-operative course. *(See SS, Preoperative care)*
- Postoperative nursing care is similar to that of any abdominal surgery, with these special points:
  1. Prevent respiratory complications. The operative area is high in the abdomen, so it will be painful for the patient to deep breathe. Encourage deep breathing. *(See NR, Deep breathing techniques)*
  2. Drainage from the Penrose drain tends to be profuse and irritating to the skin, so keep skin dry, clean, and protected with an ointment *(see NR, Ostomies, fistulas, and draining wounds)*. Montgomery straps are practical (see Fig. 5-3).
  3. *Care of the T-tube* (choledochostomy tube): The "T" is inserted into the common duct, with the tube to the outside. It is usually sutured into place, and the tube is attached to gravity drainage. The drainage bag must be kept below the level of the gallbladder.
     a. Drainage is measured and recorded (200 to 500 ml is normal for the first day, with amounts decreasing each day there-

after). Usually red or red-tinged at first, it soon becomes the color of bile.

b. Patients must be cautioned against exerting tension on the tube or kinking it.

c. The physician may order that the T-tube be clamped at intervals before its removal. Observe how the patient tolerates this. Usually the tube is removed around the seventh to tenth day after cholangiogram indicates there is no obstruction.

d. Recycled bile: if drainage has been excessive over a period of time, bile may be taken from the drainage system and returned to the patient by giving it orally mixed with fruit juice and chilled.

4. Watch for complications unique to biliary tract surgery.

a. Signs of obstruction from either stones or edema (*e.g.*, jaundice), failure of stools to return to normal color, and excessive T-tube drainage.

b. Displacement of the T-tube may be indicated by sudden change in the T-tube drainage or by leaking around it. Sudden chills, fever, and abdominal pain may indicate bile peritonitis.

GASTROINTESTINAL BLEEDING (THE GI BLEEDER)

Description

Bleeding may occur anywhere in the gastrointestinal tract and may constitute a life-threatening emergency. Vomited blood nearly always indicates bleeding above the duodenojejunal juncture, because blood that leaks into the GI tract below the duodenum rarely reenters the stomach. Common causes of upper GI bleeding include esophageal varices (usually a complication of cirrhosis of the liver), gastritis, peptic ulcer, and the use of certain drugs (*e.g.*, aspirin, steroids, and anticoagulants). Bleeding from the lower GI tract may occur as a result of any of the inflammatory conditions, including diverticulitis, Meckel's diverticulum, ulcerative colitis, and Crohn's disease. Finally, bleeding from the anorectal area occurs as a result of hemorrhoids, rectal polyps, anal fissures, and fistulas. Bleeding may result from neoplasms anywhere along the intestinal tract.

Common Diagnostic Tests

- Positive test for occult blood either in aspirated gastric contents or stool. (*See LAB*)
- Fiberoptic esophagogastroduodenoscopy and an upper GI series

to find the location of an upper GI bleed. *(See NR, Endoscopic procedures and x-ray preparations)*
- Selective abdominal angiography may be useful for the patient with a history of duodenal ulcer or active subpyloric bleeding when other studies fail to establish the site of the bleeding.
- Sigmoidoscopy, colonoscopy, barium enema, and arteriography for lower GI bleeding.
- Complete blood count, frequently repeated hemoglobin and hematocrit, type and crossmatch, coagulation studies, blood gases, and electrolyte screen; liver function tests; renal function tests *(e.g.* blood urea nitrogen and creatinine). *(See LAB)*

What to Look for

Symptoms will depend upon the source of bleeding and the rate of blood loss. You will want to ascertain the amount and color of the blood vomited or passed. When? How often?
- Vomited, bright red blood is fresh, usually from the upper GI tract, though epistaxis (nose bleed) and hemoptysis (bleeding from the respiratory tract) must be ruled out. Sudden, bright red hematemesis is characteristic of esophageal varices (look for signs of liver disease). *(See SS, Esophageal varices)*
- Vomitus with coffee-ground appearance indicates that the blood has been in contact with gastric acid for perhaps several hours (indicates upper GI bleeding).
- Melena (black tarry stools) is usually a sign of bleeding from the upper GI tract.
- Bright red blood in the stool is a sign of bleeding from the colon or anorectal area.

In Acute GI Bleeding
- Look for symptoms of shock: fallen blood pressure and rapid pulse, cold and clammy skin, hyperventilation, weakness, chills, restlessness, confusion.
- Syndromes resulting from diminished renal and liver function.
- Shock and hemorrhage will be treated first; efforts to discover the cause and exact site of bleeding will follow.

After the Acute Stage
- Check for postural hypotension (an early sign of sharply reduced blood volume and renewed bleeding). *(See NR, Postural hypotension)*

In Slow GI Bleeding
- Weakness, irritability, fatigue, pallor, and anemia.

Treatment

In Acute GI Bleeding

- An IV is started immediately with a #19 gauge needle, so that there is access to the circulation both for taking samples for blood typing, crossmatching, hemoglobin, and hematocrit, and for blood transfusions, which will be ordered.
- Monitor pulse and blood pressure q. 15 min.
- A nasogastric tube is passed, so that iced saline lavage can be started *(see NR, Gastrointestinal intubation)*. The Sengstaken-Blakemore tube may be used to stop hemorrhage from esophageal or gastric varices *(see NR, Sengstaken-Blakemore tube)*.
- Oxygen therapy may be indicated. *(See NR, Oxygen administration)*
- Angiography may be used (especially in poor surgical risks) to give vasopressin by catheter or to produce embolization by introducing Gelfoam.

After the Bleeding Has Stopped

- Continue to monitor the patient's vital signs, including checks for postural hypotension.
- Decompress the stomach with a gastrointestinal tube to suction. *(See NR, Gastrointestinal intubation)*
- Advance the diet slowly.
- Cimetidine (Tagamet) may be ordered. *(See PH, Gastrointestinal system)*
- Antacids are frequently given by nasogastric tube. Be sure to clamp tube for 30 minutes following administration of any medication. Tube may become clogged with antacid, so if allowed, follow with 30 ml water.

Surgical Intervention

(See SS, Esophageal varices; Gastric surgery; Intestinal surgery; and Anorectal conditions)

- Surgical intervention may be required if patient does not respond satisfactorily to vigorous medical therapy or if he develops a perforation with accompanying peritonitis (severe abdominal pain with boardlike rigidity and ileus). *(See SS, Peritonitis and SS, Postoperative complications, Ileus)*

Nursing Tips

- Monitor the patient carefully for signs of continued bleeding. Check vital signs q. 15 min or as frequently as patient's condition indicates. Check for postural hypotension.

- Maintain the IV. Assess the patient's respiration for signs of circulatory overload (rales or wheezing).
- Monitor urinary output carefully. Keep an accurate record of intake and output.
- Keep the nasogastric tube patent. Mark the level of the drainage on the collection bag or bottle and the time, at intervals, so that by comparison you can verify that the suction system is working properly. If it is not, notify the physician. Irrigate the tube, only if ordered, with sterile solutions.
- Empty the drainage bag or bottle every shift. Measure and record the amount as output separate from regular intake and output, which will also be monitored. Water or saline if used as an irrigant counts as intake; what is withdrawn either with syringe or by suction machine is counted as output. Describe color of drainage.
- Iced lavage with normal saline or water is intended to remove clots and to stop bleeding. Chilling constricts the blood vessels of the stomach. *(See NR, Gastrointestinal intubation)*
- Be sure that blood has been typed and crossmatched, and that it is available and up to date.
- Special mouth care: dilute hydrogen peroxide mouthwashes, lozenges, lemon-swabs, gargles, ice chips (if ordered). Water from ice chips equals half their volume *(e.g., 1 cup ice chips = $\frac{1}{2}$ cup water).*

HERNIA
ABDOMINAL HERNIA
Description

Hernia is a weakness in a wall of a cavity through which viscera may protrude.

- *Indirect inguinal hernia,* by far the most common hernia (especially in men), occurs through the inguinal ring and extends down into the scrotum or labia.
- *Direct inguinal hernia* passes through an area of muscular weakness in the abdominal wall (not through the inguinal canal).
- *Femoral hernia* descends through the femoral ring. It is more common in women than in men.
- *Umbilical hernia* results from failure of the umbilical orifice to close. It is more common in obese women and in children and blacks.
- *Ventral* or *incisional hernias* occur in areas of weakness of the abdominal wall following surgery.

Hernias are described as *reducible* (meaning that the contents can be returned to their original position), *incarcerated* or *irreducible,* and *strangulated,* in which not only is the hernia irreducible, but blood and intestinal flow through the intestine in the hernia is stopped completely. Strangulation is a medical emergency, initially as acute bowel obstruction. If the situation persists, there is danger of gangrene of the strangulated loop of bowel.

What to Look for
- Swelling or a soft outpouching, especially with increased intra-abdominal pressure *(e.g.,* from coughing or lifting).
- Pain may or may not be present. If present, it may be due to stretching of muscle and fascia.
- Severe pain, tenderness, and symptoms of obstruction (ileus, distention, and absence of flatus or defecation) indicate strangulation of the hernia.

Treatment
- Reduction of the hernia by applying gentle pressure in order to return contents of hernial pouch to original position.
- A truss (a pad made with firm material and held in place over the hernia with a belt) may be used to keep the hernia from protruding. It does not correct the problem and is not recommended by most authorities.
- *Herniorrhaphy* is the surgical repair of a hernia.
- *Hernioplasty* is the surgical repair of the hernia with reinforcement of the area with synthetic sutures or mesh for additional support.

Nursing Tips
- Coughing could damage the hernia repair. Teach the patient to splint the incision. Provide cough depressants, if indicated.
- Urinary retention may be relieved by assisting the male patient to stand at the bedside to void.
- To relieve swelling of the scrotum, elevation on a small rolled towel may be helpful. Intermittent use of a small ice bag (one that applies no pressure) may help. The patient may require a scrotal support.
- The patient who has had an umbilical or an incisional hernia repaired may have a nasogastric tube in place postoperatively to reduce intra-abdominal pressure. *(See NR, Gastrointestinal intubation)*

HIATAL HERNIA
Description
Hiatal hernia is the herniation of the stomach into the thoracic cavity through the diaphragmatic esophageal hiatus. In the *sliding hiatal hernia,* the upper part of the stomach and the esophagogastric junction intermittently ride up into the chest cavity. In the *para-*

esophageal, or *rolling, hernia* some part of the greater curvature of the stomach extrudes through a diaphragmatic defect near the esophageal hiatus. In this type there is danger of strangulated hernia. Loss of lower esophageal sphincter function permits reflux of stomach contents into the esophagus, leading to esophagitis, occasionally to esophageal ulceration or esophageal stricture, or to tracheal aspiration.

Common Diagnostic Tests

- Upper GI series with a barium swallow.
- Esophagoscopy. *(See NR, Endoscopic procedures)*
- Acid perfusion test (Bernstein test) is often positive when esophagitis is present.
- Manometric studies for evaluation of lower esophageal sphincter function, often with *p*H, motility, and acid-clearing studies.

What to Look for

- History of mild or intermittent indigestion aggravated by lying down or bending forward.
- Substernal pain that sometimes mimics heart attack.
- Dysphagia (difficulty in swallowing); regurgitation; nocturnal respiratory distress; history of transitory relief with antacids.

Treatment and Nursing Tips
Medical

- Diet: small feedings of moderately bland food, with avoidance of coffee, alcohol, and smoking.
- Weight reduction is sometimes helpful for the obese patient.
- Meals should be eaten slowly, with the patient sitting up.
- Antacids are given after meals. *(See PH, Gastrointestinal system)*
- Unless patient has an esophageal spasm, anticholinergic medications are not given because they delay emptying of the stomach and decrease esophageal sphincter tone.
- The head of the bed should be elevated at least 6 inches, which is best done by putting the legs of the head of the bed on blocks.
- The patient should avoid eating within 2 hours of bedtime; constipation and straining at stool; and corsets, girdles, heavy lifting, and leaning forward.

Surgical

- The stomach is replaced into its correct position, and the defect is repaired. The procedure is done sometimes through the chest, sometimes through the abdomen. Nursing care would be similar

to any thoracotomy (the patient will have chest tubes immediately postoperatively), or upper abdominal surgery. *(See SS, Gastric surgery and SS, Pulmonary surgery)*
- Vagotomy is sometimes done in selected cases to reduce acid reflux.

INFLAMMATION OF THE INTESTINAL TRACT
APPENDICITIS
Description

Appendicitis is an infection of the veriform appendix, a small fingerlike blind pouch attached to the cecum just below the ileocecal valve. It may be caused by a fecalith (a stonelike mass of feces) or anything that occludes the lumen of the appendix *(e.g.,* adhesions, pinworms, or inflammation).

Common Diagnostic Tests
- Complete blood count usually shows leukocytosis. *(See LAB)*

What to Look for
- Acute generalized abdominal pain that localizes in the right lower quadrant (RLQ), also called McBurney's point; rebound tenderness (tenderness after the pressure is released) at this point.
- Nausea and vomiting, constipation, anorexia, and low-grade temperature.
- Symptoms of *ruptured appendix:* Severe abdominal pain, which may be relieved at the time of rupture, followed by generalized intense pain, rigid abdomen, elevated WBC, elevated temperature, and symptoms of shock.

Treatment
- Rule out other causes of pain.
- If there is any doubt, a laparotomy is done rather than chance rupture of the appendix with resulting peritonitis.

Nursing Tips
- Postoperative care for an uncomplicated appendectomy is like that of any laparotomy.
- Appendectomy following rupture of the appendix requires the following additional elements of care:
  1. A drain will remain in place.
  2. IV fluids. *(See NR, Intravenous therapy)*
  3. Nasogastric tube (n.g. tube). *(See NR, Gastrointestinal intubation)*
  4. Large doses of antibiotics, often more than one.

5. Semi-Fowler's or Fowler's position to promote drainage into the pelvic cavity.
6. Careful assessment for symptoms of paralytic ileus (absent bowel sounds, no passage of gas or feces by rectum) and peritonitis. *(See SS, Postoperative complications)*

DIVERTICULITIS AND DIVERTICULOSIS
Description

A diverticulum is an outpouching of the intestinal wall at a point of weakness. Usually found in the sigmoid colon, diverticula are now thought to be caused by lack of bulk in the diet and by increased intraluminal pressure. The presence of several of these herniations is called *diverticulosis*. Inflammation in one or more of the diverticula is called *diverticulitis*. In making the diagnosis, carcinoma of the bowel must be ruled out. Complications resulting from diverticulitis include perforation with resulting peritonitis *(see SS, Peritonitis)*, hemorrhage, abscess, and fistula formation.

Common Diagnostic Tests

- Barium enema. *(See NR, x-ray preparations)*
- Colonoscopy and sigmoidoscopy (fiberoptic). *(See NR, Endoscopic procedures)*
- Elevated WBCs in diverticulitis.
- Selective mesenteric arteriography, if there is bleeding.

What to Look for

- Lower abdominal discomfort—particularly localized to the left lower quadrant; tenderness to palpation; and possibly a palpable mass.
- Change in bowel habits: patient may have alternating diarrhea and constipation.
- Fever (in diverticulitis)
- Signs of complications *(e.g.,* perforation with peritonitis, obstruction, and massive bleeding evidenced by bright red blood or mahogany-colored stools and a drop in blood pressure). *(See SS, Gastrointestinal bleeding)*

Treatment
Medical
Diverticulosis

- High-fiber diet, force fluids, bulk laxatives *(e.g.,* Metamucil), no anticholinergic drugs. *(See PH, Autonomic nervous system)*
- Enemas should be avoided because they increase luminal pressure and could lead to perforation.

Acute Diverticulitis

- Antibiotics.
- Bed rest.
- Nothing by mouth; IV fluids; may go to hyperalimentation. *(See NR, Intravenous therapy)*
- Nasogastric suction. *(See NR, Gastrointestinal intubation)*
- Meperidine (Demerol) is usually ordered for pain. *(See PH, Central nervous system)*
- Anticholinergic drugs may be ordered. *(See PH, Autonomic nervous system)*

Surgical

- If possible, surgical treatment should be elective. It may be indicated in case of intractability or in case of complications.
- Incision and drainage of abscesses
- Bowel resection of affected parts; may include temporary or permanent colostomy.

Nursing Tips

- See Nursing Tips for patients with intestinal surgery. *(See SS, Intestinal surgery)*

MECKEL'S DIVERTICULUM
Description

Meckel's diverticulum is a congenital sacculation usually found near, but proximal to, the ileocecal valve. When inflamed, it may lead to bowel obstruction.

What to Look for

- Symptoms may resemble appendicitis.

Treatment

- Meckel's diverticulum is treated by surgical removal.

Nursing Tips

- Nursing care is similar to that of any laparotomy.

PERITONITIS
Description

Peritonitis is an inflammation of the lining (peritoneum) of the abdominal cavity. It is most often caused by a bacterial invasion as a result of perforation or rupture of an organ into the abdominal cavity (*e.g.*, a perforated ulcer or a ruptured diverticulum, appendix, or gallbladder). It may also be caused by leakage or contamination during abdominal surgery, or by an ascending infection through the female reproductive tract (*e.g.,* salpingitis).

Common Diagnostic Tests

- X-rays: flat plate of the abdomen may show free peritoneal fluid or air in the abdominal cavity.
- Elevated WBC. *(See LAB)*
- Blood and peritoneal cultures may identify the offending organism.

What to Look for

- Abdominal pain: diffuse at first, but becoming localized in the affected area; later becoming exquisitely tender with muscle guarding, abdominal rigidity, and abdominal distention.
- Paralytic ileus and absence of bowel sounds. *(See SS, Postoperative complications)*
- Anorexia and nausea and vomiting.
- Elevated temperature, drop in blood pressure, tachycardia (rapid pulse), and rapid, shallow breathing.
- Effects of dehydration and electrolyte imbalance. *(See LAB, Electrolytes)*

Treatment

- Remove source of irritation; this may require surgical intervention.
- Control infection by using broad-spectrum, antimicrobial drug until results of cultures are available; then use specific antibiotic. *(See PH, Antimicrobials)*
- Replace fluids and electrolytes. Monitor electrolytes daily. *(See LAB and NR, Intravenous therapy)*
- Relieve pain with minimum doses of medication to prevent masking of symptoms. Use nursing comfort measures.
- Oxygen therapy may be required. *(See NR, Oxygen administration)*
- Semi-Fowlers's position: to try to localize infection in lower abdominal cavity.
- Nasointestinal tube with suction to decompress bowel. *(See NR, Gastrointestinal intubation)*

Nursing Tips

These patients are extremely ill. They require gentle, total nursing care including

- Accurate, intelligent assessment of symptoms.

- Management of nasointestinal tubes, oxygen, IV, and drug therapy.
- Comfort measures, including mouth care and fever reduction.
- Nasogastric tubes are in place for a long time and cause sore nares and throat. Lubricating ointment helps the nares; anesthetic gargles are sometimes helpful to the throat.

REGIONAL ENTERITIS (CROHN'S DISEASE)
Description
Crohn's disease (also known as regional enteritis, granulomatous ileitis or granulomatous ileucolitis) is an inflammatory process that involves all layers of the intestinal wall, especially the submucosa. Areas of normal bowel lie between inflamed segments. Most often the disease affects the ileum alone, but it may also involve the colon, and infrequently the colon only. Narrowing of the lumen of the intestine caused by thickening of the intestinal wall may lead to obstruction. Fistula formation and mesenteric abscesses are common late complications.

Common Diagnostic Tests
- X-rays of the small and large intestine. *(See NR, x-ray preparations)*
- Sigmoidoscopy. *(See NR, Endoscopic procedures)*

What to Look for
- History of chronic diarrhea. Usually three to four semi-soft stools a day, some with fat. Usually there is no blood or pus.
- Right-lower quadrant pain in an acute attack may mimic appendicitis.
- Symptoms of obstruction *(e.g.,* severe abdominal pain, distention, constipation, and vomiting).
- Abdominal fistulas and abscesses with fever, and painful abdominal masses.
- General debilitation may occur if disease has been long standing.

Treatment
Medical
- Diet: low residue, bland, high calorie, and high protein, with vitamin supplements.
- Anticholinergics, diphenoxylate (Lomotil), and tincture of opium. *(See PH, Autonomic nervous system)*
- Antibacterials for specific complications, though sulfasalazine (Azulfidine) may be given long term to prevent relapses. *(See PH, Antimicrobials)*
- Corticosteroids for acute stages. *(See PH, Endocrine system)*

- Azathioprine (Imuran), an antimetabolite, still unproved in the treatment of Crohn's disease.

Surgical
- Resection of involved bowel or bypass procedures have generally not been curative, so they are attempted infrequently. Surgery may be required to deal with complications *(e.g.,* fistulas, recurrent obstruction, and abscesses that do not respond to conservative treatment), but it is a last resort because postoperative healing is poor, and interior fistula formation commonly occurs.

Nursing Tips
- All of the nursing tips outlined under "ulcerative colitis" would apply to the nursing of the patient with Crohn's disease, except for the reference to ileostomy and the one regarding regular checks for cancer of the colon. Although colon cancer is an all too-common complication of ulcerative colitis, it is rare in regional enteritis. *(See SS, Ulcerative colitis: Nursing tips)*

ULCERATIVE COLITIS
Description
Ulcerative colitis is a condition involving inflammation of the mucous membrane of the large bowel, usually beginning in the rectum and spreading to involve the entire colon. The disease is characterized by exacerbations and remissions. The cause is unknown, though it is now believed that there may be an autoimmune basis. Patients who have had the disease over a period of years are at greatly increased risk for colon cancer.

Common Diagnostic Tests
- Barium enema may show shortening, scarring, narrowing, and ulceration of the bowel. *(See NR, x-ray preparations)*
- Proctoscopic and sigmoidoscopic examination: may include biopsy. *(See NR, Endoscopic procedures)*
- Stool culture to rule out amebic colitis and bacillary dysentery.
- Leukocytosis (elevated WBCs), anemia, and elevated sedimentation rate. *(See LAB)*

What to Look for
- Diarrhea: in an acute attack there may be 15 to 20 stools daily, containing blood, mucus, and pus.
- Abdominal cramps, sometimes with leakage of stool.
- Anorexia (loss of appetite), occasional nausea and vomiting, low-

grade fever, weakness, anemia, dehydration, weight loss, and hypoalbuminemia.
- Symptoms of complications of hemorrhage, perforation, or toxic megacolon (massive colonic dilatation that may result in rupture of the colon). Distended abdomen is symptomatic of toxic megacolon.

Treatment
Medical

- Nutrition: High-protein, high-calorie, high-vitamin, low-residue diet. Preparation for surgery may include hyperalimentation. *(See NR, Intravenous therapy)*
- Elimination: Relieve discomfort around anus by washing area frequently; use an anesthetic ointment, *e.g.,* dibucaine (Nupercaine) p.r.n.; Sitz baths.
- Medications:
  1. Opium derivatives *(e.g.,* Paregoric) for short-term use only (to decrease intestinal motility). *(See PH, Gastrointestinal system)*
  2. Kaolin or bismuth salts. *(See PH, Gastrointestinal system)*
  3. Antispasmodic drugs *(e.g.,* belladonna group) or diphenoxylate hydrochloride (Lomotil) *(see PH, Gastrointestinal system). Caution:* These drugs may be very dangerous and may precipitate toxic megacolon. At any sign of abdominal distention, stop therapy and report to physician.
  4. Antibiotics to prevent secondary infections, *e.g.,* sulfasalazine (Azulfidine), which frequently is also used long-term to help prevent relapses. *(See PH, Antimicrobials)*
  5. Corticotropin (ACTH) or adrenal steroids, very effective in treatment of acute attacks. Started IV, then p.o. May also be given rectally with great benefit, especially when disease is confined to the rectum. *(See PH, Endocrine system)*
  6. Azathioprine (Imuran) is being used; it is still under study.

Surgical

- Subtotal colectomy with ileostomy is done most frequently as emergency treatment for massive hemorrhage, toxic colitis, or perforation.
- Total colectomy with ileostomy is the procedure of choice in elective situations.
- Continent ileostomy (Kock pouch): an internal pouch is fashioned out of the terminal end of the ileum, and a one-way valve keeps stool and gas from escaping except when the patient empties it with a catheter (several times a day). *(See SS, Intestinal surgery)*

Nursing Tips

- Rest and emotional support.
- Emotional support is imperative, especially in the acute phase, during preparation for and following surgery. The frustration and exhaustion associated with the patient's symptoms cannot be over-emphasized.
- Adjustment to and acceptance of an ileostomy can be eased by intelligent, sympathetic nursing care and patient education.
- Document frequency and character of stools. Have bedpan within patient's reach. Padding may add to comfort. Room deodorizers may be needed.
- The patient in the acute phase is very ill and will require all comfort measures, including skin care, decubitus prevention, and protection of boney prominences.
- The patient, even when asymptomatic, will require medical supervision, including checks for colon cancer. If he is on long-term therapy with sulfasalazine (Azulfidine), he should have good education regarding this drug. *(See PH, Antimicrobials)*

LIVER

Description

A remarkable organ, sometimes called the body's chemical plant, the liver plays many roles, including that of synthesizer, detoxifier, and storehouse. The liver also has impressive powers of rejuvenation, a fact that has important implications for nursing care. Particularly in cases of liver failure, if the patient can be carried through the crisis he has a chance of recovery, for a time at least.

Table 5-1 highlights the effects of hepatic function disorders, which may have any one of a number of underlying causes.

Common Diagnostic Tests

- Serum bilirubin
  1. Total bilirubin: done most often. Normal: 0.01 mg/100 ml to 1 mg/100 ml.
  2. Direct or conjugated: elevated in obstruction. Normal: 0.01 mg/100 ml to 0.50 mg/100ml.
  3. Indirect or unconjugated: elevated in parenchymal cell damage. Indirect is total minus direct.
- Serum alkaline phosphatase: elevated in obstructive liver disease (also elevated in metastatic bone disease, fractures, hyperparathyroidism, and diseases in which there is osteoblastic activity). Normal values vary greatly with testing methods. *(See LAB)*

TABLE 5–1. **Liver Disorders**

Dysfunction	What Happens	What to Look for
Intrahepatic: inflammation or disorder of hepatic cells (e.g., hepatitis, cirrhosis, carcinoma). Extrahepatic: *Hemolytic jaundice* caused by too-rapid breakdown of RBCs. *Mechanical obstruction* to the flow of bile (e.g., obstruction of the common bile duct by gallstones or tumors).	Bilirubin accumulates in the bloodstream; tissues of the body, including skin and sclera, become yellowish.	Jaundice (yellowing of the skin and sclera) accompanied frequently by pruritus (itching). Dark, orange-colored urine and clay-colored stools are seen frequently.
Changes in the liver that slow circulation and cause backup pressure in the portal system, as in cirrhosis.	Hypertension of the portal circulation.	Esophageal varices, hemorrhoids, splenomegaly, ascites.
Interference with synthesis of blood clotting factors.	Bleeding tendencies.	Petechiae, easy bruising, ecchymoses, GI bleeding.
Interference with protein and carbohydrate synthesis.	Hypoalbuminemia, decreased glycogen reserves, decreased gluconeogenesis.	Generalized edema and hypoglycemia during fasting.
Interference with the conversion of ammonia to urea.	Accumulation of ammonia in the blood, causing metabolic effects on the brain (hepatic encephalopathy).	Drowsiness, confusion, disorientation, flapping tremor (asterixis), and behavioral and personality changes, with gradual depression of level of consciousness developing into coma.
Interference with the synthesis of some immune globulins.	Reduced resistance to infection.	
Interference with the liver's ability to detoxify toxic substances.	Increased risk of toxicity from alcohol and from drugs given in normal doses.	Signs of alcohol or drug toxicity. Check which drugs are hepatotoxic and which are detoxified by the liver.

- Serum glutamic-oxaloacetic transaminase (SGOT) and serum glutamic-pyruvic transaminase (SGPT) are elevated in hepatocellular disease. SGPT is found mainly in the liver, so it is especially significant. Normals: SGOT 8 to 33 U/ml; SGPT 1 to 36 U/ml.

- Prothrombin time: elevated. Normal: 12 to 14 sec. Test for differentiation between obstructive and hepatocellular disease: administration of vitamin K will normalize prothrombin time of obstructed liver, but not of cell-damaged liver.
- Blood lipids and cholesterol: usually elevated in obstructive jaundice.
- Blood ammonia levels: elevated in severe liver disease, especially following GI bleeding. Normal varies with methodology.
- Liver biopsy. *(See NR, Liver biopsy)*
- Hepatic scanning, sonography, CAT scanning, selective hepatic angiography, and peritoneoscopy. Radioimmunoassay for antihepatitis A virus (anti-HAV), hepatitis B surface antigen (HB_sAg), and hepatitis B surface antibody (anti-HB_s).

Treatment and Nursing Tips

- Bed rest in the acute phase. Sympathetic support.
- For jaundice (icterus):
  1. Best seen in the sclera (white of the eye), especially in people of colored skin.
  2. Pruritus (itching) due to icterus
     a. Avoid alkaline soaps.
     b. Keep nails trimmed to prevent scratching.
     c. Apply emollient lotions.
     d. Medications (such as Benadryl) are of limited benefit. *(See PH, Central nervous system)*
- For ascites and fluid retention:
  1. Evaluate the degree of abdominal distention.
     a. Weigh daily, at the same time and under the same circumstances.
     b. Measure abdominal girth daily. Mark the abdomen at the level at which you are measuring, so that measurement can be taken at the same place consistently.
  2. Low semi-Fowler's position will relieve pressure on the diaphragm, diminishing dyspnea. Reposition frequently.
  3. Accurate measurement of intake and output.
  4. Low-sodium diet.
  5. Total fluid intake is often restricted.
  6. Diuretics may gradually be introduced. *Caution:* hypokalemia is deadly to the damaged liver, so monitor potassium levels. *(See LAB and PH, Urinary system)*
  7. Salt-poor albumin may be given IV. *(See NR, Intravenous therapy)*
  8. Special skin care is essential: bathe with mild, nonalkaline soap and water, rinse thoroughly, and use emollient lotions, especially to massage pressure points.

9. Paracentesis may be required to relieve pressure. Usually no more than 1000 ml of fluid are removed at one time. *(See NR, Paracentesis)*

- For edema of extremities:
  1. Elevate extremities. Antiembolism stockings may be ordered.
  2. Provide comfort measures to relieve pressure on boney prominences, *(e.g., sheepskin protectors and eggcrate mattress)*.
- For bleeding tendencies:
  1. Monitor for bleeding. Describe subcutaneous bleeding, petechiae, ecchymoses (bruising), nosebleeds, and bleeding gums.
  2. Provide good mouth care. Tooth brushing should be done with a soft brush.
  3. Test vomitus and stools for occult blood, as indicated. *(See LAB)* Gastrointestinal bleeding is a frequent complication of cirrhosis. *(See SS, Esophageal varices snd Gastrointestinal bleeding)*
- Check special cautions regarding all drugs prescribed for these patients.
  1. Check for hepatotoxicity. Some common offenders are acetaminophen (Tylenol), allopurinol (Zyloprim), isoniazid (INH), and methyldopa (Aldomet).
  2. Check for drugs detoxified by the liver *(e.g., sedatives, barbiturates, and some diuretics)*; these must be used cautiously. Many physicians feel that sedatives should never be given to the patient with impaired liver function.
  3. Dosages of all drugs may have to be reduced.
- Diet is usually high in carbohydrate and protein and low in fat in the early stages of liver disease. Protein is reduced in an effort to reduce ammonia formation.
- Surgical treatment for portal hypertension: shunts to divert some blood away from the liver.
- *Liver failure* leading to *hepatic coma*: The patient may have all of the symptoms described in Table 5-1. He will require all of the treatment and vital nursing care described above. In addition:
  1. Assist in the control of fluid and acid–base and electrolyte imbalances.
  2. Protect the patient from sources of infection.
  3. Assist in the effort to reduce production of ammonia.
     a. Restrict protein intake.
     b. Attempt to remove blood from the GI tract with laxatives and enemas.
     c. Neomycin may be ordered in an effort to kill ammonia-producing bacteria. *(See PH, Antimicrobials)*
     d. Lactulose (Cephulac) may be ordered to reduce blood ammonia.

4. Watch for signs of hypoglycemia, and see that it is corrected if it occurs.

CIRRHOSIS

Description

Cirrhosis is a chronic disease of the liver characterized by destruction of normal liver tissue and the replacement of it by connective (scar) tissue that divides it into nodules. It is becoming a leading cause of death in the 25- to 65-year-age group. Cirrhosis is almost always due to the toxic effects of alcohol, though nutritional deficiencies, poisons, hepatitis, and biliary obstruction are also known to be causative factors.

Common Laboratory Tests

(See SS, Liver: common laboratory tests)

What to Look for

(See Table 5-1)

Nursing Tips

- Refer to all of the nursing tips on the management of patients with liver disorders listed above.
- Emphasize the importance of *no alcohol ingestion.*

HEPATIC TUMORS

Description

The liver is a common site of metastasis from malignancies originating elsewhere. Primary liver carcinoma is uncommon.

What to Look for

- Most often symptoms appear too late for curative treatment. They include anemia, weight loss, weakness, and jaundice (if the tumor obstructs the biliary system.

Treatment

Anticancer drugs are administered directly into the liver, and sometimes surgical removal of segments of the liver may be attempted.

LIVER ABSCESS

Description

Liver abscesses may form as a complication of infection elsewhere in the body. The offending organism is most often *Escherichia coli* but staphylococci, certain fungi, and the Protozoa *Entamoeba histolytica* (which causes amebiasis) are some of the other agents that also cause liver abscess.

What to Look for

The patient may have high fever, jaundice, and a painful and enlarged liver. He may be extremely toxic.

Treatment

Antibiotics specific for the disease organism are indicated. Surgical drainage of the abscess is often required.

VIRAL HEPATITIS

Description

Viral hepatitis is an inflammation of the liver with cell damage and necrosis. It is caused by a virus.

- Type A hepatitis—hepatitis A virus (HAV), or "infectious hepatitis"—is a milder disease than type B. It is spread largely by the fecal–oral route, though it may be transmitted parenterally through serum and blood products.
- Type B hepatitis—hepatitis B virus (HBV), hepatitis B surface antigen (HB_sAg), or hepatitis-associated Antigen (HAA)—was formerly known as "serum hepatitis." It is a more severe infection, and has a longer incubation period, than type A. Although it is most commonly transmitted parenterally by contamination by blood and blood products, it may be spread by exposure to any body secretion, including saliva and seminal fluid. It is a particular threat in hemodialysis units, as well as to those receiving blood transfusions—particularly hemophiliacs; to drug addicts; and to male homosexuals. People may be carriers without symptoms of disease.
- Type non-A, non-B, still under study, designates any of what are believed to be possibly several hepatitis-causing viruses, which are neither type A or type B. It has been found in patients who have had repeated blood transfusions.
- Inadequately cooked shellfish, when infested, is a source of infection for both type A and type B viruses.

Most patients recover from viral hepatitis with little residual damage. A few go on to develop chronic hepatitis or even fulminant hepatitis with fatal, massive liver necrosis.

What to Look for

Before the jaundice appears:
- Nausea, vomiting, anorexia, diarrhea, and a distaste for cigarettes.

- Malaise, weakness, unusual fatigue, and muscle tenderness.
- Headache, fever, and sometimes upper respiratory symptoms.
- Hives, pruritus, and edema.
- Darkened urine and clay-colored stools just before jaundice appears.
  Jaundice stage:
- Gastrointestinal symptoms may decrease.
- Weight loss.
- Liver enlargement and tenderness.
- If hepatitis is severe, any of the symptoms listed in Table 5-1 may be seen.

Common Diagnostic Tests

The following are in addition to the common diagnostic tests described under the general treatment of liver disorders. *(See SS, Liver: common diagnostic tests)*
- Negative serum HB_sAg in type A hepatitis.
- Positive serum HB_sAg in type B hepatitis.
- Lymphocytosis is seen in WBC differential.

Treatment

- Hepatitis B immune globulin (HBIG) may be given as soon as possible to anyone who has been exposed by contact with the blood or mucous membranes of a person believed to have hepatitis type B. Needleprick innoculation is a common mode of exposure in health care workers who handle blood.
- Immune serum globulin (ISG), given within a few days after exposure to hepatitis virus A, has proven quite effective in preventing infection or reducing its severity.

Nursing Tips

- All of the nursing tips outlined in the treatment of general liver disorders apply. *(See SS, Liver: nursing tips)*
- Bed rest is usually ordered.
- High-carbohydrate diet.
- Isolation (if hospitalization is required). *(See NR, Isolation technique)*
  1. Type A: private room; blood and enteric precautions.
  2. Type B: blood precautions only, in most cases. For the incontinent patient, one with diarrhea, or an infant, isolation with blood and enteric precautions would be required.
  3. Type non-A, non-B: Private room; blood and enteric precautions.
- Scrupulous hand washing should be carried out by the patient, his

family, and the staff. Everyone should understand the infectiousness of this disease and how to prevent its spread. All bodily secretions are considered infectious, particularly the blood of the type B hepatitis patient.

- Extra care should be exercised to avoid contaminating the outside of specimen containers. All specimens should be marked "HEPATITIS" in large letters before sending them to the laboratory.
- Prognosis is generally good, but the course of and recovery from viral hepatitis is discouragingly long. Emotional support is an important element in this patient's care.
- Drug rehabilitation programs should be strongly encouraged for the drug addict.

OBSTRUCTION OF THE INTESTINAL TRACT

Description

Obstruction occurs when intestinal contents either cannot pass or cannot pass in a normal way because of partial or complete closing of a section of the lumen of the intestine.

Causes of mechanical obstruction include tumors (malignant or benign) within or adjacent to the intestinal tract and carcinoma of the bowel. Polyps, adhesions, strangulated hernias, volvulus (twisting of the bowel on itself), intussusception (the telescoping of one segment of the bowel into another—seen most often in children), impacted feces, foreign bodies, or a mass of parasitic worms may also lead to obstruction.

Paralytic (adynamic) ileus represents a failure of normal peristalsis. It may occur as a complication of peritonitis or as a result of handling of the bowel during surgery, of acute illness, of spinal cord lesions, or of embolism or thrombosis of one of the mesenteric arteries or their branches. *(See SS, Postoperative complications, paralytic ileus)*

Common Diagnostic Tests

- Flat plates (x-rays) of the abdomen.
- Small barium enema with great care because of the danger of perforation. *(See NR, x-ray preparations)*
- Hemoglobin and hematocrit elevated with dehydration. *(See LAB)*
- Leukocytosis (elevated WBCs) may indicate strangulation. *(See LAB)*
- Serum sodium, potassium, and chloride may be depressed because of continued vomiting. *(See LAB)*
- BUN (blood urea nitrogen) may be elevated because of decreased renal perfusion secondary to hypovolemia. *(See LAB)*
- Stools for occult blood. *(See LAB)*

What to Look for

Symptoms will vary according to whether the obstruction is partial or complete, whether it is high or low in the gastrointestinal tract, and whether there is interference with the blood supply to the affected part. In general, symptoms of obstruction high in the gastrointestinal tract appear more suddenly and are more severe. A careful nursing history will include information about the patient's eating patterns, stool, vomiting, and distention.

Small Bowel Obstruction

- Increased peristalsis and borborygmi (loud, gurgling bowel sounds heard on auscultation or even without benefit of stethoscope).
- Cramping upper abdominal pain.
- Vomiting: frequent, may be projectile, starting with semi-digested food, next becoming watery, then bile colored, and finally becoming dark and fecal in odor.
- Signs of dehydration, electrolyte imbalances. *(See LAB, Electrolytes),* shock, and peritonitis. *(See SS, Postoperative care)*
- Abdominal distention occurs later.
- Abdominal muscle guarding or rebound tenderness may indicate strangulation or perforation.

Large Bowel Obstruction

- Symptoms usually appear insidiously (except in the case of volvulus).
- Abdominal distention.
- Vomiting and pain are usually less severe than in upper intestinal obstruction.
- Failure to pass gas or stool, if obstruction is complete. Irregular, small stools common if obstruction is partial.
- Absent bowel sounds in paralytic ileus. *(See SS, Postoperative complications, paralytic ileus)*

Treatment

- Intestinal decompression with suction to a nasointestinal tube, most frequently the Miller-Abbot double-lumen tube or the Cantor single-lumen tube. Gastric suction through a Levine tube may be sufficient. *(See NR, Gastrointestinal intubation)*
- Maintain fluid and electrolyte balance. *(See LAB, Electrolytes)*
- Antibiotics may be ordered. *(See PH, Antimicrobials)*
- Surgical relief of mechanical obstruction if conservative measures fail. Surgery may involve lysis (cutting) of adhesions, bowel resection with re-anastomosis, or colostomy—possibly temporary—with

further correction of the problem planned for a time when the patient is in better condition.

Nursing Tips

- Careful assessment includes
  1. Observation and recording of character and amount of emesis, bowel sounds, passing of flatus or stool, and level of pain or discomfort.
  2. Measurement of abdominal girth to assess distention. Mark level at which you are measuring on the abdomen with magic marker so that you can measure at the same place each day.
  3. Daily weights before breakfast on the same scale to assess hydration.
  4. Vital signs every 4 hours (an elevated temperature may indicate peritonitis).
- Maintain gastric or intestinal suction.
- Record intake and output accurately. Remember that vomitus and drainage from the GI tract are counted as output and recorded separately.
- Good skin care. The patient may be both dehydrated and very toxic.
- Good mouth care.
- Analgesics are used sparingly because of constipating side-effects.
- Maintain Fowler's or low Fowler's position to relieve respiratory distress caused by distention and to promote drainage.

PANCREAS

Description

The pancreas is an elongated, fish-shaped gland that lies behind the stomach, the head attached to the duodenum, the tail reaching the spleen. In addition to the hormones insulin and glucagon, the pancreas produces amylase, which is needed for the digestion of carbohydrates, trypsin for the digestion of proteins, and lipase for the digestion of fats. These are secreted into the duodenum through the papilla of Vater.

ACUTE PANCREATITIS
Description

Acute inflammation of the pancreas is most commonly associated with biliary tract disorders, alcoholism, trauma during surgery of adjacent organs, some infectious diseases (*e.g.,* mumps), some drugs, and hyperparathyroidism. Progress from edema to hemorrhage to necrotic pathological changes in the pancreas occurs as the disease advances. Seriousness of the symptoms and the incidence of mortality increase accordingly. The formation of pseudocysts and pancreatic abscesses are serious complications.

Common Diagnostic Tests

- Serum amylase is elevated, particularly in first 24 hours.
- Urinary amylase in 2-hour specimen is elevated.
- Fat globules in stool.
- Serum lipase elevated, usually longer than serum amylase.
- Serum bilirubin elevated if common bile duct is obstructed. *(See LAB)*
- Hyperglycemia (elevated blood sugar) may occur.
- Serum calcium may decrease. *(See LAB)*
- Elevated WBC; hematocrit (Hct) may increase. *(See LAB)*
- Cholangiography may be used to determine whether biliary tract is normal. *(See NR, x-ray preparations)*
- Duodenum intubation and aspiration to examine pancreatic juices. *(See NR, Gastrointestinal intubation)*

What to Look for

- Severe abdominal pain, usually generalized in the upper quadrants, with radiation to the back.
- Nausea and vomiting.
- Fever, developing during the first few days.
- Symptoms of shock may develop in severe attacks.
- Jaundice, if the biliary tract is obstructed.
- Stools may be pale, bulky, foul smelling, and high in fat content.

Treatment

- Relief of pain, usually with meperidine (Demerol) *(see PH, Central nervous system)*. *Caution:* Morphine sulfate is contraindicated because it contracts the sphincter of Oddi.
- Reduce pancreatic secretion by continuous gastric suction through a nasogastric tube, keeping the patient n.p.o. *(see NR, Gastrointestinal intubation)*. Anticholinergic drugs were formerly an accepted part of treatment, but their usefulness is now under question.
- Maintain fluid and electrolyte balance with appropriate IV therapy and electrolyte monitoring. *(See NR, Intravenous therapy and LAB, Electrolytes)*
- Treat shock, if present.
- Calcium gluconate may be ordered. *(See PH, Endocrine system)*
- Hyperglycemia may be treated with insulin. *(See PH, Endocrine system)*

- Antibiotics may be ordered for specific reasons. *(See PH, Antimicrobials*
- Diet, when resumed, should be low in fat and protein and high in carbohydrates; intake of coffee should be limited; alcohol should be avoided.
- Cysts and abscesses are usually drained surgically.

Nursing Tips

- Assume nursing responsibilities for treatment outlined above, including the administration of medications and the management of IV therapy and nasogastric suction. Accurate measurement of intake and output is extremely important.
- Frequent, careful assessment of the patient's condition is essential. He is seriously ill.
- Provide all comfort measures, including back care, mouth care, and skin care. (If patient is jaundiced, pruritus may be relieved by washing with water only, using emollient lotions.)
- Patient will be more comfortable sitting up, with some flexion at the waist. He will require bed rest in the most acute stage of his illness and may need assistance in position changes.

CHRONIC PANCREATITIS

Description

Chronic pancreatitis results in marked fibrous scarring associated with calcification of the pancreas and is most often associated with chronic alcoholism. It may also occur after repeated attacks of acute pancreatitis or may be associated with biliary tract problems. With progressive destruction of the gland, digestion of both fat and protein is impaired. Diabetes mellitus may result due to destruction of the islets of Langerhans.

Common Diagnostic Tests

- 24-hour urine amylase may be elevated.
- Serum amylase and lipase show variable elevations.
- Secretin test for pancreatic function.
- Flat plate of the abdomen to show pancreatic calcification.
- Sonogram, CAT scan. *(See NR, Scans)*
- Pancreatic angiography.
- Endoscopic examination. *(See NR, Endoscopic procedures)*

What to Look for

- Pain in the upper abdomen—which may be dull or severe, persistent or intermittent—usually radiating to the back.
- Nausea and vomiting.

- Fatty and foul smelling stools.
- Weight loss and malnutrition.
- Evidence of diabetes mellitus. *(See SS, Endocrine, Diabetes mellitus)*

Treatment

- Control of pain, though the need for analgesics frequently leads to drug addiction.
- Abstinence from alcohol; avoidance of caffeine.
- Diet low in fat. Small meals.
- Control of diabetes mellitus, if it exists. *(See SS, Diabetes mellitus)*
- Medications
  1. Pancreatic extract, *e.g.,* pancreatin (Viokase), before meals.
  2. Antacids, fat-soluble vitamin supplements, and calcium may be given.
- Treatment of underlying gallbladder disease, if this is believed to be the cause of the pancreatitis.
- Operative procedures that attempt to reduce pressure and back-flow of pancreatic juices into the pancreas may be tried.

Nursing Tips

- Provide emotional support for the patient who is frequently in great pain over a long period of time. Chronic pancreatitis is a debilitating disease that frequently is made more difficult by problems of underlying alcoholism and problems of diabetes control.
- Patient and family must be educated as to the absolute necessity of the patient's abstinence from alcohol.

PEPTIC ULCER

Description

Peptic ulcer is a sharply defined break in the mucosal lining of any part of the gastrointestinal tract that is exposed to acid pepsin. Most commonly (between 80% to 85% of the time) peptic ulcers are found in the duodenum just beyond the pylorus. Ulcers may penetrate the mucosa, submucosa, or muscle wall of the lower end of the esophagus, stomach, or duodenum, or they may appear at the site of an anastomosis between intestine and stomach.

While the etiology is not fully understood, the following are thought to be contributing factors: stress and anxiety, high-pressure personality type, familial predispositions, blood group 0, smoking, alcohol, coffee, and usage of ulcerogenic drugs, *e.g.,* acetylsalicylic acid (aspirin), indomethacin (Indocin) phenylbutazone (Butazolidin), the steroids, and iron preparations.

Hemorrhage and perforation are complications caused by penetration of the ulcer. Pyloric obstruction may be caused by scarring or edema around the pylorus caused by the ulcer. Perforation, pyloric obstruction, and failure of the ulcer to heal after intensive medical treatment are usually indications for surgical treatment.

Gastric ulcers differ from duodenal ulcers in that, while usually benign, there is a significant incidence of underlying cancer, they are less likely to heal quickly, and they are more frequently treated surgically.

Common Diagnostic Tests

- X-ray: barium studies of the upper gastrointestinal tract. *(See NR, x-ray preparations)*
- Endoscopic studies of the upper gastrointestinal tract, often with biopsy or cytological examination of washings to rule out malignancy. *(See NR, Endoscopic procedures)*
- Gastric analysis (analysis of gastric content aspirated by means of a nasogastric tube) for the following
  1. Blood, either gross or occult. *(See LAB, Testing for occult blood)*
  2. Acid concentration (basic acid output—BAO).
     a. Elevated in duodenal ulcer.
     b. Normal or depressed in gastric ulcer or cancer.
     c. Excessively high acid secretion and an elevated serum gastrin level in *Zollinger-Ellison* syndrome (caused by a gastrin-producing adenoma of the pancreas).

What to Look for

- Pain: gnawing, boring epigastric pain that is temporarily relieved after ingestion of food or antacids.
  1. With duodenal ulcer, pain usually returns 3 or 4 hours after eating and frequently occurs in the middle of the night.
  2. With gastric ulcer, pain may return within 1 hour after eating, rarely occurs at night, and may be relieved by vomiting.
- Bleeding: vomiting of blood (often coffee ground in appearance) and passing of tarry stools; fatigue and symptoms of anemia may be signs of slow oozing of blood. *(See SS, Gastrointestinal bleeding)*
- Pyloric obstruction: vomiting, which may or may not be preceded by feeling of nausea, may be projectile, and if persistent, may lead to alkalosis; anorexia; nausea.
- Perforation: very sudden onset of severe, sharp abdominal pain, a rigid and boardlike abdomen with decreased or absent bowel sounds, and symptoms of shock and peritonitis. *(See SS, Peritonitis)*

Treatment

Medical

- About 85% of ulcers respond to conservative treatment.
- Drug therapy
  1. Cimetidine (Tagamet): synthetic hydrogen receptor antagonist believed to be dramatic breakthrough in ulcer treatment. *(See PH, Gastrointestinal system)*
  2. Antacids *(e.g.,* Maalox, Gelusil, Amphojel): frequently given every hour while patient is awake, then 1 to 3 hours after eating and at h.s. while patient is hospitalized. *(See PH, Gastrointestinal system)*
  3. Anticholinergics, *e.g.,* propantheline bromide (Pro-Banthine): decrease gastric motility by suppressing vagal activity; may be ordered at h.s. to slow emptying of stomach at night; controversial because of side-effects. *(See PH, Autonomic nervous system)*
- Diet: small frequent feedings; avoid acid-stimulating foods such as coffee, tea, cola, alcohol, and spices.
- Care of hemorrhage. *(See SS, Gastrointestinal bleeding)*

Surgical

- Emergency: closure of an area of perforation.
- Elective: for recurrent ulcers, bleeding episodes, pyloric obstruction, or intractable ulcer (one failing to respond to medical treatment, frequently gastric ulcer).
- Procedures: usually pyloroplasty and vagotomy. (Resection and gastroenterostomy are seldom performed today as treatment for peptic ulcer.)

Nursing Tips

- Try to provide mental and physical rest in the acute stage.
- Try to help patient find ways to reduce stress in his life.
- Review the pharmacology *(PH)* section of this handbook for important tips concerning administration of cimetidine, antacids, and anticholinergic drugs. Teach patient to avoid medications containing aspirin and to look for it in over-the-counter drugs.
- Postoperative care. *(See SS, Postoperative care and Gastric surgery)*
- Total gastrectomy (done for Zollinger-Ellison syndrome) terminates production of intrinsic factor needed for the absorption of vitamin B_{12}. Vitamin B_{12} injections (cyanocobalamin injection, U.S.P.) will be required for life to prevent pernicious anemia. *(See PH, Cardiovascular system and SS, Pernicious anemia)*
- Dumping syndrome: a vasomotor and gastrointestinal disturbance

associated with eating that follows subtotal gastric resection with gastroenterostomy. It is believed to be caused by the rapid emptying of stomach contents into the small intestine. *(See SS Gastric surgery, nursing tips)*

PILONIDAL CYSTS

Description

A pilonidal cyst is found in the sacrococcygeal region, usually at the upper part of the intergluteal fold, and is believed to be caused by a developmental defect in which epithelial tissue is trapped below the skin. Hair is often present, protruding from the cyst. It is usually asymptomatic until late adolescence or early adult life; however, then trauma may cause an inflammatory reaction, which results in swelling, abscess formation, and draining sinuses or fistulas.

Treatment

- Antibiotic therapy: until inflammation is controlled.
- Incision and drainage of an abscess.
- Surgical excision of the cyst and sinuses.

Nursing Tips

- Surgical techniques vary as to how the wound is closed. Post-operative orders will vary accordingly.
- Analgesics are usually needed only during the first 24 hours.
- Early ambulation is usually encouraged, though patients are advised not to undertake strenuous activities until healing is complete.

SURGERY (GASTROINTESTINAL)
GASTRIC SURGERY
Description

Presently, surgical removal is the only cure for carcinoma of the stomach, though other therapies are under investigation. *Total gastrectomy,* which includes total removal of the stomach and anastomosis of the esophagus to the jejunum, is rarely done because of the high incidence of postoperative complications.

Partial gastrectomy (see below) involves removal of part of the stomach. Excision of nearby organs may be required, but an attempt is made to restore the gastrointestinal tract to as near normal functioning as possible. If metastasis appears to be widespread, bypass procedures may be attempted as a palliative measure.

The goal of surgery for peptic ulcer is to reduce acid secretion either by interference with the vagus nerve or by removal of part of the stomach containing parietal cells, which are acid producing, or the antrum of the stomach, where gastrin (which stimulates acid production) is formed.

Gastric surgical procedures (Fig. 5-4) include the following:

- *Vagotomy* (resection of the vagus nerve): decreases acid secretion, but also may slow stomach emptying, causing symptoms of fullness, abdominal distention, and flatus. Therefore, *pyloroplasty*—increasing the pyloric opening—may also be done to aid in gastric emptying.
- *Selective parietal cell vagotomy:* Only vagal supply to body and fundus is removed, denervating acid-secreting cells. Stomach emptying will remain normal.
- *Vagotomy plus antrectomy:* vagotomy with removal of antrum, which is where gastrin (which is acid stimulating) is secreted.
- *Partial gastrectomy:* with or without vagotomy
    1. *Billroth procedure I:* the body, antrum, and pylorus of the stomach are removed, and the stomach remnant is anastomosed to the duodenum (gastroduodenostomy). Postoperative problems include the dumping syndrome, anemia, weight loss, and marginal ulcers.
    2. *Billroth procedure II:* same as with Billroth I, except that stomach remnant is anastomosed to the jejunum behind the transverse colon (retrocolic gastrojejunostomy). Sequelae similar to Billroth I.

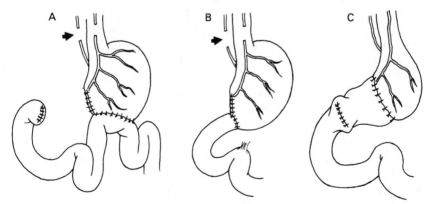

FIG. 5-4. *Gastric surgery. A. Truncal vagotomy with Billroth II subtotal distal gastrectomy. B. Truncal vagotomy with Billroth I gastroduodenal anastomosis. C. Segmental gastric resection with pyloroplasty.* (Hardy JD: Rhoads' Textbook of Surgery, 5th ed, pp 843, 845. Philadelphia, JB Lippincott, 1977)

Nursing Tips

Preoperative Care

- If surgery is not being done on an emergency basis, general preparation of the patient will include attention to his nutritional status, and correction of anemia (with blood transfusions) and electrolyte imbalances, if present.
- Nasogastric tube to low intermittent suction or continuous low suction (if available) if gastric sump tube (*e.g.,* Salem or Venrol) is used. *(See NR, Gastrointestinal intubation)*
- General preoperative teaching and preoperative care. *(See SS, Preoperative care)*

Postoperative Care

- General postoperative care. *(See SS, Introduction, postoperative care)*
- Patient will have nothing by mouth (n.p.o.) for first days and will require special mouth care with rinses, gargles, and lubricants.
- Intravenous fluids. *(See NR, Intravenous therapy)*
- Nasogastric tube to low intermittent suction or continuous low suction (if gastric sumptube is being used) for 3 or 4 days after surgery. Ascertain that equipment is working properly and that tube is patent. *(See NR, Gastrointestinal intubation)*
- *Caution:* Danger of disturbing the suture line dictates that one *never* irrigates the n.g. tube without an order. (If ordered, it must be with a small amount (30 ml) of normal saline, very gently.) *Never* attempt to move the n.g. tube. If its patency is in question, have the patient change his position and cough with his incision splinted. If this does not correct the situation, notify the surgeon.
- Drainage from the n.g. tube will be bloody for the first 24 hours, will gradually become dark red, then coffee ground, and finally greenish yellow in color. Appearance of bright red blood after the first 12 hours should be called to the attention of the physician immediately.
- After peristalsis has returned, the patient will be allowed gradually increasing amounts of fluid p.o., even while the n.g. tube is still in place.
- The n.g. tube may be clamped at intervals to test for the amount of residual stomach contents as an indication of when to remove it. After removal, look for signs of distention.
- After total gastrectomy there will be little n.g. drainage because there are no stomach secretions and the stomach's storage function has been eliminated.
- Accurate intake and output is essential. Remember that drainage

from the n.g. tube is counted as output and recorded separately. Account for irrigation fluid.

- Diet after the n.g. tube is removed is gradually advanced. Patient should be cautioned to eat slowly.
- Semi-Fowler's position is maintained postoperatively to promote drainage.
- Since patient will have high abdominal incision, special attention should be paid to the prevention of respiratory complications. Assist him with deep breathing techniques. *(See NR, Deep breathing techniques)*
- The patient with total gastrectomy will also have chest tubes. *(See NR, Chest tube drainage)*

Long-Term Postoperative Implications

- The patient who has had total gastrectomy will require injections of Vitamin B_{12} (cyanocobalamin injection, U.S.P.) throughout the rest of his life because of his lack of the intrinsic factor. Those with partial gastrectomy may require some Vitamin B_{12} supplements and should have regular checks for anemia. *(See PH, Cardiovascular system)*
- *Dumping syndrome:* a fairly common sequela to gastric surgery. Patient may have feeling of fullness and nausea 5 to 40 minutes after eating, followed by sweating, pallor, headache, and dizziness. Two or three hours after a meal (particularly one high in carbohydrates) the patient has a hypoglycemic reaction with weakness, sweating, anxiety, and tremors. Patient teaching includes
  1. Lie down immediately after eating.
  2. Small, frequent meals should be eaten slowly in a semi-recumbent position.
  3. Fluids should be taken between, *not* with, meals.
  4. Anticholinergic medications may help by slowing gastric emptying. *(See PH, Autonomic nervous system)*

INTESTINAL SURGERY
Description

Bowel resection: The goal is the removal of a section of diseased or obstructing bowel, with anastomosis (rejoining) of the two healthy ends and the resumption of normal bowel function.

Cecostomy (Fig. 5-5): An opening is made into the lower right colon (the cecum), and a tube is introduced to decompress the bowel. Attention must be paid to the care of the skin around the tube because drainage will be liquid and will include digestive enzymes.

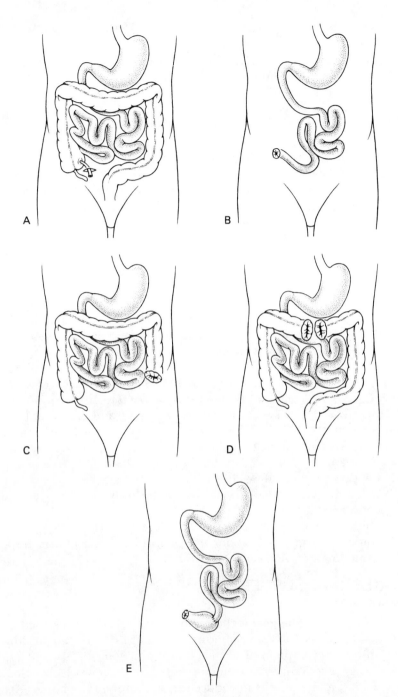

FIG. 5-5. *Types of ostomies. A. Cecostomy, B. Ileostomy with proctocolectomy. C. Colostomy with abdominal perineal resection. D. Double-barrel colostomy. E. Continent ileostomy (Kock pouch).*

Colostomy: An opening of some portion of the large bowel is made onto the skin, thereby forming an abdominal anus (with no sphincter control). The consistency of the feces will depend upon how much reabsorption of fluids has taken place. Fecal material from a colostomy in the ascending colon will be quite liquid; feces from a colostomy in the descending or sigmoid colon (in the left lower quadrant of the abdomen) will normally be soft formed. Regulation of evacuation of a colostomy in the descending or sigmoid colon is often achieved by regular diet, activity, and irrigation *(see NR, Ostomies, fistulas, and draining wounds)*. If regulation is achieved the patient will need to cover the stoma with a cap but may not need to wear a bag most of the time.

A *temporary colostomy* may be done if there is a possibility that the lower bowel will heal with rest *(e.g.,* in severe diverticulitis and recto-vaginal or recto-vesical fistula). There will be two openings in a *double-barrel colostomy* or *loop colostomy:* the proximal opening (on the side closest to the small intestine) will drain fecal material, the distal one, mucus (see Fig. 5-5). The surgeon will close the colostomy and re-anastomose the two ends when he deems it appropriate. The proximal opening is the functional one.

Permanent colostomy: a permanent diversion of fecal contents to the skin, usually done for carcinoma of the colon or rectum or both. *(See SS, Oncology)*

Loop colostomy or loop transverse colostomy: may be permanent or temporary. Because it can be done quickly with minimal trauma, it is done frequently in an emergency situation *(e.g.,* diverticulitis, cancer, and bowel perforation or obstruction). A loop of transverse colon is brought up to the skin. Then a stomal support, such as a glass rod, rubber catheter, or butterfly bridge, is put in place until the bowel adheres to the abdominal wall (usually in 5 to 7 days). A painless incision is made in the colon wall usually 24 to 48 hours later to allow for fecal drainage. In effect this is a double-barrel colostomy (see above) with two openings.

Colostomy with abdominal perineal resection (Fig. 5-5): usually done for carcinoma near the rectum *(see SS, Oncology)*. A colostomy is formed, and the complete anus and rectum are resected, leaving a wide perineal wound that may heal slowly and become infected easily. Drains may be left in place. Packing, which the surgeon will remove after about 24 hours, may fill the cavity. Some surgeons leave the wound open.

• Expect copious serosanguineous drainage from the perineal wound. Be alert for fresh hemorrhage, edema, and infection. The surgeon will do the first dressing.

- Medicate for pain, which may be especially severe in the first 24 hours.
- Patient may have the sensation of wanting to have a bowel movement due to pressure from the packing.
- Cotton pants may be worn to hold the perineal dressing in place. A "T" binder, if used, should be snug enough that it doesn't rub up and down.
- After the packing is removed, the perineal wound may require the following:
  1. Perineal irrigations several times a day, using meticulous aseptic technique. Specifics, including type of irrigating solution, depth of insertion, and size of irrigating catheter, will be ordered.
  2. Sitz baths, ordered to stimulate circulation, promote healing, and cleanse. Be aware that the patient may feel faint. Protect and assist him accordingly.
- Position the patient on a foam rubber ring or turned on his side so that he is off the perineal wound.

Ileostomy (Fig. 5-5): The end of the ileum is brought out to the skin. Ileostomy is usually associated with proctocolectomy (removal of the colon and rectum) or colectomy for carcinoma *(see SS, Oncology)* or for ulcerative colitis. It is sometimes done as a temporary diversion of the feces. It differs from colostomy in that the feces are liquid and extremely irritating to the skin around the stoma; therefore special efforts are required to protect the skin *(see NR, Ostomies, fistulas, and draining wounds)*. There is no regularity of evacuation, so an appliance must be worn at all times. It is emptied several times a day, usually when the patient voids. Irrigations are, of course, unnecessary. If a rectal stump is left, the patient may have periodic discharge of mucus from the rectum. The patient with an ileostomy should wear an identifying bracelet with his name, his doctor's name, and the hospital emergency number.

Continent Ileostomy (Kock Pouch): Using a loop of ileum, a pouch is devised to serve as a reservoir for fecal effluent to be discharged from the ileostomy. A nipple or valve is formed that prevents leakage from the stoma. The patient discharges the fecal contents of the pouch several times a day by temporary insertion of a catheter through the nipple valve into the pouch.

Ileal conduit: The ileum is resected, and a segment is separated from it. One end of the segment is closed, and the other end is brought to the skin to form an ileal stoma (anastomosis of the two ends of the resected ileum reinstates its continuity). Ureters are implanted in the ileal segment, forming a diversion for urine when conditions require bypassing or removal of the urinary bladder.

Nursing Tips
Preoperative Care

- Review general preoperative care and teaching. *(See SS, Preoperative care)*
- General preparation of the patient, if time permits, with attention to nutritional status (hyperalimentation may be required), anemia (blood transfusions p.r.n.), and electrolyte balance.
- Diet: high calorie, low residue, or clear liquid diet for several days preoperative in most cases. Nothing by mouth (n.p.o.) if there is a question of obstruction or perforation.
- Bowel preparation
  1. Enemas (may include a neomycin solution).
  2. Intestinal antibiotics: to suppress flora in bowel. Neomycin or sulfonamides (succinylsulfathiazole) are usually ordered. *(See PH, Antimicrobials)*
- Nasogastric tube to low intermittent suction or low continuous suction if gastric sump tube is being used. *(See NR, Gastrointestinal intubation)*
- An indwelling catheter is usually ordered preoperatively for the patient undergoing lower abdominal surgery. *(See NR, Urinary bladder catheterization and drainage)*
- Psychological support.
- When the stomal therapist visits the patient who is to have an ostomy (at the request of the surgeon), she may mark an appropriate site for placement of the stoma.
- A visit from a member of the local ostomy association may be arranged.
- Preparation for the closure of a temporary colostomy:
  1. Patient is usually admitted 2 days preoperatively.
  2. Clear liquid diet.
  3. Antibiotics: systemically and, in irrigations of colostomy and distal stoma, frequently. *(See PH, Antimicrobials)*
  4. Preparation of both stomas:
     a. Colostomy irrigations b.i.d.
     b. Rectal enemas: be sure to apply pouch to distal stoma to receive enema solution.
     c. Irrigations of distal stoma with patient sitting on the toilet. (Irrigation will be expelled through the rectum).

Postoperative Care

- General principles of postoperative care and assessment for symptoms of complications, including auscultation for bowel sounds.

Their presence indicates the return of peristalsis. *(See SS, Intro-duction, postoperative care)*
- Management of nasogastric or nasointestinal suction. *(See NR, Gas-trointestinal intubation)*
- Accurate intake and output.
- Progressive diet after the return of peristalsis.
- Prevention of contamination of the abdominal wound by feces when ostomy is present. Protect the incision with oiled silk, plas-ticized skin drape, or plastric wrap over the dressing.
- Care of the ostomy *(see NR, Ostomies, fistulas, and draining wounds)*: The color of the stoma should be dark pink to red. Blanching or deep red could indicate interference with the blood supply and should be reported. If patient complains of pain, check the pouch, open it, and release gas p.r.n. Report if pain is unrelieved.
- Care of the perineal wound, in addition to the ostomy and the abdominal wound, in the patient with abdominal perineal resec-tion. *(See colostomy with abdominal perineal resection)*
- Patients with ileostomy should take oral medications in liquid form for quick absorption.
- Intelligent and thoughtful emotional support for the patient with an ostomy, as he adjusts to his new body image. Emphasize the need for self-care and a return to normal living.
- *Management of complications associated with colostomy.*
  1. Odor and gas: Avoid gas-producing foods. Use charcoal tablets and other antiflatulents p.o. or bismuth subgallate or bismuth subcarbonate p.o. to reduce odor. These are best taken only occasionally, after eating odor- or gas-producing foods. *Caution:* Reversible deterioration of mental ability, confusion, and central nervous system symptoms may be side-effects of prolonged use of bismuth preparations.
     a. Deodorants may be used in the pouch. Irrigation of the co-lostomy and cleanliness of the appliance help reduce odors. Gas may be passed by opening bag.
  2. Erratic function: Control with well-regulated diet. Be aware of drugs that may cause diarrhea *(e.g.,* ampicillin and tetracycline).
  3. Bleeding: A small amount at the stoma site is rather common. Any appreciable amount should be reported to the surgeon.
  4. Obstruction: Patient may have cramping, abdominal pain, and nausea and vomiting. Notify the surgeon.
  5. Herniation around the colostomy: May be a special problem because forcing an irrigating tip into the herniated loop of bowel may lead to perforation.
  6. Perforation: Symptoms include acute onset of pain around the

stoma, swelling and fever, and diffuse abdominal pain. Perforation constitutes a surgical emergency.

7. Prolapse of the colostomy: Seen most often in the distal, nonfunctioning stoma of a transverse loop colostomy.

- *Management of complications of ileosotomy* (the following are in addition to those associated with colostomy).
  1. Acute or chronic dehydration:
     a. Fluid balance must be maintained.
     b. Measure and record intake and output accurately. (Remember to count drainage from the ileostomy as output.)
     c. A urine output of less than 30 to 50 ml/hr should be reported to the physician.
     d. Antidiarrheal agents may be required at first when output from the ileostomy may be excessive.
  2. Breakdown of the parastomal (around the stoma) skin from contact with the irritating liquid feces from an ileostomy:
     a. Careful skin prep (no cuts) preoperatively.
     b. Well-fitting appliance. Stoma should protrude about 2 cm so that it won't discharge directly onto the skin. The stoma size will change during the first 6 weeks, so it should be measured every time it is changed.
     c. Appliance should be changed every 2 or 3 days or often enough to avoid leakage. Leakage should be suspected if patient complains of burning or itching around the stoma. Change appliance immediately.
  3. Blockage of the stoma: May be indicated by sharply diminished output associated with nausea and abdominal cramps. Note type of discharge from the stoma. Food particles may indicate impaction. A clear discharge may indicate another type of obstruction. Notify the surgeon.

Neurological System

CHRONIC ORGANIC BRAIN SYNDROME

Description

Chronic organic brain syndrome is a term commonly used to describe all senile dementia in older adults. When this deterioration of mental abilities occurs before the age of 65, it is called presenile dementia or Alzheimer's disease and is characterized by diffuse brain atrophy. There is no known cause, although high aluminum levels have been found in brain tissue. Vascular dementia, caused by vascular insufficiency, causes most chronic organic brain syndrome, especially the senile dementias. Specific degenerative diseases such as late-stage syphilis, alcoholism, or brain tumors may also cause chronic organic brain syndrome.

Common Diagnostic Tests

- CAT Scan. *(See NR, Scans)*
- Lumbar puncture for cerebrospinal fluid if infection or syphilis is suspected.

What to Look for

- Deterioration of memory and intellectual ability.
- Disorientation as to time and place.
- Confusion in recognizing family and friends.
- Depression in early stages.
- Emotional and personality changes.
- Physical deterioration due to failure to eat, falling, and improper body hygiene.

Treatment

- There is no known cure for Alzheimer's disease.
- Vascular dementia sometimes is helped if the blood supply to the

brain is increased. Carotid endarterectomy and cerebral artery by-pass surgery may be helpful.
- Haloperidol (Haldol) given on a round-the-clock schedule is very effective in calming agitation. *(See PH, Psychotropics)*

Nursing Tips

- Symptoms of Alzheimer's disease increase gradually.
- Early symptoms of dementia may depress or agitate the patient because of the realization that he is unable to function well.
- Darkness frequently increases anxiety and restlessness. Restraints often only make it worse. Putting the patient in a wheelchair by the nurse's station at night will frequently calm a confused patient.
- It is best to avoid barbituates and hypnotics, *e.g.,* flurazepam hydrochloride (Dalmane), with confused or agitated patients. *(See PH, Central nervous system)*

INCREASED INTRACRANIAL PRESSURE

Description

Increased intracranial pressure (IICP) results from increases in any of the three components within the skull: the brain, blood, and cerebrospinal fluid. The skull, being nonflexible, cannot accommodate such internal expansions.

Space-occupying lesions, such as brain tumors, abscesses, or hematomas, are common causes of IICP. Head injuries, brain surgery, or hemorrhage also result in IICP. If the pressure is not relieved the patient may die from cerebral anoxia (lack of oxygen reaching brain tissue due to compressed arteries) or from heart or respiratory failure resulting from the pressure on the vital center controlling these functions.

Common Diagnostic Tests

- Skull x-rays: especially in head trauma.
- CAT scan: the preferred technique in diagnosing intracranial clots, tumors, cerebral edema, and aneurysms. *(See NR, Scans)*
- Angiography: done to study blood supply to brain and tumors.
- Brain scan: for cerebral blood flow study. *(See NR, Scans)*
- EEG: reflects seizure activity. *(See NR, Electroencephalogram)*
- Lumbar puncture: done primarily to obtain specimens of cerebrospinal fluid. Contraindicated when IICP is known to exist because of possible brain shift, which leads to herniation and death.
- Neurological examination: to identify neurological impairments, which help locate affected brain area.

What to Look for

- Restlessness and headache. These often are the first signs of IICP and are followed by a decrease in the level of consciousness (LOC).
- Pupil reactions. Changes in the pupils, especially if unilateral, indicate significant pressure effects within the brain. The development of a unilateral, fixed dilated pupil is an *Emergency* situation. Check (the use of a flashlight is helpful) to see that the patient has coordinated eye movements and that the pupils
  1. Are equal in size.
  2. Constrict when exposed to light.
  3. React equally to light.
  4. Dilate after covering the eyes for a few minutes.
- Changes in rate and depth of respirations. This often begins as a slight irregularity. Thus it is important to observe respirations for at least a minute.
- Increase in systolic blood pressure.
- Bradycardia.
- Any sudden muscle weakness, paralysis, or difficulty with verbal responses.
- Seizures. *(See SS, Seizures)*
- In a cerebral hemorrhage the neurological impairments slowly worsen, rather than remaining constant as in a cerebral thrombosis.
- Stiff necks are usually associated with subarachnoid hemorrhages and with meningitis.
- There is usually a slow progression of signs and symptoms with a brain tumor. Edema of the optic disc (papilledema) with accompanying double or blurred vision is an early indication of IICP.
- Malignant tumors of the breast and lung frequently metastasize to the brain.
- Metastatic tumors comprise 50% of all brain tumors.

Treatment

- *No narcotics.* Sedatives (phenobarbitol) are used occasionally.
- IV line for immediate access for medication.
- Steroids and osmotic diuretics, which reduce cerebral edema. *(See PH, Endocrine system)*
- Antifibrinolytics, *e.g.,* aminocaproic acid (Amicar), to prevent rebleeding in case of an aneurysm.
- Anticonvulsants, *e.g.,* phenytoin (Dilantin). *(See PH, Central nervous system)*
- Antihypertensives, *e.g.,* diazoxide (Hyperstat). *(See PH, Cardiovascular system)*

- Surgery for tumors, clots, and repair of aneurysms.
- Chemotherapy and radiation for tumors. *(See SS, Oncology and PH, Antineoplastics)*

Nursing Tips

- Keep an open airway. Position an unconscious patient on his side or semi-prone, but never fully prone. Keep suction equipment immediately available. Tracheostomy or endotracheal tube may be required.
- Head of bed should be at 30° to 45° angle unless contraindicated by vertebral fractures. This aids venous return from head, which decreases cerebral volume.
- Always check unconscious patients for contact lenses. *(See SS, Eye-patient care)*
- Neurological assessment, blood pressure, pulse, and respiration should be taken every 15 minutes (four times) every 30 minutes (four times), and then every hour, or as frequently as indicated by the patient's condition *(see SS, Assessment)*. During the 24 hours following even mild head injuries the patient should be awakened every 1 to 2 hours for neurological check. This assessment, to be valid, requires that everyone use the same criteria.
- Patients who are rendered unconscious by head injuries have an increased incidence later of headaches, vertigo, irritability, impaired mental abilities, and seizures.
- Take seizure precautions: tape a padded tongue blade or soft airway to the head of the bed or bedside stand. Pad siderails the full length of the bed, and have suction equipment immediately available.
- Take temperatures every 4 hours. Continuing changes in temperature signify that the temperature-regulating center of the brain is affected. Hypothermia blankets are useful in lowering body temperature, which decreases cerebral edema. *(See NR, Hypothermia blanket)*
- Patient with IICP should be in a quiet environment. Avoid bright lights and strictly limit visitors.
- Coughing, vomiting, or straining of any type should be avoided.
- Avoid use of restraints, if possible, since restraints will often increase agitation.
- Monitor IV therapy carefully to avoid fluid overload.
- Carefully observe and record intake and output every hour and specific gravity every shift.

INFECTIONS
ACUTE BACTERIAL MENINGITIS
Description

Acute meningitis is an inflammation of the meninges of the brain or spinal cord caused by bacteria. Bacterial infections in the central nervous system (CNS) usually spread from an infection originating elsewhere in the body. Often this follows an ear or sinus infection, craniotomy, or head injury.

Common Diagnostic Tests

- Lumbar puncture for cerebrospinal fluid to determine causative agent.
- Blood cultures to determine causative agent. *(See LAB)*
- Nose and throat cultures to determine causative agent. *(See LAB)*

What to Look for

- Sudden, severe headache, temperature elevation, photophobia (sensitivity to light), and a stiff neck that prevents pressing the chin onto the chest.
- Kernig's sign: difficulty in extending the lower leg when the thigh is flexed on the abdomen.
- Brudzinski's sign: involuntary flexion of the legs when the neck is bent.
- Rash in meningococcal meningitis.
- Dehydration.
- Signs and symptoms of increased intracranial pressure (IICP). *(See SS, Increased intracranial pressure)*
- Changes in level of consciousness that may lead to coma.

Treatment

- IV antibiotics specific for causative organism. *(See PH, Antimicrobials)*
- Anticonvulsants, *e.g.,* phenytoin sodium (Dilantin). *(See PH, Central nervous system)*
- IV therapy to prevent dehydration. *(See NR, Intravenous therapy)*
- Isolation, in accordance with communicable disease regulations. *(See NR, Isolation technique)*

Nursing Tips

- Sterile technique is always important in suctioning patients. The direct extension of bacteria from the nasopharyngeal area to the brain is possible following a craniotomy or head trauma.

- Attempt to provide a quiet and dark room because of increased sensitivity to light and noise.
- Hypothermia blankets are effective in controlling body temperature. *(See NR, Hypothermia blanket)*
- All secretions from mouth, nose, and ears should be disposed of promptly and carefully.

ACUTE VIRAL ENCEPHALITIS

Description

Acute encephalitis is a viral infection that causes inflammation of the cord and brain tissue. It results from a direct viral infection in the brain and cord, or from tissue hypersensitivity occurring as a toxic complication of a viral disease elsewhere in the body, such as measles or chicken pox. An epidemic form commonly called "sleeping sickness" is carried by mosquitos and occurs primarily in warm weather.

Common Diagnostic Tests

- No direct tests exist.
- Lumbar puncture for cerebrospinal fluid is used to rule out bacterial infection, such as meningitis.
- CAT scan to rule out mass lesions (*e.g.,* tumors). *(See NR, Scans)*

What to Look for

- A sudden onset of fever, headache, vomiting, and lethargy. Muscle weakness, tremors, and difficulty in speech may also occur.
- This disease may rapidly progress to coma and death within 24 to 48 hours, or the coma may last for several weeks (as in sleeping sickness).

Treatment

- There is no specific antiviral medication.
- Care is directed toward reducing fever, providing adequate nutrition and hydration, and relieving headache.
- If the patient becomes comatose, an IV, indwelling urinary catheter, and nasogastric tube may become necessary. *(See NR, Intravenous therapy; Urinary bladder catheterization and drainage; and Gastrointestinal intubation)*

Nursing Tips

- Monitor temperature and make neurochecks as frequently as indicated by patient's condition. *(See SS, Assessment, neurological)*

- Hypothermia blankets are useful to control temperatures. *(See NR, Hypothermia blanket)*
- Maintain as quiet an environment as possible.
- Patient may become disoriented and restless; padded siderails should be used.
- Seizures are always a possibility in inflammation of the brain. *(See SS, Seizures)*

MULTIPLE SCLEROSIS

Description

Multiple sclerosis is a disease characterized by sclerotic areas that form in a random pattern on the myelin sheath that covers nerve fibers in the brain and spinal cord. The symptoms vary depending on the location of the sclerotic areas. It is a chronic disease that has periods of exacerbation and temporary remission. Emotional upsets and any illness tend to intensify the symptoms. The cause is unknown, but a viral origin is suspected.

Common Diagnostic Tests

- Lumbar puncture: cerebrospinal fluid often has increased protein.
- Tests are conducted to rule out other possible causes of symptoms (*e.g.* bone marrow biopsy *(see NR)* to exclude pernicious anemia and a CAT scan *(see NR, Scans)* to eliminate brain tumor).
- Classic symptoms increase with time and are considered sufficiently distinctive to permit confirmation of the disease.

What to Look for

- Unusual fatigue, weakness, and clumsiness, especially of arms and legs, often resulting in gait irregularity.
- Double vision and other ocular problems.
- Numbness, particularly on one side of the face, sometimes with mild pain.
- Decreased bladder control; possible incontinence in advanced cases.
- Slight speech disturbance.
- Elevated levels of creatine phosphokinase (CPK). *(See LAB)*

Treatment

- No specific curative treatment is known.
- Steroids are given in acute exacerbations. *(See PH, Endocrine system)*
- Exercise (especially swimming) and daily physiotherapy to improve muscle tone is beneficial.

Nursing Tips

- No two patients exhibit the same group of symptoms, which often move from one body area to another. However, usually one side of the body is more affected than the other.
- The symptoms may subside and then recur in a more severe form.
- The disease usually progresses to total disability.
- Since these patients are very easily fatigued, just eating may be an exhausting experience.
- Bladder and respiratory infections are often a recurring problem.
- A medical identification bracelet should always be worn to show that this person has multiple sclerosis.

Sources of Information

- The Multiple Sclerosis Society, 205 E. 42nd Street, New York, N.Y. 10017

MYASTHENIA GRAVIS

Description

Myasthenia gravis is a chronic disease of sporadic muscle weakness that varies from mild to life threatening. The muscles of the face, mouth, and throat are primarily affected. The cause is unknown, but it is thought to be an autoimmune disease.

Common Diagnostic Tests

- Edrophonium chloride (Tensilon) is given subcutaneously. If the patient has myasthenia gravis, weak muscles become normal immediately, but this effect only lasts for 5 to 10 minutes.
- Neostigmine methylsulfate (Prostigmin) is given subcutaneously. If the patient has myasthenia gravis, weak muscles become normal within 45 minutes, and this effect lasts for several hours.

What to Look for

- Ptosis (drooping of the upper eyelid).
- Diplopia (double vision).
- Difficulty in chewing, swallowing, and breathing.

Treatment

- Cholinergic drugs, *e.g.,* pyridostigmine (Mestinon), treat symptoms by acting as a temporary muscle stimulant.
- Coricosteroids, *e.g.,* prednisone, are often effective as a long-term treatment for autoimmune diseases. Steroids block immune mechanisms. *(See PH, Endocrine system)*

Nursing Tips

- Cholinergic medications must be taken on a schedule that is individualized for each person. Thus a hospitalized patient with myasthenia gravis should keep medication at the bedside for self-administration in order to keep strictly to the prescribed schedule.
- When dysphagia (difficulty in swallowing) is a problem, the medication should be taken about 30 minutes before a meal.
- The patient should fully understand when medication is to be taken and the consequences of improper dosage. Undermedication produces myasthenic crisis and overmedication produces cholinergic crisis. Both crises result in increased severity of basic symptoms, including a marked inability to swallow or breathe.
- A tracheotomy set and suction equipment must be on the unit, and its location known to all the staff, in case of a crisis of either type.
- Any patient with muscle weakness should have a call light adapted for this problem.
- Upper respiratory infections (URI) are dangerous because muscle weakness limits coughing ability to clear airway of secretions.
- Fatigue and physical or emotional stress should be avoided because these aggravate the symptoms.
- A medical identification bracelet must be worn to signify that this person has myasthenia gravis.

Sources of Information

- The Myasthenia Gravis Foundation, 230 Park Avenue, New York, N.Y. 20017

PARKINSON'S DISEASE

Description

Parkinson's disease is a chronic, progressive disorder associated with a malfunction of the neurochemical process in the brain that results in a lack of dopamine. Dopamine is used in a location near the center of the brain that regulates physical movement of the body. Physical stability is thus affected, and as the condition worsens the patient is bedridden and unable to speak or eat.

Common Diagnostic Tests

- Parkinson's disease is determined by observing classic symptoms of involuntary tremors (often the first symptom), rigidity, and slowness of movement.

What to Look for

- Stooped posture, stiff and slow muscle movement, and resting tremors.

- Fixed facial expression and nodding of the head.
- Bradykinesia: a slowing of body movements.
- Speech is slurred and muffled.
- Mental processes are not usually affected, although depression is common.

Treatment

- Levodopa. *(See PH, Central nervous system)*
- Sinemet (a levodopa compound). *(See PH, Central nervous system)*
- Anticholinergic drugs, *e.g.,* trihexyphenidyl (Artane). *(See PH, Central nervous system)*
- Physiotherapy.

Nursing Tips

- Although it is not a cure, levodopa is extremely effective in controlling the symptoms of Parkinson's disease. There are serious side-effects that can be debilitating. Nausea and vomiting often occur for periods of up to several months after the medication is started. An antiemetic drug, *e.g.,* trimethobenzamide hydrochloride (Tigan), may be ordered to control this *(see PH, Gastrointestinal system)*. It is helpful to give levodopa after a meal or with an antacid.
- Orthostatic hypotension may occur as a side-effect in the beginning months of treatment. Be sure the patient wears elastic stockings to help control this, and that he changes position slowly to prevent vertigo.
- An anticholinergic, trihexyphenidyl (Artane) *(see PH, Central nervous system),* is often used in conjunction with levadopa. Under no circumstances should anticholinergic drugs be stopped suddenly because severe tremors and rigidity may occur.
- Mental confusion may occur as a side-effect of medications used to control Parkinson's disease.
- Constipation is a common problem because of decreased intestinal motility. A diet high in fibers and liquids should be encouraged.
- A daily schedule of exercise is extremely important to prevent muscle rigidity. A physiotherapy referral is helpful for specific exercises that improve balance and walking.

SEIZURES (CONVULSIONS)

Description

A seizure is a brain function disorder that causes changes in the level of consciousness (LOC) with involuntary motor and sensory responses. The effect may vary from minor to severe dysfunctions. A temporary abnormality, such as hypoglycemia, uremia, cerebral anoxia, drug overdose, or alcohol withdrawal, may cause transient seizures that disappear when the underlying condition is corrected. Idiopathic epilepsy is the name given recurrent seizures that occur spontaneously, and which have no readily identifiable cause. Frequently lesions in the brain are associated with epilepsy. There are four common types of seizures.

- *Grand mal seizures* comprise 90% of all seizures and are characterized by loss of consciousness with severe, generalized motor and sensory dysfunction.
- *Jacksonian seizures* have an initial localized motor dysfunction that tends to spread in a continuous pattern to adjacent areas of the body. Changes in consciousness may occur.
- *Petit mal seizures* are momentary changes in LOC; these are rarely seen after the age of 20.
- *Psychomotor seizures* are periods of physical behavior that the patient is unable to control, and are characterized afterward by amnesia.

Status epilepticus describes continuous grand mal seizures that occur in rapid succession without the patient regaining consciousness—*this requires immediate medical attention.* Such seizures are frequently the result of the abrupt discontinuation of anticonvulsant medication.

Post-traumatic epilepsy frequently follows severe head injuries, and may occur within the first few days or several months later. The prognosis for remission is good in cases appearing in the first few days or weeks.

Common Diagnostic Tests

- CAT Scan. *(See NR, Scans)*
- Angiograms.
- EEG *(See NR, Electroencephalogram)*
- EKG *(See NR, Electrocardiogram leads and how to place them)*
- Neurological examination.
- Blood sugar. *(See LAB)*
- BUN *(See LAB)*
- Electrolytes. *(See LAB)*
- Lumbar puncture: contraindicated when there is increased intracranial pressure.

What to Look for

Observation and recording of seizure activity is extremely important. You may be the only witness. Be sure to describe any injuries that result from the seizure. Document as accurately as possible, recording the following information:

- *Duration:* how long the seizure lasted and any activity or specific sensation (aura) that preceded it.

- *LOC*: if unconscious, the length of time and the mental state when consciousness returned. Did sleep follow, and for how long?
- *Motor activity:* describe as "tonic movements" (contraction of muscles causing rigidity) and "clonic movements" (alternating contraction and relaxation of muscles, producing jerking spasms). Did muscle activity start in one area of the body and move to another, and was it unilateral or bilateral? Were the teeth clenched? Was there frothing at the mouth? Did incontinence occur? Describe the respirations and whether there was cyanosis. Were the eyes open or closed, or in an unusual position?

Treatment

- Maintain an airway and prevent aspiration of secretions. If the teeth are not clenched insert a bite stick. *Never force entry.* Try to keep the patient on his side. When the seizure is over, mouth suctioning may be necessary if the LOC is depressed.
- Never leave patient alone during a seizure.
- Protect the patient from injuring himself, but restrain his movements only as much as is necessary. Pay particular attention to preventing head injury. It may be possible to put a blanket under his head or to cradle it in your lap. If he has fallen onto the floor do not try to get him into bed until the seizure is over.
- Start an IV as soon as possible.
- Anticonvulsants, *e.g.,* phenytoin sodium (Dilantin) and diazepam (Valium), are given. *(See PH, Central Nervous System)*

Nursing Tips

- Be familiar with patient's history and laboratory results so that you are alert to possibility of seizures.
- Seizures associated with alcohol withdrawal usually appear within 48 hours after cessation of drinking.
- Those patients with a history of seizures or a predisposing condition must have seizure precautions. These include a padded tongue blade or soft airway taped to the bedside stand or the head of the bed, and immediately available suction equipment. If it is indicated by the frequency and severity of seizures, padded siderails should be used the full length of the bed. Temperatures should be taken rectally to avoid thermometer breakage in the mouth.
- The highest incidence of seizures is at night and in the early morning.
- Once a patient has a seizure, chances increase that others will occur.

- Anticonvulsant medication must be given on schedule. If the patient is n.p.o. for any reason, the physician must be aware of this so medications can be given parenterally.
- When a seizure occurs, the patient's roommate may be the only witness. Ask him for information about the seizure.
- If possible, try to provide some privacy during a seizure. This can be an extremely upsetting experience for other patients.
- Patients with epilepsy should wear bracelets identifying the problem.

SPINAL CORD TRAUMA

Description

Spinal cord trauma may be caused by fracture of the vertebrae with direct damage to the cord or by indirect damage from compression, primarily caused by a tumor or a ruptured intervertebral disc.

Fractured vertebrae constitute a major cause of injury. The effects of the injury occur throughout the body below the point of the spinal cord damage. This may be only a brief loss of neurological function, such as occurs from spinal cord concussion.

Varying degrees of paralysis result from compression and laceration. Initially, cord damage generally results in flaccid paralysis and areflexia (loss of reflexes). As the edema decreases there may be spastic paralysis and some return of reflexes.

Permanent loss of voluntary and involuntary movement results from transection of the cord.

Additionally, cervical cord damage affects respiratory function.

Common Diagnostic Tests

- Myelograms (to view distortions of spinal cord).
- Spine x-rays.
- Neurological examination.

What to Look for

- Spinal shock, which results in an immediate loss of all functions below the level of injury. This occurs within minutes and is the result of direct injury or edema of the spinal cord. It is transient but may last weeks to months. There is no voluntary or involuntary elimination of urine or stool. A major risk is the possibility of overdistention of the bladder, which may cause it to rupture. Impactions, abdominal distention, and paralytic ileus are the effects of spinal shock on the bowel.
- Respiratory failure, which occurs when injury is above the third cervical vertebra. The patient can live only by means of a respi-

rator. When damage occurs below the third cervical vertebra or in the upper thoracic vertebrae area, respiratory problems, caused by edema compressing the cord, often occur within the first few days. A tracheostomy may be necessary. These patients are very susceptible to pneumonia.

- Bladder dysfunction, high incidence of urine retention after spinal cord trauma. A *flaccid* or *autonomous bladder* with dribbling incontinence because of overdistention. There is an increased incidence of infection of stagnant urine. A *spastic* or *reflex bladder* empties spontaneously with no controlling influence to regulate it.
- A flaccid bowel has no sphincter control. A reflex bowel has sphincter control.
- Autonomic hyperreflexia: a sudden, severe increase in blood pressure due to damage of the sympathetic nerves. It is most frequently seen in those patients with injury at the T_6 (sixth thoracic vertebra) level or above. It is usually the result of a distended bladder or impacted rectum. *This is a medical emergency.* Notify the physician *immediately.* If possible, sit the patient up after relieving distention or impaction.
- Pressure sores are the most preventable complication. They are difficult to heal and slow down rehabilitation.
- Muscle spasms, which are involuntary contractions of muscles. Spasms develop after cord shock has subsided. They occur most often following high cord injury, and are frequently severe.
- Any changes in neurological function must be carefully monitored and recorded. A decrease in function should be reported to the physician immediately.

Treatment

- Steroids to reduce spinal cord edema. *(See PH, Endocrine system)*
- Analgesics for pain that often occurs at site of injury or disease. *(See PH, Central nervous system)*
- Crutchfield tongs or halo traction for cervical fractures.
- Skeletal traction to keep the vertebral column in proper alignment. *(See NR, Traction)*
- Laminectomy for decompression, especially with increased neuro deficit, or to remove bone or disc fragments. *(See SS, Orthopedics)*
- Surgical stabilization of vertebral column (*e.g.,* through fusion or the use of stabilizing rods).

Nursing Tips

- In cervical injuries, aspiration due to a decreased ability to cough must be anticipated. Suction equipment should always be immediately available. An emergency tracheotomy set should be at the bedside whether or not there is a tracheostomy.

- The severity of signs and symptoms *immediately* following an injury is not always a reliable indicator of the eventual extent of permanent damage.

- Return of function within a few days after an initial loss of all function indicates that the patient was in spinal cord shock. There may also be a return of involuntary movements, stimulated by such things as pinching the skin. However, this should not be confused with the return of voluntary movements, the lack of which, after several months, indicates permanent damage.

- Although spinal cord shock effects are temporary, any resultant edema of the cord may cause permanent damage. It is extremely important to maintain proper body alignment whenever edema exists.

- Turning every 2 hours is a necessity. This should be accomplished by log rolling with a pull sheet. Use three people to do this properly. Patients with a spinal cord injury need to avoid all movement and flexion of the spinal column. Movement of the head must also be avoided.

- Skin care, proper body alignment, and range of motion (ROM) exercises four times a day are immediate needs from the onset of injury. Also, footboards and wrist splints should be used to prevent contractions. Heels should never rest directly on the mattress. Circulation is decreased and, with no sense of feeling, pressure sores may develop. It is just as important to relieve pressure points when the patient is sitting in a chair as when he is lying on a bed. Teach the patient to raise his buttocks off the seat for 20 seconds every 15 minutes. If the arms are too weak to do this, assistance is necessary.

- There is often pain at the level of injury. Occasionally patients experience acute pain in paralyzed areas, although physiologically it is not possible to feel it.

- Be sure the patient has a usable nurse's call signal available (such as a whistle for someone not able to move their hands). All nursing personnel must know what it is. The more helpless the patient is, the greater his fear of being left unattended.

- Intake and output recording is extremely important.

- Flaccid bladders lack the stimulus to empty and will continue to distend. Never catheterize more than 300 ml from a distended bladder; wait 15 minutes and remove the remainder in amounts of 300 ml at 15-minute intervals. Sudden decompression of a distended bladder in a patient with injury to nerve tracts may cause sudden, severe hypotension. Permanent indwelling catheters are often necessary, or ileoconduit surgery may be performed.

- In reflex bladders there is a loss of the sensation of a full bladder. The bladder will empty by reflex activity, which the patient will be unable to consciously control. Catheterization should be done every 4 to 6 hours *(see NR, Urinary bladder catheterization and drainage)*. Intake is carefully monitored, with less fluid in the evening. Total daily intake should not exceed 2000 ml.

- Self-catheterization should be taught if the patient is capable of managing this procedure. Hopefully, the individual will begin to recognize secondary symptoms of a full bladder, such as headache or sweating. Pressing down on the abdomen or tapping on it at this time may initiate urine flow. Bethanechol chloride (Urecholine) p.o. may help stimulate voiding. Catheterization for residual urine must be done after each reflex voiding until there is a regular pattern of less than 100 ml. When this is accomplished, catheterization for urine residual is done only once or twice a week.

- Urinary tract infection (UTI) must be treated immediately. Renal failure is the most common cause of death in the patient with impaired bladder function. The urine specific gravity must be done daily *(See LAB)*, and the urine must be kept acidic to decrease the possibility of UTI. Urine cultures are done weekly *(see LAB)*, and colony counts of 50,000 and above are treated. The patient must know the signs and symptoms of UTI (foul-smelling urine, flulike symptoms, and an elevated temperature).

- Demineralization of bones occurs after long periods of immobilization and results in urinary stone formation. Fluid intake of 1800 to 2000 ml should be maintained to help prevent this occurrence.

- A flaccid bowel has no sphincter control. Therefore, a permanent colostomy is sometimes done.

- Bowel training for those with a reflex bowel and sphincter control problem begins with a diet high in fiber and daily stool softeners. A regular time of day is selected, and a bowel movement is stimulated with gentle manual evacuation of the rectal vault. Suppositories or enemas should be used only when absolutely necessary.

- In both bowel and bladder training a nursing-care plan is imperative; an inflexible routine and schedule must be maintained.

Orthopedics

AMPUTATION

Description

Complications of peripheral vascular disorders and diabetes, trauma, malignant bone tumors, osteomyelitis, and congenital defects may be indications for amputation of all or part of an extremity.

The following are common abbreviations indicating the level of amputation: B.K. (below the knee), A.K. (above the knee), B.E. (below the elbow), and A.E. (above the elbow). A Syme amputation removes the foot at the ankle joint including the malleoli.

Long-range goals following amputation include proper fit of the prosthesis and rehabilitation of the patient both physically and psychologically.

Common Diagnostic Tests

- X-rays, bone scans. *(See NR, x-rays and scans)*
- Arteriography and oscillometric readings for evaluation of circulatory status.
- Doppler. *(See NR, Ultrasound)*

What to Look for

Preoperative

- Changes in skin temperature, color, and pulses in both the affected and unaffected extremities. Assess when limb is in both elevated and dependent position.
- Signs of gangrene: color changes (redness to black); skin may appear dry and wrinkled, especially in diabetes and peripheral vascular disease. *(See SS, Diabetes and SS, Arterial occlusive diseases of the lower extremities)*

Postoperative

- Watch for signs of hemorrhage, infection, and edema; later, watch for irritation on the stump (stumps of patients with diabetes or vascular problems are subject to wound separation and decubitus formation).

Treatment

- Closed amputation (flap method): skin flap covers the stump.
- Open amputation: stump is left open to provide for drainage, especially when there is vascular impairment. Skin traction may be applied. The wound is closed 4 or 5 weeks later.
- Level of amputation is determined by adequacy of circulation, considerations regarding type of prosthesis that may be used, and future usefulness of part.

Nursing Tips

Preoperative

- Psychological preparation if there is time, capitalizing on what patient *will* be able to do. Emotional support both pre and postoperatively, allowing patient to go through grieving process.
- Prosthetist (the person who creates and supervises the use of the prosthesis) may visit, if requested by surgeon.
- Exercises initiated and supervised by physiotherapist.
  1. Pushups to strengthen triceps in preparation for crutch walking.
  2. Use of the trapeze.
  3. Isometric abdominal-tightening exercises.
  4. Muscle-setting and joint-mobilizing exercises of both shoulders, in an upper-extremity amputation.
  5. Practice in transferring (moving) from bed to chair.

Postoperative

- Hemorrhage is the greatest danger.
  1. Assess frequently for oozing on dressing (mark it). A portable wound suction system, such as Hemovac, may be used immediately postoperatively.
  2. *Caution:* Bright red bleeding is not normal. Apply pressure dressing and elevate stump by raising foot of bed. Notify surgeon immediately.
  3. Keep large blood pressure cuff at bedside for emergency use as a tourniquet in case of sudden hemorrhage.
  4. Check vital signs frequently, especially during first 48 hours, for signs of shock and hemorrhage. *(See SS, Postoperative care)*

- Prevent edema, which occurs most during first 24 hours postoperatively. Heavy cast or pressure dressing is applied in surgery.
  1. Elevate stump of leg by elevating foot of bed. (Avoid contractures. Pillows are *never* placed under an A.K. stump, and only if knee is extended for a B.K. one).
  2. Ice bags to part, only if ordered.
- Pain relief
  1. "Phantom limb sensation" is common; it lessens with activity and weight bearing.
  2. "Phantom limb pain" is uncommon; a burning, crushing kind of pain, it may be lessened by weight bearing, if allowed. Other treatment may include whirlpool, massage, injection of stump with local anesthetic, sympathectomy, and transcutaneous nerve stimulation (TNS).
  3. Neuroma, in which there is scar formation on severed nerves, may cause great pain and require excision.
  4. Frequently, patients who have had gangrene feel surprisingly little pain after amputation.
- Infection
  1. Suspect infection if a bad odor comes from stump dressing or cast or if patient's temperature elevates.
  2. Treatment may include antibiotics, elevation of the stump (by elevating foot of bed in leg amputation), hot packs, incision and drainage, and possible reamputation at a higher level.
- Exercise program: usually initiated by physiotherapist, it will commonly include the following objectives:
  1. Prevent contractures, particularly of hip, knee, and elbow.
     a. Prone position with head turned away from the affected side for 30 minutes three or four times a day.
     b. Traction, trochanter rolls, and firm mattress to keep body in alignment while patient is in bed.
     c. No prolonged sitting; no pillow under knee or under A.K. stump.
     d. Avoid abduction of the hip.
     e. Range of motion (ROM) exercises. *(See NR, Range of motion exercises)*
  2. Prepare for use of prosthesis, for crutch walking, and for transferring to a wheelchair (if patient is not to get prosthesis).
  3. Assist in developing balance.
- Stump care
  1. Stump treatment will depend upon the patient's condition and the requirements of the anticipated prosthesis. Approaches include

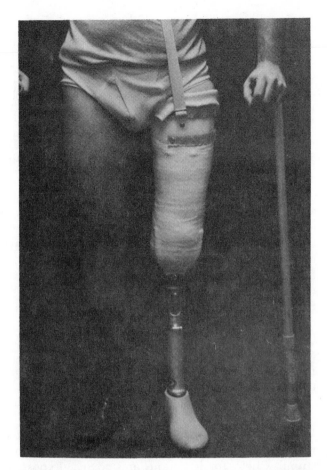

FIG. 5-6. *Immediate, temporary prosthetic fitting (pylon) used following amputation.*
(Courtesy of the Prosthetic Research Study, Veterans Administration Con-
tract V663P-784)

   a. Compression dressing with elastic bandage.
   b. Skin traction for open amputation, with closure later.
   c. Immediate temporary prosthesis (pylon): plaster cast with
      prosthetic extension and artificial foot (Fig. 5-6).
2. Stump is bandaged after wound has healed to shrink and shape
   the stump to a tapered, rounded, smooth end in preparation
   for the prosthesis (Fig. 5-7).
   a. A clean elastic bandage or stump shrinker should be used
      each day.
   b. While the joint above the amputation is extended, the band-

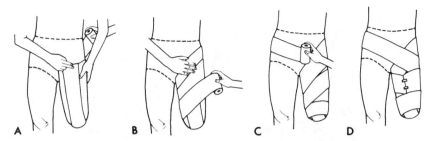

FIG. 5-7. *Method for bandaging an above-the-knee amputation stump.*

age should be wrapped smoothly, applying even, moderate tension to all parts of the stump. Rewrap as needed to maintain continuous pressure. Avoid tourniquet-like effect caused by too much pressure or circular turns (use oblique, modified figure eight pattern).

3. Stump conditioning: (ordered by physician)
   a. Check stump every day for minor irritations and edema (indications that wrapping has been done incorrectly).
   b. Gentle massage to increase circulation; this may be started 5 to 7 days postoperatively.
   c. Push stump against harder and harder surfaces in preparation for artificial lower extremity.
4. To maintain good condition of stump, patient teaching includes the following:
   a. Wash stump with soap and water every night. Rinse and dry thoroughly. Use a mirror to observe incision and entire stump. Check for irritations and edema. Expose to air and sun when possible.
   b. Stump socket should be washed every night and left open to air.
   c. Stump socks and stump wrapping should be clean every day. Wash and dry flat. Sock should be made of wool. Have several on hand so that there is time for thorough drying between washings. Never wear a mended sock.
   d. Avoid wearing shoes with unevenly worn heels.
   e. Stump may shrink for up to 2 years after surgery, so prosthesis will need adjustment, as it will in growing children.
5. Rigid dressing technique with immediate temporary prosthesis (pylon) (Fig. 5-6)
   a. Plaster cast on the stump, with prosthetic extension, that fits into the socket in the cast and into an artificial foot; provides for almost immediate mobility, and decreases edema and pain.

b. Cast will be changed at intervals two or three times before stump is measured for prosthesis.

c. Controlled, progressive ambulation is allowed, but too much weight bearing can cause disruption in healing.

d. *Caution:* If cast comes off, wrap stump immediately with an elastic bandage and notify the surgeon. Edema could develop very rapidly.

e. Pylon is removed from socket when patient is in bed.

f. Check skin condition around cast.

g. Severe or increasing stump pain or odor coming from cast should be reported.

ARTHRITIS

Description

Arthritis is defined as an inflammation of a joint (frequently the lining), in which there is usually pain and often eventual structural change. Usually due to excessive joint use or trauma, it may also be due to metabolic, collagenic, vascular, infectious, or neoplastic disorders. In this reference, we will consider osteoarthritis and rheumatoid arthritis. Elements of nursing care of patients with inflamed joints have many commonalities, regardless of the etiology of the arthritis.

OSTEOARTHRITIS

Description

Osteoarthritis is a degenerative joint disease, characterized by destruction of the joint cartilage and overgrowth of bone, causing impaired function. Sometimes called hypertrophic arthritis, it is usually associated with the aging process, but may be secondary to trauma or other causes.

Common Diagnostic Tests

- X-ray shows characteristic narrowing of joint space and osteophyte or spur (boney outgrowth) formation.
- Sedimentation rate and aspirated synovial fluid are usually normal.

What to Look for

- Gradual onset of joint pain after exercise and stiffness following inactivity, with gradual limits in motion.
- Joint tenderness, with gradual joint enlargement.
- Crepitus (joint noise on motion caused by diseased cartilage, bone, or joint lining).

- Heberden's nodes (hard nodules and enlargement of the distal finger joints).
- Joint involvement tends to be localized in one or a few joints. Most commonly affected are distal finger joints, the hips, the knees, and the spine.

Treatment

- Rest the affected joints (may involve use of cane, crutches, traction, or splints).
- Weight reduction in obese patients.
- Moist heat to the affected joint; physiotherapy.
- Progressive exercises, especially isometrics.
- Nonsteroid anti-inflammatory drugs (*e.g.*, salicylates). *(See PH, Analgesic antipyretics, anti-inflammatory agents, drugs for gout)*
- Analgesics for relief of pain. *(See PH, Analgesic antipyretics, anti-inflammatory agents, drugs for gout)*.
- Interarticular corticosteroids: very effective for occasional use in acute inflammatory flare-ups.
- Surgery, joint replacement: total hip replacement has been very successful, total knee replacement, less so. *(See SS, Orthopedics, joint replacement)*

Nursing Tips

- Encourage activity as long as possible. Avoidance of emotional strains or activities that precipitate flare-ups (*e.g.*, lifting) is important.
- Provide emotional support for patient with chronic disorder.
- Encourage compliance with prescribed treatment.
- Follow specifics of care following surgical treatment, such as for total hip replacement. *(See SS, Orthopedics, total hip replacement)*

RHEUMATOID ARTHRITIS
Description

Rheumatoid arthritis (RA) is a chronic, systemic disease characterized by exacerbations and remissions. It is manifested usually by symmetrical involvement of peripheral joints, starting within inflammation of the synovium (lining of the joint) and maybe progressing to destruction of the joint. Generalized symptoms may be present. Although the cause is still unknown, increasing evidence points to autoimmunity as a factor. A disease usually of moderately young adults (around 35 to 40 years of age), it is three times more common in women than in men.

Common Diagnostic Tests

- Complete blood count (CBC). *(See LAB)*
- Hemoglobin depressed; usually below 10 g/100 ml. *(See LAB)*
- Elevated WBC. *(See LAB)*
- Sedimentation rate elevated. *(See LAB)*
- Rheumatoid factor (RF): presence of RFs helps confirm diagnosis if clinical picture is present.
- Synovial fluid aspirated from joint: viscosity poor, WBCs elevated.
- Characteristic histological appearance of RA nodules
- X-rays of the joints.

What to Look for

- History of abrupt onset of inflammation in multiple joints or of gradual progressive joint involvement. May be accompanied by low-grade fever, fatigue, anorexia, and weight loss.
  1. Morning stiffness, gradually diminishing with activity.
  2. Pain and tenderness of joints, usually symmetrical involvement.
  3. Soft swelling of joint with redness, warmth, and subcutaneous nodules (rheumatic nodules) found especially over boney prominences.
  4. Hands often show involvement of proximal interphalangeal or metacarpophalangeal (knuckle) joints, or both, with deformity of the fingers, muscle wasting, and ulnar deviation of fingers (fingers drift away from thumb).
  5. Involvement of wrists, feet, ankles, and elbows is also typical, though other joints may also be involved.
- If disease process continues, end result may be instability and subluxation (partial or incomplete dislocation) of joints.
- Systemic changes may include pulmonary changes that must be differentiated from carcinoma (*e.g.,* pleural effusion, fibrosis, nodules), pericarditis, leg ulcers due to vasculitis, enlargement of the spleen, and carpal tunnel syndrome.

Treatment

The goal is to prevent deformity and disability.

Drug Therapy

- Nonsteroid anti-inflammatory drugs (NSAID).
  1. Acetylsalicylic acid (Aspirin) in high doses, which must be continued even during periods of remission. Enteric coated aspirin (Ecotrin) may be ordered for h.s. *(See PH, Analgesic antipyretics, anti-inflammatory agents, drugs for gout)*

2. Ibuprofen (Motrin), naproxen (Naprosyn), indomethacin (Indocin), phenylbutazone (Butazolidin), or others may be tried. *(See PH, Analgesic antipyretics, anti-inflammatory agents, drugs for gout)*

- Specific drugs
  1. Gold salts: *e.g.*, gold sodium thiomalate (Myochrysine).
  2. Penicillamine (Cuprimine).
  3. Antimalarial agents: *e.g.*, hydroxychloroquine (Plaquenil) and chloroquine phosphate (Aralen).
  4. Immunosuppressant drugs: *e.g.*, Azathioprine (Imuran).
  5. Cytoxic agents: cyclophosphamide (Cytoxan) or methotrexate, which is sometimes tried as a last resort. *(See PH, Antineoplastics)*
  6. Corticosteroids. *(See PH, Endocrine system)*
     a. Used systemically only in acute flare-ups, not for long-term use.
     b. Intra-articular injections may relieve pain and improve mobility in selected joints.

Physiotherapy

- Exercise program is devised by physiotherapist based on patient's condition. Program will avoid strain on joints and may emphasize isometrics and hydrotherapy.
- Heat treatment: moist heat preferred; may include moist hot packs, warm tub baths, and warm paraffin applications (usually done before exercises).
- Cold applications may be tried when heat increases pain.

Rest for Inflamed Joints; General Body Rest

- Bed rest may be indicated in acute stages, though exercises should be continued. Avoid flexion contractures by not placing any pillows under the patient's knees or large pillows under his head. Have him lie prone several times a day.
- Splints or traction may rest inflamed joints and provide proper alignment.
- Orthopedic shoes may help decrease metatarsophalangeal joint pain on weight bearing.

Surgery

- Synovectomy: may produce pain relief and prevent tissue destruction.
- Arthrodesis: fusion of a joint to provide stability.
- Joint replacements (*e.g.*, total hip replacement). *(See SS, Orthopedics, total hip replacement)*

Nursing Tips

- Provide emotional support for the patient who is undergoing pain and potential body changes that may be deforming and disabling. Use a positive approach, working with the patient's hope to live as normal a life as possible.
- Stress faithful adherence to the individualized rehabilitation program.
- Help patient develop plan to avoid stress and to rest before he becomes tired. Joint pain for longer than 1 hour following an activity indicates that the activity should be restricted or eliminated.
- Occupational therapist may provide specific tips regarding ways to protect joints while performing activities of daily living, including use of self-help devices.
- Provide patient education regarding prescribed medications and their potential side-effects.
- Local arthritis associations may be sources of both information and support.

Sources of Patient Information

- National Institute of Arthritis, Metabolism and Digestive Diseases, National Institutes of Health, Bethesda, MD, 20205.
- Arthritis Foundation, 3400 Peachtree Rd. NE, Suite 1101, Atlanta, Georgia, 30326. Telephone (404) 266–0795. Excellent booklets and pamphlets for patients are available, including "Rheumatoid Arthritis—Handbook for Patients" and "Arthritis—the Basic Facts."

FAT EMBOLISM

Description

Following injury particularly of the long bones and the pelvis, fat cells leave bone and go into the blood stream, causing occlusion of small blood vessels in distant organs, especially the lungs, brain, and kidneys. Most common in young adults, the onset of this syndrome may appear 12 to 36 hours after trauma or up to three weeks later.

Common Diagnostic Tests

- Arterial blood gases (ABGs). *(See LAB)*
- Chest x-ray.
- Urinalysis for fat.
- Elevated serum lipase.

What to Look for

- Sudden, steady rise in pulse, respiratory rate, and temperature.
- Respiratory distress and dyspnea.
- Bizarre mental symptoms: confusion, disorientation, mild agitation, and coma (related to reduced oxygen to brain).
- Petechiae over the anterior aspect of the chest, shoulders, conjunctival sacs, and buccal membranes.

Treatment

- Oxygen therapy. *(See NR, Oxygen administration)*
- Elevate head of bed if no signs of shock are present.
- Controlled volume ventilation with positive end expiratory pressure (PEEP).
- Steroids. *(See PH, Endocrine system)*
- Low-molecular-weight dextran. *(See NR, Intravenous therapy)*
- Heparin. *(See PH, Cardiovascular system)*
- Antihyperlipemics.
- IV fluids; blood transfusions. *(See NR, Intravenous therapy)*

Nursing Tips

- Try to prevent fat embolism by gentle, proper handling of injured part.
- Never massage.

FRACTURES

Description

A fracture is a break in a bone. An *open* or *compound fracture* is one with a wound, through which a fragment of bone may or may not be protruding. It is always considered infected. *(See SS, Orthopedics, open fracture)*

Common Diagnostic Tests

- X-ray
- Scan. *(See NR, Scans)*
- Routine urine and blood work preoperatively; may include type and crossmatch.
- Hemoglobin and hematocrit are usually repeated 3 or 4 days postoperatively.
- Serum calcium may be ordered. *(See LAB)*

What to Look for

- Pain at the site, which increases with pressure or movement.
- Deformity of the part.

1. Muscle spasm may cause shortening of a limb.
2. Change in contour or alignment.
- Swelling: usually rapid over fracture; there may be some bruising.
- Numbness, tingling, and occasionally paralysis.
- Abnormal mobility.
- Crepitation: grating sound when ends of bones move against each other.
- Signs of visceral (internal) injury, for example
  1. Hemoptysis (bloody sputum), as a result of injury to lungs caused by fractured ribs.
  2. Oliguria or anuria or blood in the urine, caused by injury to urethra or bladder by fractured pelvis. (Oliguria or anuria are also seen in shock.)
- Signs and symptoms of complications. *(See nursing tips)*

Treatment

- Reduction: replacement of bone fragments into normal position.
  1. Traction: may be temporary before internal fixation of fracture or may be the definitive treatment. (Skeletal traction requires surgical placement of pin.)
  2. Closed reduction (without surgery).
  3. Open reduction: surgical reduction with use of plates, nails, screws, wires, and rods for stabilization.
- Immobilization (to maintain reduction).
  1. Splints.
  2. Cast or cast brace. *(See NR, Cast brace; Cast care)*
  3. Continuous traction. *(See NR, Traction)*
  4. Internal fixation with plates, nails, screws, and so forth.
  5. External fixation device. *(See NR, External fixation device)*
  6. Bandages of muslin or elastic *(e.g.,* Velpeau's bandage for fracture of scapula, clavicle, and humerus).
- Rehabilitation, including physiotherapy, and training to resume activities of daily living.

Nursing Tips

(See also NR, Traction; NR, Casts; SS, Fat embolism; and SS, Open fractures)

Preoperative

- Prep with antibacterial scrub may be ordered. Shaves are usually done in the operating room.
- Acquaint patient with traction equipment.
- Have patient practice voiding in recumbent position to make it easier postoperatively.

Postoperative

- Turn patient to the unaffected side, unless otherwise ordered.
- Early ambulation is desirable when possible (must be ordered by physician).
- Watch for urinary retention.
- Be alert for complications; try to prevent them.
  1. Shock and hemorrhage. *(See SS, Postoperative care)*
     a. Assess vital signs frequently until stable.
     b. Check dressing or cast for evidence of bleeding. Run your hand underneath to be sure blood is not pooling there.
     c. Look for changes in the circumference of the limb (swelling).
     d. Blood loss may be high, especially in fracture of the femur. Blood volume should be replaced appropriately.
  2. Anemia
     a. Hemoglobin and hematocrit usually ordered 3 or 4 days postoperatively. Blood transfusions or iron supplements may be ordered.
  3. Fat embolism *(See SS, Fat embolism)*
  4. Infection (especially common following open fractures)
     a. Maintain sterile technique when dressing wound.
     b. Provide regular pin care, as ordered or according to hospital policy, when patient has skeletal traction or external fixation.
  5. Circulatory impairment: constitutes a medical emergency; if unrelieved, it can lead to permanent disability *(e.g.,* Volkmann's contracture).
     a. Check affected limb every 2 hours or as ordered for color, pulses, and skin temperature, especially in first 24 hours posttrauma or postoperatively. If there is any doubt about presence of pulses, use a Doppler.
     b. Pain usually decreases after reduction. Any increase should be reported immediately. Pain, paresthesia (tingling, numbness, difference in sensation), pallor (blanching—usually indicates arterial impairment; cyanosis, venous impairment), peripheral pulselessness, any abnormal coolness, or difficulty in movement should be reported immediately.
  6. Thrombophlebitis *(See SS, Postoperative care)*
     a. Watch for pain, redness, and swelling, especially along a vein.
     b. Prevent it by encouraging exercises, early ambulation, and use of antiembolism stockings according to surgeon's order.

7. Disseminated intravascular coagulation (DIC)
8. Neuro impairment
   a. Check for sensory disturbances and loss of motion.
   b. The area over the peroneal nerve (3 inches below the knee on its outer aspect) must be kept free from pressure.
9. Problems of immobilization
   a. Renal calculi and urinary tract infections. *(See SS, Urinary system and the prostate, urinary calculus and urinary tract infections)*
   b. Respiratory problems *(e.g.,* hypostatic pneumonia). *(See SS, Pneumonia and NR, Deep breathing techniques)*
   c. Decubitus: inspect all pressure areas, especially heels and coccyx. Keep heels from resting on the bed. *(See MNS, Decubitus ulcer prevention and treatment)*
   d. Contractures
      1) Hip: lower head of bed several times a day to permit extension of the hip.
      2) Knee tends to flex when there is pain in the hip. Do not support the knee with a pillow.
10. Muscle spasm
    a. Prevent spasm with frequent position changes and by keeping pressure off the limb.
    b. Skeletal muscle relaxants, *e.g.,* carisoprodol (Soma), chlorzoxazone (Paraflex), and methocarbamol (Roboxin), may be ordered.
    c. Benedryl at bedtime may also be helpful. *(See PH, Central nervous system)*
- Other complications of fractures include non-union, delayed union, malunion, and avascular necrosis (death of tissue due to decreased blood supply—rather common in capsular fractures of the femur, and the reason for use of replacement head of the femur).

HIP FRACTURES
Description
Intracapsular hip fractures occur within the hip joint or capsule, near the head or through the neck of the femur. *Extracapsular* fractures are those occuring outside the joint and capsule in the area of the greater or lesser trochanter. They may be referred to as *trochanteric* fractures.

These "hip" fractures—occuring most often in the elderly—require special management because of frequently concurring medical, physical, and age-related problems. Early ambulation and restoration of daily living activities, when possible, are high priorities in treatment.

Common Diagnostic Tests

(See Fractures, common diagnostic tests)
- Usually also include typing and crossmatching blood and reservation of packed cells.
- Hemoglobin and hematocrit may be frequently repeated.

What to Look for

- Affected leg is usually shortened and externally rotated.
- Pain and inability to move the leg.
- Slight pain in the groin or the inner side of the knee—may be the only symptoms of an impacted fracture.

Treatment
Preoperative (To Reduce Pain and Muscle Spasm)

- Buck's extension traction, especially for subcapital fractures.
- Russell's traction, for intertrochanteric or subtrochanteric fractures. *(See NR, Traction)*
- Trochanter rolls to maintain alignment of leg (Fig. 5-8).
- Anticoagulant therapy may be initiated. *(See PH, Cardiovascular system)*
- Antibiotics usually ordered. *(See PH, Antimicrobials)*

Surgical

- Internal fixation of the reduced fracture with nails, screws, plates, and pins.
- Replacement of the femoral head with a prosthesis; used frequently in intracapsular fractures where nonunion and avascular necrosis are frequent complications of internal fixation techniques.
- Total hip replacement is done occasionally. *(See SS, Orthopedics, total hip replacement)*

Nursing Tips

(See SS, Fractures; nursing tips and NR, Traction)
- Specifics of patient care must be ordered by the surgeon, but the following are general principles for care of patient who has had internal fixation of a hip fracture:
  1. Antiembolism stockings will be ordered.
  2. Turning
     a. Initially, patient may usually be turned gently to the unaf-

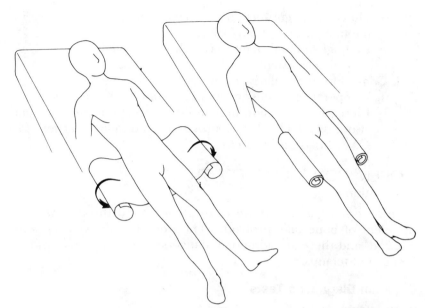

FIG. 5-8. *Method of making trochanter rolls to support the patient's legs and prevent them from rotating outward.* (Lewis LW: Fundamental Skills in Patient Care, 2nd ed, p 208. Philadelphia, JB Lippincott, 1981)

fected side with a pillow between the legs to maintain abduction of the affected leg. Eventually, turning to the affected side will be permitted.

3. Position affected leg, as ordered. Use trochanter roll (Fig. 5-8) or sandbags to maintain alignment. Prevent hip and knee flexion deformities by lowering head of bed several times a day; no pillow under knees.

4. Exercise: quadriceps setting, arm and shoulder strengthening (use of overhead trapeze), range of motion, and isometric muscle exercises of the abdomen and gluteal muscles usually are encouraged.

5. Early transfer to chair with weight on unaffected leg.
   a. Knee should be flexed at 90° angle while patient is in the chair.

6. Early ambulation with a walker, usually with no or only partial weight bearing.

7. See *Nursing Tips* under *Total Hip Replacement* for the patient with a prosthesis. *(See SS, Orthopedics, total hip replacement)*

- Prevention of complications.
  1. Bleeding is rather common.

    a. Closed drainage suction (*e.g.*, Hemovac) may be in place for the first 24 to 48 hours.

    b. Hemoglobin and hematocrit will be repeated.

    c. Packed cells usually are kept on reserve.

2. Confusion, particularly in the elderly, is common.

    a. Preoperatively assess mental awareness and orientation.

    b. Increased confusion may indicate stress reaction, but may also indicate blood loss, stroke, or medication reaction. *(See MNS, Disoriented patients)*

OPEN (COMPOUND) FRACTURES

Description

In an open fracture there is an open wound through which a fragment of bone may protrude. The wound is always considered infected, and there are additional dangers of osteomyelitis, gas gangrene, and tetanus.

Common Diagnostic Tests

- X-ray and scans. *(See NR, Scans)*
- Routine urine and blood work, preoperatively; may include typing and crossmatching.
- Wound culture for bacteria and sensitivity. *(See LAB)*

Treatment

- Wound is cleaned and debrided in the operating room.
- Reduction and stabilization of the fracture—increasingly, external fixation is being used. *(See NR, External fixation device)*
- Wound may be left open until there is no sign of infection.
  1. Frequent sterile dressing changes will be required.
  2. Wound and skin precautions must be followed. *(See NR, Isolation technique)*
  3. Wound will be closed later by suture or grafts.
- Tetanus prophylaxis.
- IV antibiotics.

Nursing Tips

- Check distal pulses. Observe for circulatory and neuro impairment. *(See Fractures: nursing tips)*
- Check vital signs every 4 hours. Watch for temperature elevation, a sign of infection.
- *(See nursing tips under SS, Fractures, NR, Traction, and NR, External fixation device)*

GOUT

Description

Gout is a purine metabolism disorder in which there is an accumulation of uric acid in the blood (hyperuricemia). It is characterized by acute inflammation of joints with tophi (subcutaneous urate deposits) formation in and around them. Kidney stone formation leading to chronic renal disease may also occur. Primarily a genetic defect in purine metabolism, hyperuricemia may also occur secondarily in other situations in which there is an overproduction or underexcretion of uric acid (*e.g.*, in leukemia, multiple myeloma, and psoriasis, after prolonged use of particularly the thiazide diuretics, and in certain cancer chemotherapies). Duration and degree of hyperuricemia will affect whether symptoms appear.

Common Diagnostic Tests

- Urate crystals are found in synovial fluid aspirated from joint cavity.
- X-rays of affected joints—in chronic disease these show tophi and destructive joint disease.
- Serum urate levels elevated.

What to Look for

- Sudden onset of acute, exquisite pain accompanied by redness, warmth, swelling, and tenderness in one or more joints (most commonly the great toe or the knee), usually lasting a few days with treatment (gouty arthritis).
- Fever, chills, and malaise may be present.
- Tophi may ulcerate and leave draining sinuses. Permanent deformity and disability of joints and history of more frequent attacks are symptoms of chronic gout, which may develop if patient is not on prophylactic therapy.
- Signs and symptoms of renal stones. *(See SS, Urinary calculus)*

Treatment
Acute Attacks

- Colchicine, given IV or p.o. at first signs of impending attack every 1 to 2 hours until pain is relieved or until nausea, vomiting and diarrhea appear.
- Nonsteroid anti-inflammatory drugs, *e.g.*, indomethacin (Indocin), phenylbutazone (Butazolidin), and ibuprofen (Motrin). *(See Analgesic antipyretics, anti-inflammatory agents, drugs for gout)*

- Narcotics and analgesics may be needed until other therapies provide relief. *(See PH, Central nervous system, analgesics)*
- Rest, cradle to keep bedding off of joint, and elevation of part.
- Force fluids to promote urate excretion.

Prophylactic Treatment (Between Attacks)

- Uricosuric medications: increase excretion of uric acid, *e.g.*, probenecid (Benemid) and sulfinpyrazone (Anturane). *(See PH, Analgesic antipyretics, anti-inflammatory agents, drugs for gout)*
  1. Salicylates should not be used with either probenecid or sulfinpyrazone because they antagonize their uricosuric effects. Acetaminophen (Tylenol) may be used.
  2. Force fluids to prevent high concentration of urinary urates.
  3. Sodium bicarbonate may be ordered to maintain alkaline urine.
- Allopurinol (Zyloprim) inhibits uric acid synthesis. *(See PH, Analgesic antipyretics, anti-inflammatory agents, drugs for gout)*

Nursing Tips

- During acute attack relieve pain, administer medications as ordered, monitor the effect of colchicine (if ordered), protect affected joint, and force fluids.
- Patient teaching to prevent recurrent attacks include the following tips:
  1. Slow weight reduction is recommended for the obese patient to reduce strain on joints. He should avoid fasting (because it increases serum uric acid).
  2. Patient should avoid foods or situations that precipitate attacks. Foods high in purine (*e.g.*, organ meats, shellfish, anchovies, sardines, and meat extracts) are usually to be avoided.
  3. Alcohol is usually restricted to one or two cocktails a week.
  4. Patient should wear comfortable shoes with toe room.
  5. Patient should understand the importance of taking his medications as prescribed. He should also be aware of possible side-effects and special precautions associated with them.

JOINT REPLACEMENT
TOTAL HIP REPLACEMENT
Description

In total hip replacement (THR) two component parts bound firmly in place with bone cement are implanted in place of the acetabulum and the femoral head and neck. Performed primarily to relieve pain, THR may also restore function to patients with diseased or injured hip joints (*e.g.*, from arthritis or aseptic necrosis of the femoral head).

Infection in, and dislocation of, the affected hip are serious complications of THR.

Common Diagnostic Tests

- X-rays.
- Preoperative urine and blood work, include typing, and cross-matching, and prothrombin time.
- EKG may be ordered.

Treatment

- Surgical replacement of hip joint with synthetic components.
- Intravenous antibiotics may be started 24 hours before surgery and continued several days postoperatively. *(See PH, Antimicrobials)*
- Anticoagulants may be ordered prophylactically to prevent pulmonary embolism. *(See PH, Cardiovascular system)*

Nursing Tips

Preoperative

- Infection is a dreaded complication; report any sign of any infection. If infection occurs, surgery may be postponed.
- Skin must be clean and in perfect condition. Antibacterial scrubs of the operative area and antibacterial showers with shampoo are usually ordered. Shave is usually done in operating room, unless otherwise ordered.
- Specific preparation for what is to be expected postoperatively with THR should accompany general preoperative teaching. *(See SS, Preoperative care)*

Postoperative

- General postoperative care. *(See SS, Postoperative care)*
- Blood loss is usually relatively large; replacement may be expected. Be sure blood is on reserve, if ordered. Hemoglobin and hematocrit are frequently ordered for the postoperative evening and the following morning.
- Closed-wound suction drainage unit is frequently in place (*e.g.,* Hemovac). This must be monitored carefully. Report if drainage exceeds 100 ml/4 hours.
- Check dressings frequently for amount of drainage. So that you will have a basis for comparison, outline area of visible drainage and record time on the dressing with a marking pen.
- Full-length antiembolic stockings, overhead frame, and trapeze are usually ordered. Provide heel pads to protect heels.
- Ice bags may be ordered for immediate postoperative use.

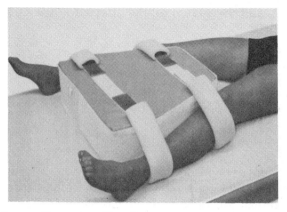

FIG. 5-9. *Abductor pillow.* (Farrell J: Illustrated Guide to Orthopedic Nursing, p 138. Philadelphia, JB Lippincott, 1977; courtesy, Zimmer Co.)

- Positioning and limitations of movement are prescribed specifically for the patient by the surgeon. The goal is to prevent dislocation of the affected hip by maintaining it in a position of abduction (outward from the midline) and avoiding rotation and acute hip flexion. The following tips will usually apply:
  1. Abduction splint or wedge (triangle pillow) is placed between patient's legs (Fig. 5-9). Straps should be applied loosely enough so that there is no pressure over the peroneal nerve (3 inches below knee on outer aspect). Traction or pillows between legs are other ways of maintaining abduction. *(See NR, Traction)*
  2. Use trochanter roll (see Fig. 5-8) to prevent too much external rotation of the femur. Toes should point upward.
  3. Flexion of hip to 90° angle is seldom permitted at first, though raising head of bed to 45° may be allowed.
     a. When sitting is permitted (for brief time at first), seat of chair or wheelchair should be raised with a pillow. Another pillow should be placed between legs. Legs must not be crossed.
     b. Provide an elevated toilet seat.
  4. When placing patient on the bed pan, assist him, have him use the trapeze, and keep his hip in partial flexion. Hyperextension is a common cause of prosthesis dislocation.
  5. To prevent adduction of the operated hip when transferring patient from bed to chair, assist him to exit with the side that was operated on leading. Do not let him pivot toward the surgical side. When returning to bed, the side that was operated on leads.

6. Turning or "tilting" (only about 45°) toward the unoperated side should be done with two people assisting. Use splint or hard pillow to maintain abduction.
7. Exercises as ordered are usually started preoperatively by the physiotherapist, with emphasis on transferring techniques and walking, hip, knee, and ankle exercises.
8. Amount of weight bearing is prescribed individually. Patient should wear well-fitting shoes or slippers with nonskid soles.
9. Lying prone with feet over end of bed several times a day or night (to prevent hip flexor tightness) may be ordered by the surgeon 4 or 5 days postoperatively.

Postoperative Complications

- In addition to signs of general postoperative complications (*see SS, Postoperative care and Postoperative complications*), watch for
  1. Temperature elevation and redness or discharge at the wound site, common indications of infection.
  2. Inability to rotate the hip internally or externally, inability to bear weight, shortening of the affected leg, and increased pain: all symptoms of prosthesis dislocation.

TOTAL KNEE REPLACEMENT
Description

Total knee replacement is indicated when chronic pain and deformity limit joint function, usually as a result of degenerative joint disease (*e.g.*, arthritis). *(See SS, Arthritis)*

Treatment and Nursing Tips

Postoperative: orders vary, but the following would usually apply.
- Knee is immobilized in a nearly extended position with
  1. Light cast, which may be split and further spread p.r.n. to relieve pressure. *(See NR, Cast care)*
  2. Knee immobilizer: made of heavy canvas material, heavy metal stays, and Velcro straps and buckles that may be adjusted. There may be prescribed periods of removal.
- Elevate the knee to reduce swelling by elevating foot of bed. Heart should be below the level of the elevated part. Protect heel from pressure.
- Closed-wound suction (*e.g.*, Hemovac) may collect up to 500 ml drainage in first 24 hours, but it is usually removed after approximately 48 hours or when drainage has ceased.
- Ice bags to be propped against the sides of the knee are frequently ordered.

- Elastic stocking for the uninvolved leg is usually routine.
- Ambulation and exercise as ordered, with quadriceps-setting exercises a priority.

LAMINECTOMY, DISC EXCISION, SPINAL FUSION

Description

Laminectomy, or surgical removal of the lamina (the flattened part on either side of the arch of a vertebra), may be done in any case where exploration of the nerves or spinal cord in indicated, including trauma, suspected tumor, hematoma, or herniated intervertebral disc.

Spinal fusion may be done with laminectomy to stabilize the spine by fusing the spinous processes with a bone graft usually taken from the iliac crest but sometimes from the tibia.

A *ruptured* or *herniated intervetebral disc* is frequently the cause of pressure on either the spinal cord or a spinal nerve, and may be removed.

In the cervical spine, the disc is often removed by anterior approach so that no laminectomy is required.

What to Look for
Preoperative

- Pain, paresthesia, and muscle spasm. Record history so that there is a baseline for postoperative evaluation.
- Function and movement of extremities, bladder, and bowels.

Postoperative

- Following *cervical disc excision,* hoarseness and inability to cough effectively may be the result of recurrent laryngeal nerve damage. Slight hoarseness is normal, but any increase should be reported. Sore throat and difficulty in swallowing are fairly common. Sudden return of pain may mean the spine has become unstable.
- Following *lumbar disc excision,* check vital signs frequently. Check dressing for signs of hemorrhage. Check lower extremities for sensation, movement, color, and temperature. Check for urinary retention, bowel control, or sensation.

Nursing Tips
Cervical Disc Excision With or Without Cervical Laminectomy

- Cool, mist vaporizer is frequently ordered.
- Support patient's head as he gets up. Apply cervical brace or soft collar to support head and neck, if ordered.

Lumbar Laminectomy With or Without Spinal Fusion
Preoperative

- Teach "log rolling" (turning body as a unit), deep breathing *(see NR, Deep breathing techniques),* and muscle-setting exercises.

Postoperative

- Two people turn the patient as a unit (log rolling). Patient's knees should be flexed with pillow between them. Turn sheet may be used.
- Position according to surgeon's orders, usually with a pillow under the head and with slight knee flexion, while patient is on his back. Back must be kept in alignment in all positions.
- Relieve pain and anxiety with analgesics, as ordered. *(See PH, Central nervous system, narcotic analgesics)*
- Early ambulation is usually encouraged. Patient requires assistance in keeping back straight and in rising smoothly. Keep the bed elevated.
- Watch dressing for signs of hemorrhage or leakage of cerebrospinal fluid (more common following spinal fusion). Check any clear drainage for glucose with a Dextrostix. Cerebrospinal fluid contains glucose, normal urine does not. Report apparent leakage of cerebrospinal fluid immediately.
- Lumbar brace is frequently ordered.
- Recovery following spinal fusion takes longer than recovery from laminectomy or disc excision and requires the following additional elements of care:
  1. Monitor vital signs frequently postoperatively.
  2. Closed drainage suction (*e.g.,* Hemovac) is frequently in place. Notify surgeon if drainage exceeds 100 ml every 3 to 4 hours.
  3. Care for the site of graft removal.
  4. Bed rest 2 or 3 days postoperatively is usually ordered. Prolonged sitting should be avoided.

MENISCECTOMY AND LIGAMENTOUS REPAIR OF THE KNEE

Description

The meniscus (a crescent-shaped cartilage) attaches to the top of the tibia and provides for wider weight distribution between the tibia and femur. Its removal or partial removal is done for tears that cause pain, locking (limitation of motion), or persistent swelling, Repair of torn ligaments may or may not accompany meniscectomy.

What to Look for

- Pain and swelling, usually severe at onset, following injury.
- Quadriceps atrophy may develop if condition persists.

Nursing Tips

- Orders concerning amount of flexion and weight bearing vary with the surgery. The following tips usually apply:
  1. Compression dressing usually used. Only elastic wrap should be redone. Any sign of drainage should be reported to the surgeon immediately.
  2. Immobilization splint or cast may be applied. *(See NR, Cast care)*
  3. Elevate limb postoperatively.
  4. Quadriceps strengthening exercises may be ordered. Straight leg raising with weights is often prescribed.
  5. Postoperative pain with exercise is not uncommon.
  6. Watch for complications (*e.g.*, thromboembolism, infection, decreased muscle strength, and recurrent effusions).

OSTEOMYELITIS

Description

Osteomyelitis is an inflammation of the bone, particularly the marrow, often caused by *Staphylococcus aureus*, although other organisms may be involved. The infection may enter the bone directly from an open wound or an adjacent infection, or it may be blood borne.

The infection causes a bone abscess, which results in dead bone tissue called a *sequestrum.* Nearby joints may also become involved. If the disease process continues and fails to respond to antibiotic therapy, it becomes chronic osteomyelitis, in which all involved bone and cartilage must be removed before the infection can be brought under control and healing can take place.

Common Diagnostic Tests

- Elevated WBC almost always present. *(See LAB)*
- Sedimentation rate elevated. *(See LAB)*
- Blood cultures occasionally positive. *(See LAB)*
- Specimens are taken of aspirated material from bone or nearby joint for culture and sensitivity (C and S).
- X-rays may or may not show bone involvement.
- Bone scans reveal marked increase in uptake of radionuclear material.

What to Look for

Acute Osteomyelitis

- Fever and sudden pain in affected bone.
- Swelling and tenderness over bone and painful movement of adjacent joint.
- Later development of swelling over the bone and joint.

Chronic Osteomyelitis

- Persisting or recurring bone abscesses.
- Sudden rises in temperature and new painful areas on bones or joints may indicate extension or formation of secondary abscesses.

Treatment

- Antibiotic therapy: immediate and long term, directed against causative organism. It is usually given IV or IM before bone necrosis has taken place but may also be instilled directly into the wound. *(See PH, Antimicrobials)*
- Sensitivity of organism to antibiotic must be tested periodically.
- In addition, chronic osteomyelitis may require the following treatment:
  1. Sequestrectomy: removal of sequestrum and surrounding new bone (involucrum), sometimes in sufficient amounts to form a saucerlike cavity.
  2. Immobilization to decrease pain and muscle spasm.

Nursing Tips

- Bones and joints require gentle handling. They may be very painful.
- Dressing changes may be frequent. Scrupulous sterile technique is required.
- Wound and skin isolation precautions are often required.

Respiratory System

CHRONIC OBSTRUCTIVE PULMONARY DISEASE

Description

Chronic obstructive pulmonary disease (COPD), or chronic obstructive lung disease (COLD), may result from the following conditions:

- *Chronic bronchitis,* a constant inflammation of the bronchi that produces large amounts of heavy mucous secretions. Permanent dilatation of one or many bronchi is called *bronchiectasis.*
- *Asthma,* a spasm of the bronchi as a result of an allergy, an infection, or emotional upset. The lungs are unable to empty out used air, and thus cannot completely fill with new air. *Status asthmaticus* refers to an asthmatic episode that lasts hours to days and is resistant to therapy.
- *Emphysema,* in which the elasticity of the lungs diminishes and they are no longer able to effectively perform their principal function of exchanging oxygen for carbon dioxide. Ultimately they are destroyed by inflammation and infection. Emphysema is often associated with chronic bronchitis.

Common Diagnostic Tests

- Chest x-ray.
- Arterial blood gases (ABGs). *(See LAB)*
- Pulmonary function tests.
- Lung scan with flow studies. *(See NR, Scans)*

What to Look for

- Nature of respirations: shallow, rapid, and labored. Note whether shoulders, neck, or abdominal muscles are used in breathing, especially when exhaling.
- Color of skin: a very pink skin color indicates oxygen retention. Cyanosis indicates an oxygenation failure.

- Jugular vein distention (JVD): a sign of right-sided heart failure, often associated with respiratory distress.
- Cerebral anoxia demonstrated by restlessness and confusion.
- Clubbing of the fingers is common in some types of long-standing pulmonary disease (*e.g.,* pulmonary fibrosis)
- Cough.
- Chest sounds.
- Symptoms of upper respiratory infection (URI).

Treatment

- Inhalation therapy with the introduction of bronchodilator drugs, *e.g.,* epinephrine and isoproterenol hydrochloride (Isuprel). *(See PH, Respiratory system)*
- Water by mouth, nebulizer, or vaporizer to aid in liquifying mucous secretions.
- Medications, *e.g.,* steroids (prednisone) *(see Endocrine system),* bronchodilators (Aminophylline) *(see PH, Respiratory system),* and antibiotics *(see PH, Antimicrobials).*
- Oxygen: administration must be carefully monitored with blood gases *(see NR, Oxygen administration).* Never give more than 2 liters (per minute) without a physician's order.

Nursing Tips

- The normal stimulus to increase the depth of breathing is an increase in the carbon dioxide (CO_2) level in the blood. Patients with severe COPD become habituated to a high CO_2 level, and their resultant lack of stimulus to breathe produces insufficient oxygen (O_2), called hypoxia. A secondary stimulus then takes over, based on the sensing of hypoxia. If this hypoxia is relieved by giving the patient high concentrations of O_2, the secondary stimulus does not function and the patient may breathe too slowly or even cease to breathe. This results in further buildup of CO_2, which may rapidly lead to coma, called CO_2 narcosis. Thus, either too little or too much oxygen will be harmful, and the flow rate must be carefully monitored.
- At the beginning of each shift, check patients receiving oxygen for correct liter flow. Also, oxygen must pass through humidification. Be sure that the water bottle is kept full. Extension tubing should enable the patient to move about the room without taking the oxygen on and off.
- Sedatives, tranquilizers, hypnotics, and narcotics should be avoided because they suppress respiratory drive and cough reflex and thereby may be fatal.

- Instruct patients in the use of hand nebulizers: teach them to blow out as much air as possible, place the nebulizer in the mouth, inhale slowly, and then exhale through pursed lips. Caution about the overuse of nebulizers, which decreases their effectiveness and may aggravate arrythmias, which are very common with COPD.
- Damaged lungs display a high degree of infection; normal lungs are seldom infected. Antibiotics generally should not be started until after a sputum for culture is obtained and a specific antibiotic is selected *(see LAB)*. It is best to collect a sputum specimen shortly after the patient awakens and coughs it up. It can also be obtained during a respiratory therapy treatment, when the patient may find it easier to produce sputum. Document the volume, consistency, color, and odor of sputum collected during each shift. Do not allow it to collect at the bedside for longer than 24 hours.
- Teach the emphysema patient abdominal breathing by placing one of his hands on his chest and one on the abdomen. In abdominal breathing the abdomen moves while the chest remains immobile.
- Breathing through pursed lips prolongs the time it takes to exhale. This enables the patient to perform the actions requiring the greatest exertion *(e.g.,* sitting up in bed or moving to a chair) while exhaling.
- Milk and milk products thicken mucous secretions and should be avoided.

MOUTH AND NECK
LARYNGECTOMY
Description

Total laryngectomy removes the thyroid cartilage, vocal cords, and epiglottis. This is the surgical treatment for cancer of the larynx. It results in a permanent tracheostomy and a loss of normal speech. The ability to smell is also lost. Occasionally a partial laryngectomy is done when the cancer is limited to one vocal cord. In such a case there is no permanent tracheostomy and the voice, while husky, is recognizable.

Common Diagnostic Tests

- Laryngoscopic examination to visualize the lesion.
- Chest x-ray to rule out metastases.

Nursing Tips
Preoperative

- These patients are facing the loss of their voices and may be extremely depressed. Encourage family and close friends to be with the patient.

- Establish a method of communication (*e.g.*, magic slate or picture cards).
- It is imperative that the physician and nurse confer regarding the planned surgery and the necessary patient education. The equipment that will be in use following surgery needs to be explained (*e.g.*, laryngectomy tube, nasogastric tube, or suctioning).
- Plan to have the patient return after surgery to a room adjacent to the nurse's station.

Postoperative

- Answer call light *immediately,* and check patient every 15 minutes until he is competent in self-care.
- Keep an extra tracheostomy or laryngectomy tube (with its obdurator) taped to the head of the bed. A laryngectomy tube is shorter and wider than a tracheotomy tube, but the care is the same *(see NR, Tracheostomy care)*. Be sure the tube is the proper size. After several weeks the laryngectomy tube may not be needed because the stoma will remain open.
- The skin around the suture line may be very delicate from radiation therapy, so be very gentle in cleaning the area.
- A humidified tracheostomy mask is necessary in the immediate postoperative period. Later a humidifier in the room helps relieve tracheal dryness. *(See NR, Oxygen administration)*
- The possibility of an airway obstruction always exists with these patients. If this occurs, suction the tracheostomy, bag with oxygen, and call the physician. If a tube is in place, remove the inner cannula, clean and replace, and bag to ventilate.
- Small, implanted catheters in the surgical area are attached to Hemovacs or suction machines to remove blood and fluid, lessen edema, and promote healing. Notify the surgeon if they appear to be obstructed. It is very important to chart output and description of drainage each shift. By the third postoperative day there should be less than 50 ml of drainage.
- An n.g. tube may be used *(see NR, Gastrointestinal intubation)*. It is inserted by a physician because of the danger of penetrating a suture line. Remember, after a laryngectomy there is no longer any connection between the mouth and nose and the lungs. The appearance of any food particles in the tracheostomy indicates that a fistula has formed between the esophagus and trachea.
- Suction only as needed; no tracheal suctioning is to be performed without an order. Emphasize the importance of coughing up secretions. Teach the patient how to suction, using sterile technique and sitting in front of a mirror. *(See NR, Tracheostomy care)*
- Spend as much time as possible with the patient. Help with com-

munication by magic slate and picture card. Be certain the call light is always in reach and note pads and pencils are provided.

- Frequently, severe depression occurs after surgery with the full realization of loss of voice. Contact "Lost Chord" group through the American Cancer Society to arrange a visit from a functioning laryngectomee.
- An identification bracelet should be worn noting that the person is a laryngectomee.
- Cardiopulmonary resuscitation (CPR) for a person with a neck stoma involves mouth to stoma resuscitation. There is no need to seal off the mouth and nose.

RADICAL NECK DISSECTION
Description

Radical neck dissection is done for malignancies in the mouth and throat that extend to the lymph nodes and tissue in the neck. It includes removal of lymph nodes, muscle, nerves, and blood vessels, and may include a tracheostomy.

Common Diagnostic Tests

- Laryngoscopic examination, chest x-ray, and thyroid scan to determine any metastases.

Nursing Tips
Preoperative

- The patient and the family need a great deal of emotional support preoperatively. Disfigurement after surgery may be severe. Encourage a family member to be with the patient as much as possible before and after surgery.
- Prepare the patient for the possibility of a tracheostomy. Establish a method of communication (*e.g.*, magic slate or picture cards). Also, discuss the use of suctioning and explain the procedure. Explain that secretions can often be removed by forceful coughing and deep breathing.
- If the use of a nasogastric tube is a possibility, explain its use to the patient and family. *(See NR, Gastrointestinal intubation)*
- Demonstrate arm exercises useful in preventing shoulder drop, which occurs after resection of neck muscles. Have patient go through the exercises.
- Explain that the surgical dressings may be thick and very bulky.

Postoperative

- If the patient returns from surgery with a tracheostomy, be sure an extra tracheostomy tube of the *same size* is included in an emergency tracheostomy set kept *always* at the bedside.

- Do not perform tracheal suctioning without an order. There is a danger of penetrating suture lines.
- Keep humidifier in use after a radical neck dissection to minimize breathing difficulty.
- The possibility of airway obstruction always exists with these patients. If this occurs, suction, bag with oxygen, and call for a physician. If the tracheostomy tube is in place, remove inner cannula (if present), clean and replace, and bag to ventilate.
- Check the dressings hourly for the first 24 hours. Always keep them uncovered by gowns. Carotid artery blowout begins as a small amount of bright red bleeding at the surgical site and massive hemorrhage follows. Call the physician *immediately* when any amount of bright red bleeding is observed. Keep surgical packing material at the bedside.
- Small, implanted catheters in the surgical area are attached to Hemovacs or a suction machine to remove blood and fluid, lessen edema, and promote healing. Notify the physician if they appear to be obstructed. It is very important to chart their output, along with a description of drainage, each shift. By the third postoperative day, there should be less than 50 ml of drainage.
- Mouth care is especially important to eliminate foul taste and odor. Use irrigations, but be careful of surgical incisions. One commonly used solution is one part of hydrogen peroxide to five parts of water. If this is too irritating, increase the water.
- Difficulty in swallowing saliva is a common aftereffect. Patients need many tissues.
- Support the neck when moving the patient.
- An n.g. tube for feeding and hyperalimentation may be used *(see NR, Gastrointestinal intubation and NR, Intravenous therapy)*. Nasogastric insertion must always be done by a physician because of suture line hazards. The n.g. tube may be clamped off in a few days to see if the patient can swallow. An elevated head of bed makes swallowing easier. If a permanent feeding tube is left in place, the patient and family need instruction in its use.
- Initially, support of the arm and shoulder should be done with a sling.
- Arm exercises should be used to prevent shoulder drop, which occurs after resection of neck muscles.
- A carotid artery is often included in the resection. Some lightheadedness occurs until collateral circulation is established. Support and observe the patient carefully when he is getting in and out of bed and ambulating.
- Observe respirations before and after giving narcotics.
- Radiation of the mouth and neck is often done *(see SS, Oncology: nursing tips)*. An extremely dry mouth, sore throat, difficulty swal-

SYSTEMS AND SPECIALTIES

lowing, and a loss of taste may occur. Popsicles are soothing to a sore mouth; sucking citrus candy helps relieve the symptoms of a dry mouth, as does the use of synthetic saliva (*e.g.,* Xero-lube).

- Radiation skin reactions tend to be severe. Patients should wear loose collars to avoid skin friction. The use of an electric razor decreases the chances of cuts, which are prone to infection.
- Teeth should be examined prior to mouth radiation because unhealthy teeth increase the risk of jaw infection. Slow tissue healing follows tooth extraction after radiation.

PNEUMONIA

Description

In pneumonia the alveoli (small chambers) of the lung become inflamed and fill with an exudate. As this process continues, the lung tissue becomes consolidated, and inspired air is unable to contact blood for gas exchange. Pneumonias are generally referred to by their causative agents (*e.g.,* pneumococcal, gram-negative, staphylococcal, and viral). Pneumococcal pneumonias usually follow upper respiratory infections (URI). Staphylococcal and gram-negative pneumonias are frequently complications of other diseases in weak and debilitated patients. Viral pneumonias occur suddenly without any pre-existing condition.

Common Diagnostic Tests

- X-ray of chest.
- Sputum culture. (*See LAB, cultures*)
- Blood culture. (*See LAB, cultures*)
- Arterial blood gases (ABGs). (*See LAB*)

What to Look for

- A high temperature, which may be accompanied by chills.
- Chest pain, which, if severe, may indicate pleurisy.
- Coughing, which may produce thick or greenish yellow sputum.

Treatment

- Antibiotics specific for organisms involved. (*See PH, Antimicrobials*)
- Antitussives, expectorants (*see PH, Respiratory system*), and antipyretics (*see PH, Analgesic antipyretics, anti-inflammatory agents, drugs for gout*).
- Analgesics. (*See PH, Analgesic antipyretics, anti-inflammatory agents, drugs for gout*)
- Isolation, depending on causative agent. (*See NR, Isolation technique*)

- Oxygen, if indicated, and humidification of room. *(See NR, Oxygen administration)*
- Increased fluids, p.o. or IV.

Nursing Tips

- The causative agent needs to be identified before the antibiotics are started. Thus, it is of utmost importance that blood and sputum cultures are obtained as soon as possible.
- Use common sense in the choice of roommate if isolation is not required. It is preferable to have patients with pneumonia in a private room.
- Patients who require suctioning of the upper respiratory tract are especially susceptible to pneumonia. Always use strict sterile technique when suctioning any patient. *(See NR, Nasopharyngeal suctioning)*
- Be alert to possible reactions to antibiotics, and check for fungal infestations after several days of antibiotic use. These appear in the mouth or vagina as patches on the mucosa.
- Bath blankets placed under and above these often diaphoretic patients help absorb moisture.
- Even though it is often painful for these patients to turn and cough, insist that this be done. Mucous plugs can easily form, blocking airways and resulting in atelectasis (lung collapse).

PNEUMOTHORAX

Description

A pneumothorax is a condition in which air enters the pleural space. It may occur as the result of a leak in the lung (spontaneous pneumothorax) or an opening in the chest wall. When air is admitted into the pleural space it tends to collapse the lung or to prevent its full expansion. A tension pneumothorax occurs if the air becomes trapped within the pleural space, causing pressure within the space to exceed atmospheric pressure. A mediastinal shift may then result, in which the heart and other organs within the mediastinum shift toward the opposite side of the chest. This disturbs the normal function of the heart and of the healthy lung.

Common Diagnostic Tests

- Chest x-ray with inspiratory and expiratory films.

What to Look for

- Sudden, sharp chest pain with a lack of chest movement on one side, frequently occurring after severe coughing. This is followed

by anxiety, dyspnea, tachycardia, and possibly a fall in blood pressure.
- Tension pneumothorax and mediastinal shifts are *extreme emergencies* because shock and cardiac failure may occur within minutes.

Treatment
- Thoracentesis. *(See NR, chest tube drainage)*
- Chest tubes. *(See NR, chest tube drainage)*
- Oxygen. *(See NR, Oxygen administration)*
- Analgesics. *(See PH, Analgesic antipyretics, anti-inflammatory agents, drugs for gout)*
- Surgical correction of a leak within the lung.

Nursing Tips
- Because the patient is usually extremely apprehensive, stay with him as much as possible.
- Patients are usually most comfortable with the head of the bed elevated.
- Chest tubes cause pain, and the pain often continues for several days after their removal. Pain relief is imperative.
- Pneumothorax may be a complication of chronic obstructive pulmonary disease. *(See SS, Chronic obstructive pulmonary disease)*

PULMONARY EMBOLISM

Description
Pulmonary embolism is generally the result of a thrombus that originates in the venous system (most often in the deep veins of the legs or pelvis) or in the heart. Part of the thrombus breaks off and becomes an embolus (an embolus called a "fat embolus" may also occur after a long-bone fracture) *(see SS, Fat embolism)*. The embolus moves into the pulmonary circulation, blocking one or more arteries, thus becoming a pulmonary embolism. An infarction with necrosis of lung tissue results because of curtailment of blood supply. If sufficient arterial blood supply to the lungs is obstructed by an embolism, sudden death results.

Common Diagnostic Tests
- Lung scan. *(See NR, Scans)*
- X-ray.
- Arterial blood gases (ABGs). *(See LAB)*
- Prothrombin time (PT) and partial thromboplastin time (PTT). *(See LAB)*

What to Look for

- The intensity of the symptoms indicates the severity of the obstruction.
- Common symptoms are dyspnea, sudden chest pain with increased pain on inspiration, diaphoresis, tachycardia, weakness, cough (perhaps hemoptysis), and mildly elevated temperature.
- A positive Homans' sign (pain in calf of leg when foot is dorsiflexed) may be the first indication of deep-vein thrombosis.
- Large emboli usually begin in veins above the knee.
- Low PO_2 levels on blood gases.

Treatment

- *Immediate treatment is necessary.*
- IV for vein access. *(See NR, Intravenous therapy)*
- Oxygen. *(See NR, Oxygen administration)*
- Analgesics. *(See PH, Central nervous system)*
- Anticoagulants, *e.g.,* heparin and warfarin (Coumadin). *(See PH, Cardiovascular system)*

Nursing Tips

- Prevention should be the first consideration. Hospitalized patients must be assessed daily for any indication of deep-vein thrombosis.
- Pain, inflammation of the lower calf or thigh, and a positive Homans' sign should be reported immediately to the physician.
- Elastic stockings should be used; they should fit well and should extend to just below the knee. They can be removed twice a day for 5 to 10 minutes.
- These patients are usually on anticoagulants for many days. Be aware of any unusual bleeding. Daily PT and PTT are done. Be sure physician is notified of daily results.
- A cough pillow (a firm surface) pressed against the chest helps relieve some of the chest pain that occurs with coughing or other chest movement.

PULMONARY SURGERY

Description

Pulmonary surgery includes exploratory thoracotomy and resection of all or part of a lung. A resection is most frequently performed for removal of cancer, but it may also be necessary following a lung abscess or bronchiectasis.

The following are types of pulmonary surgery: a pneumonectomy is the removal of a lung; a lobectomy is the removal of a lobe; a segmented resection is the removal of one of the lung segments; and a wedge resection is a small, superficial removal of lung tissue.

Common Diagnostic Tests

- Chest x-ray, which includes tomography to check for any lesions.
- Sputum for cytology.
- Pulmonary function tests and blood gas studies. *(See LAB)*
- Bronchoscopy with biopsy. *(See NR, Endoscopic procedures)*

Nursing Tips
Preoperative

- Encourage smokers to stop smoking at least 2 weeks before surgery to help decrease mucus production and increase oxygen saturation of lungs.
- Patients may routinely go to an intensive care unit (ICU) after chest surgery. If this is the case, arrange for an ICU nurse to visit the patient and orient him to ICU procedures and equipment. Assess how receptive a patient is before scheduling the visit or conference.
- Patients and family members should be told about oxygen equipment, possible use of a ventilator, n.g. tubes, IVs, chest tubes, and the frequency of nursing checks of vital signs.
- Demonstrations of turning, coughing, and deep breathing, along with range of motion (ROM) and arm exercises *(see NR, Range of motion exercises)*, should be done several times. Have the patient return the demonstration. Explain that coughing and deep breathing are most effective in a sitting position. Sputum will probably be bloody at first. During the first 24 hours after surgery there will be little rest because of the necessity of maintaining circulatory and respiratory efficiency.
- Patients should be aware that, although pain is to be expected, narcotics will be given to minimize severe discomfort.

Postoperative

- In any postoperative patient, respiratory change is an important indicator of physical status. Restlessness, disorientation, or change in the level of consciousness (LOC) can indicate respiratory distress. Frequent blood gas tests are usually ordered.
- Congestive heart failure and pulmonary edema are possible complications of a pneumonectomy.
- Hemorrhage may first become evident by a drop in blood pressure and tachycardia. Mark with a pencil the drainage on a bandage at the beginning of each shift. Increases will be obvious.

- Chest tubes must be milked each hour. When two tubes are in place the anterior tube removes air, the posterior tube removes serosanguineous fluid. Chest tubes are usually not used after a pneumonectomy. *(See NR, Chest tube drainage)*
- Oxygen therapy after pulmonary surgery is critical because of the possibility of inadequate ventilation. *(See NR, Oxygen administration)*
- Suctioning is important to maintain an open airway if the patient is unable to expectorate mucus. *(See NR, Nasopharyngeal suctioning)*
- Intravenous fluids are given slowly, as little as 10 ml per hour after pulmonary surgery. Be sure an IV pump is used. Fluid overload and cardiac arrythmias can develop. *(See NR, Intravenous therapy)*
- A central venous pressure (CVP) line may be used following pulmonary surgery to monitor cardiac performance and establish infusion rates *(see NR, Central venous pressure)*. However, intra-arterial catheters have replaced CVP lines in many hospitals and this procedure is usually done only in intensive care units.
- Hourly intake and output, including the output of chest drainage, is done for the first 24 hours.
- Positioning orders should be specifically written.
- Turning, coughing, and deep breathing must be done hourly for the first 24 hours. Then the period may be extended to every 2 hours or 4 hours. Note the color of the sputum, which can be an early indication of infection, if it changes from bloody to nonclear mucus.
- When the patient is told to cough and deep breathe, the nurse should splint the chest by placing one hand on the front incision line and the other on the back incision line.
- Passive (with support) exercises involving the arm and shoulder on the affected side should begin as soon as consciousness is regained. These are done every 4 hours, they should be changed gradually to active (independent) exercises. Encourage use of the arm on the affected side by placing the bedside table on that side.
- Pain is usually severe and continues for the first 24 to 48 hours and may continue after the chest tubes are removed. Medicate the patient to keep him comfortable and cooperative when required movements are to be performed. Check the quality of respirations before and after giving narcotics.
- Check the dressings and surrounding tissue every hour for the first 24 hours and then as indicated. Subcutaneous emphysema first becomes apparent as edematous tissue that "crackles" when touched.
- A patient should not lie on the unoperated side following a pneumonectomy. This is because the weight of accumulated fluid in the

empty chest cavity could break through the sutures and flood the remaining lung.

PULMONARY TUBERCULOSIS

Description

Tubercle bacilli most commonly gain access to the lung, and an inflammatory reaction occurs that produces a tubercle (nodule). If the body's resistance is high calcification occurs, and the disease is arrested at this stage. If the disease progresses, purulent material forms within the tubercle, the tubercle eventually breaks down, a cavity forms, and the disease spreads into adjacent tissue.

Common Diagnostic Tests

- Tuberculin intradermal test (PPD intermediate): considered positive if in 48 hours an induration (swollen area) of 10 mm or more appears at the site of test.
- Chest x-ray
- Sputum culture: it often takes 4 to 8 weeks to produce a positive growth of acid-fast bacilli (AFB). *(See LAB, Cultures)*

What to Look for

- Fatigue, weight loss, elevated temperature (late in the day), chronic cough, and hemoptysis. These symptoms usually occur only when the disease is well advanced.

Treatment

- Modern treatment is dominated by drug therapy, rather than extended sanatorium care.
- Principal drugs used are ethambutol (Myambutol), isoniazid (INH), and rifampin. *(See PH, Antimicrobials)*

Nursing Tips

- Today, most patients with tuberculosis are treated as outpatients by their physicians. Those seen in hospitals have advanced disease or are diagnosed while hospitalized for other reasons.
- Respiratory isolation is ordered until the patient's AFB smears are negative, usually after 1 to 2 weeks of therapy. This could be longer in some cases.
- If there is a productive cough, teach the patient to cover his mouth, place used tissue in a disposable bag, and wash his hands afterwards.
- Be prepared to give the patient information about the medication

and review it with him. Emphasize the necessity of taking the medication daily.

- It is important that adequate rest and a good diet be maintained. Ask the dietician to talk to the patient.
- The family needs as much education as the patient. Be sure the family members understand the treatment and have been tested for tuberculosis themselves.

Urinary System and the Prostate

Description

The urinary system consists of the kidneys, the ureters, the bladder, and the urethra. Peristaltic waves propel the urine down the ureters from the kidneys, where urine is formed, to the urinary bladder, which provides temporary storage for it. (Bladder capacity in the normal adult is 250 to 400 ml.) Urine is then expelled through the urethra. Reflux, or backward flow, of urine is abnormal at any stage of its excretion.

- Common disorders of the urinary system are usually the result of obstruction, neoplasms, calculi, or infection or interrelationships among them.
- In glomerulonephritis, the inflammatory process in the glomeruli has an autoimmune basis.
- Absorption of nephrotoxic substances (*e.g.*, gentamicin or the sulfonamides), vascular changes such as those in hypertension, and some systemic diseases (*e.g.*, diabetes, and systemic lupus erythematosus) may damage the kidneys.
- Any marked decrease in circulation of blood to the kidneys may cause renal shutdown.
- Injury to the kidneys and bladder may also be the result of trauma.
- Dialysis, both peritoneal dialysis and hemodialysis, and kidney transplant have revolutionized the treatment of end-stage renal disease in recent years. Because they are done in specialized units or centers, they are not included in this quick reference. The reader is directed to any one of several more complete references, some of which are included in the bibliography at the end of this section.

Nursing Tips

Nursing management of the patient with urinary tract or prostate disorders includes

- Careful assessment.
- Accurate specimen collection.
- Some urine testing.
- Preoperative and postoperative care specific to the patient with genitourinary surgery.
- Special attention to fluid management (particularly urinary drainage), comprehensive nursing care for the patient in renal failure, and awareness of the possibility of drug toxicity because of failing renal function.

CARCINOMA OF THE BLADDER

Description

The incidence of carcinoma of the bladder has increased rapidly in recent years, especially among males over 50 years of age. Some predisposing factors are exposure to carcinogens (*e.g.*, cigarette smoking and aniline dyes) chronic cystitis, bladder papillomas, and schistosomiasis. *(See SS, Oncology)*

Common Diagnostic Tests

- Cystoscopic examination, including bimanual examination of the bladder and biopsy of tumor or bladder wall.
- Intravenous pyelograms (IVP). *(See NR, x-ray preparations)*
- Voiding cystourethrograms (VCUG).
- Urinary cytology: Clean-catch specimen obtained about 3 hours after patient has voided; it must go directly to laboratory.
- Ultrasonic probe. *(See NR, Ultrasound)*
- Computerized axial tomography (CAT scan). *(See NR, Scans)*

What to Look for

- Gross, painless hematuria.
- History of recurring urinary tract infections, with dysuria (pain), burning, and frequency of urination.
- Pain in the back, hips, or legs may be signs of metastasis.
- Generalized symptoms of carcinoma. *(See SS, Oncology)*

Treatment

- Transurethral resection with multiple biopsies and fulguration of early lesions or simple papillomas.

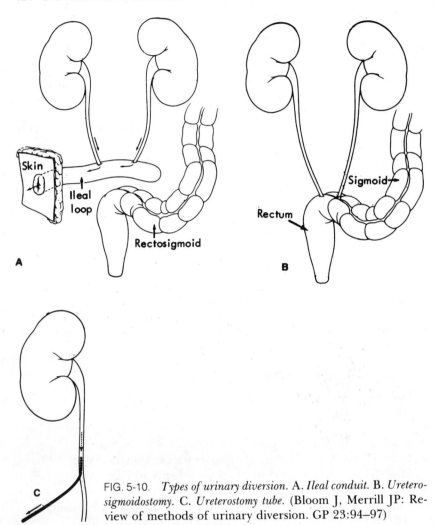

FIG. 5-10. *Types of urinary diversion. A. Ileal conduit. B. Uretero-sigmoidostomy. C. Ureterostomy tube.* (Bloom J, Merrill JP: Review of methods of urinary diversion. GP 23:94–97)

- Cystoscopies with biopsies: repeated every 3 to 6 months for 1 to 2 years to check for recurrence.
- Cystectomy (removal of part or all of the bladder with or without adjacent organs): partial, total, or radical depending upon progress of the disease. Total or radical cystectomy will require urinary diversion.
- Urinary diversion (Fig. 5-10) when required
  1. Cutaneous ureterostomy: ureter(s) brought to abdominal wall.

2. Ileal conduit (ureteroileostomy): ureters are implanted into a loop of ileum, which is brought out to form an ileostomy. The two ends of ileum are anastomosed to reinstate normal continuity. *(See NR, Ostomies, fistulas, and draining wounds and SS, Gastrointestinal surgery)*
3. Ureterosigmoidostomy: ureters are implanted into the sigmoid colon, and urine is allowed to drain it. Urine is expelled with feces through the rectum.

- Radiation: may be complicated by very severe cystitis, rectal fistula, irritation of the rectum with accompanying diarrhea, or bladder spasms. *(See SS, Oncology)*
- Chemotherapy: Thiotepa bladder instillations for superficial low-grade cancers or papillomas. *(See SS, Oncology, Nursing tips for patients on chemotherapy)*

Nursing Tips
For Partial Cystectomy (Segmental Resection)

- Adequate urinary drainage may require cystostomy tube as well as Foley catheter at first.
- Reduced bladder size may require patient to void every 20 to 30 minutes. Bladder capacity will gradually increase.
- Fluids must be forced.
- Provide emotional support.

For Ureterosigmoidostomy

- Preoperative: low-residue diet, bowel prep with enemas and Neomycin. *(See PH, Antimicrobials)*
- Postoperative: watch for complications (*e.g.*, infection, electrolyte imbalance, and acidosis). Try to prevent them.
- Immediately postoperative: sterile rectal tube to drain urine and prevent reflux of urine into ureters.
- Perineal exercises: frequent practice tightening anus and perineum as though to prevent urination or bowel movement.
- Patient should void through the rectum every 2 or 3 hours.
- In addition to the nursing tips offered in *SS, Oncology* for the general care of the patient with radiation therapy the following are usually ordered:
  1. Force fluids.
  2. Low-residue diet.
  3. Stool softeners.
  4. Decrease intestinal motility (*e.g.*, with Lomotil). *(See PH, Gastrointestinal system)*

5. Antispasmodics; they may relieve symptoms. *(See PH, Autonomic nervous system)*
6. Thiotepa bladder instillation
   a. Medication is instilled into the bladder by catheter. This is usually done by physician in the operating room.
   b. Patient must retain the medication for 2 hours, so he may return to the floor with a clamped catheter.
   c. Repositioning patient every 15 minutes helps medication reach all areas of the bladder.
   d. Follow physician's orders regarding the unclamping of the catheter or its removal.

For Ileal Conduit

(See SS, Intestinal surgery and NR, Ostomies, fistulas, and draining wounds)

(See SS, Oncology, nursing care of the patient receiving chemotherapy or radiation)

KIDNEYS

Description

The kidneys, each one made up of approximately one million nephrons, receive about 25% of the blood volume circulated with each contraction of the heart. This means that approximately 1200 ml of blood circulate through the kidneys per minute. Each day approximately 180 liters of filtrate are formed, of which only 1½ liters are normally excreted as urine, the rest being reabsorbed by the tubules. The normal adult urinary output is therefore approximately 1500 ml/24 hr, or 1 ml/min. The kidneys' functions include maintenance of homeostasis (the body's balance of fluids and electrolytes), excretion of the end products of metabolism, regulation of arterial blood pressure through the renin–angiotensin system, and production of erythropoietin (a hormone), which stimulates bone marrow to increase red blood cell production.

Common Diagnostic Tests
Urinalysis
- Glucose, ketones, albumin, bacteria, RBCs, WBCs, and casts are abnormal substances. *(See LAB)*
- Specific gravity and osmolality: to measure concentrating and diluting function of the kidney. *(See LAB)*
- pH
- Twenty-four hour urine collections: to determine volume of urine

excreted, and to measure specific amounts of electrolytes and other substances *(e.g.,* creatinine and protein). *(See LAB)*
- Urine for culture and sensitivity (C and S): obtained by "clean-catch" technique or catheterization. *(See LAB)*

Tests for Kidney Function
- Phenolsulfonphthalein (PSP) excretion tests
  1. PSP is injected IV. It is excreted at the proximal tubules at a rate proportional to renal blood flow.
  2. Urine specimens are collected at specified intervals.
  3. Factors such as incomplete emptying of the bladder, low urine volume, liver disease, and congestive heart failure may interfere with accuracy of test.
- Concentration and dilution tests: see hospital lab manuals for specifics.
  1. Fishberg concentration test: after fluids have been restricted for a specific period of time, urine specimen is collected to test kidneys' ability to concentrate urine.
  2. Addis concentration test: fluids are restricted, and timed urine is analyzed for quantitative RBCs, WBCs, casts, and protein.
  3. Dilution test: fluids are forced up to specified amount in short time span. Timed urine's specific gravity is tested to evaluate urine-concentrating power of kidneys. *Caution:* Prolonged dehydration or forced fluids may be hazardous to azotemic patients (those with elevated nitrogenous waste products—especially urea—in the blood).

Blood
- Blood urea nitrogen (BUN):normal BUN is 8 mg/dl to 18mg/dl. Elevated in renal failure, obstructive uropathy, decreased blood flow to the kidneys, and increased protein catabolism. Not as reliable an index of impaired renal function as serum creatinine. *(See LAB)*
- Serum osmolality. *(See LAB)*
- Serum creatinine: normal serum creatinine is 0.6 mg/dl to 1.2 mg/dl. This is the most reliable index of renal and glomerular function. *(See LAB)*
- Serum electrolytes. *(See LAB)*
- Serum creatinine and creatinine clearance test. *(See LAB)*

X-rays
- Flat plate of the abdomen or kidney, ureter, and bladder (KUB): for discovering location of calculi or abnormalities of renal contour

that suggest tumors, hydronephrosis, and so forth. *(See NR, x-ray preparations)*

- Intravenous pyelogram (IVP) *(see NR, x-ray preparations):* after preparation of the bowel and the use of a laxative or enema to clear the GI tract, patient is given IV dose of radiopaque organic iodide dye. Its excretion in the urine allows visualization of the urinary tract. *Caution:* This procedure is contraindicated for the patient who is allergic to iodine. Question each patient regarding possible sensitivity to iodine before preparation begins.
- Retrograde pyelogram *(see NR, x-ray preparations):* contrast dye is introduced by catheter that has been passed through the urethra, the bladder, and the right or left ureter into a renal pelvis. (This is especially useful in locating site of obstruction.)
- Nephrotomogram: combines techniques of IVP with tomography for more detailed visualization of the kidney at different levels. Useful if small tumors are suspected.
- Renal arteriogram (aortogram or angiogram): to outline renal blood supply.

Radioisotope Studies

- Renogram with radioisotope: to evaluate renal blood flow, renal function, and ability to excrete urine.
- Renal scan *(see NR, Scans)* may show outline of functioning renal tissue and location and shape of kidneys.

Ultrasound

- Ultrasound differentiates cystic disease from renal tumor. *(See NR, Ultrasound)*

Retrograde Renal and Ureteral Brush Biopsy
Renal Biopsy (Closed Percutaneous Needle Biopsy)

(See NR, Renal biopsy)

- Performed with the aid of ultrasound equipment or CAT scanner to position needle.

Computerized Axial Tomography (CAT Scan)

(See NR, Scans)

- Differentiates renal masses or injury.

ACUTE RENAL FAILURE
Description

Classified according to etiology, acute renal failure (ARF) is described as a rapid deterioration in renal function accompanied by azotemia (the buildup of nitrogenous wastes in the blood) and, usually, oliguria (urinary output below 500 ml/24 hr.)

- *Prerenal failure* may be precipitated by hypovolemia caused by cardiovascular failure, shock, hemorrhage, or burns or by any factor outside the kidneys that decreases renal blood flow, and therefore reduces glomerular perfusion.
- *Renal failure* is caused by disorders within the kidney itself (*e.g.*, primary renal diseases such as glomerulonephritis and pyelonephritis), systemic diseases (*e.g.*, diabetes and systemic lupus erythematosus (SLE), or acute tubular necrosis caused by transfusion reactions or the absorption of nephrotoxic substances (e.g., the aminoglycosides—gentamycin, neomycin—and sulfonamides).
- *Postrenal failure* is caused by damage to the kidney from obstruction to the flow of urine as a result of calculi, neoplasms, or prostatic enlargement.

Obstetrical complications, such as separation of the placenta, severe pre-eclampsia, eclampsia, and septic abortion, may also precipitate ARF.

The clinical course of reversible failure is marked by an oliguric phase that may last 1 to 2 weeks following the causative event, followed by a diuretic phase. Gradual recovery may require 3 to 12 months.

Common Diagnostic Tests

- BUN and serum creatinine: elevated. *(See LAB)*
- Blood chemistry and blood gases *(see LAB)*: watch for elevated potassium and decreased sodium. Decreases in *p*H and serum bicarbonate may lead to acidosis.
- Hemoglobin and hematocrit and complete blood count. *(See LAB)*
- Urinalysis: proteinuria, RBCs, WBCs, and casts may be present. Specific gravity usually remains around 1.010. *(See LAB)*
- Diagnostic studies to ascertain cause and degree of renal failure. *(See SS, Kidneys)*

What to Look for

- Urinary output is suddenly markedly decreased, though following burns and trauma output may be up to 2 to 3 liters/day. Period of diuresis may follow oliguric phase.
- Signs of fluid retention—sacral, periorbital or peripheral edema—and signs of congestive heart failure (*e.g.*, moist rales and distended neck veins). *(See SS, Congestive heart failure)*
- Pallor, suggesting anemia.

- Signs and symptoms of acidosis, hyperkalemia, and hyponatremia. *(See NR, Intravenous therapy, electrolyte imbalances)*
- Signs and symptoms of uremia: acidosis, uremic frost on the skin with accompanying pruritus, headaches, visual disturbances, and nausea and vomiting.

Treatment

- Goal is to maintain good fluid and electrolyte balance until renal cells can recover.
- Fluid intake to replace current daily loss (measured output plus 500 ml/day allowance for insensible loss).
- Low- or nonprotein, high-calorie, restricted potassium, high-carbohydrate diet. (Hard candy and butterballs are often provided.)
- Intravenous glucose, especially if nausea and vomiting are present.
- Correction of electrolyte imbalances
  1. Sodium polystyrene sulfonate (Kayexalate), a resin exchange is mixed with water or sorbitol and given p.o., by nasogastric tube, or rectally to treat hyperkalemia.
  2. IV glucose and insulin or calcium gluconate: temporary treatment for hyperkalemia. *(See PH, Endocrine system)*
  3. IV sodium bicarbonate: to correct acidosis and to lower serum potassium.
  4. Aluminum hydroxide: to bind phosphate. *(See PH, Gastrointestinal system)*
- Prevent or control infection with good hand washing technique and antibiotics, if indicated.
- Dialysis: peritoneal dialysis or hemodialysis, if indicated.

Nursing Tips

- Manage fluid and electrolyte balance.
- Monitor fluid intake and output carefully.
  1. Indwelling catheter with urometer may be needed to measure hourly urinary output. Frequent tests for specific gravity will be ordered.
  2. Fluctuations in body weight are probably the most accurate index of fluid retention: 1 lb = 500 ml; 1 kg (2.2 lb) = 1000 ml.
  3. During the oliguric stage a 0.2 kg to 0.5 kg ($\frac{1}{2}$ lb to 1 lb) daily loss is expected.
  4. Obtain patient's cooperation in meeting severe fluid restrictions. One method is for nursing staff to assume responsibility for offering all fluids; no fluids are to come on tray. Daily allowance is divided. Even sips of water taken with oral medications must be counted.

- Monitor for physical signs and laboratory results that might indicate fluid overload, acidosis, hyperkalemia, or hyponatremia. *(See NR, Intravenous therapy, electrolyte imbalances)*
- Fluid imbalances are particularly dangerous in the diuretic phase.
- Good supportive care.
  1. Oral hygiene, pulmonary hygiene (turn, cough, and deep breathe), decubitus prevention *(see MNS, Decubitus ulcer prevention and treatment)*, and excellent skin care.
  2. Relieve the itching of uremic dermatitis with dilute vinegar baths (2 tablespoons vinegar to 1 pint of water), antipruritic lotions, and antihistamines. Trim finger nails to prevent scratching.
  3. Protect patient from injury: may require padded side rails and tongue blade. *(See SS, Seizures)*
- Safe drug administration: drug toxicity is more likely with decreased renal function. Dosages must be adjusted.
- Awareness and prevention, where possible, of complications, such as cardiac failure and arrhythmias, convulsions, hemorrhage, and infection. Reverse isolation may be required.
- Emotional support and reassurance.

CHRONIC RENAL FAILURE
Description

Chronic renal failure is the end stage of irreversible renal disease, which over an extended period of time progresses from renal insufficiency to uremia. The changes seen in uremia affect all systems of the body and are caused by retention of the end products of metabolism, and disturbances in fluid, electrolyte and acid–base balances.

Common Diagnostic Tests

- BUN, serum creatinine: elevated. *(See LAB)*
- Hemoglobin and hematocrit. *(See LAB)*
- Serum electrolytes: elevated potassium and decreased calcium and sodium are common. *(See LAB)*
- Arterial blood gases (ABGs).
- Urinalysis and tests for renal function. *(See SS, kidneys, common diagnostic tests)*

What to Look for

- Anemia, a classic symptom; pallor, weakness.
- Hypertension.
- Edema or dehydration, depending upon status of renal function.

- Symptoms of acidosis: hyperventilation, headache, lethargy, drowsiness, stupor, and coma.
- Volume and character of urinary output may vary with progress of the disease.
- Cardiac problems.
  1. Chest pain and pericardial friction rub, indicating pericarditis.
  2. Congestive heart failure, (rales and distended neck veins). *(See SS, Congestive heart failure)*
- Electrolyte imbalances, particularly hyperkalemia. *(See LAB, and NR, Intravenous therapy, electrolytes imbalances)*.
- Anorexia, weight loss, mucosal ulcerations of the mouth, stomatitis, urine odor to breath, nausea and vomiting, diarrhea, and evidence of GI bleeding, further contributing to anemia and dehydration.
- Pruritus (itching), area of ecchymosis, excoriations, uremic frost.
- Neurological manifestations *(e.g.,* headache, lethargy, confusion, convulsions, muscle weakness or irritability, and paresthesia).
- Amenorrhea, infertility, sexual dysfunction.
- Signs of hyperparathyroidism or other thyroid abnormalities. *(See SS, thyroid)*
- Signs of infection due to decreased resistance.

Treatment

- Goal of conservative management is to preserve existing renal function; to treat symptoms of uremia; to maintain acid–base, fluid, and electrolyte balances; to prevent complications; and to provide maximal psychological and physical comfort.
- Diet: low in protein, low in potassium, and high in carbohydrates.
- Fluids replaced: 500 ml more than 24-hour output. 500 ml represents insensible loss (through respiration, perspiration, or stools).
- Aluminum hydroxide antacids to bind phosphorus in GI tract. *(See PH, Gastrointestinal system)*
- Management of hypertension with medications, *e.g.,* methyldopa (Aldomet) and propranolol (Inderal). *(See PH, Cardiovascular system)*
- Diuretics may be ordered.
- Diazepam (Valium) and phenytoin (Dilantin) may be given IV to control seizures.
- Oxygen therapy may be required. *(See NR, Oxygen administration)*
- Iron and folic acid supplements may be ordered *(see PH, Cardiovascular)*. Antiemetics may be required to relieve nausea and vomiting.
- Androgen therapy may stimulate RBC production.
- Dialysis, with efforts to minimize blood loss during treatments.
- Kidney transplant in selected patients.

Nursing Tips

- See those for nursing the patient in acute renal failure. *(See SS, Acute Renal Failure)*

GLOMERULONEPHRITIS
Description

Acute glomerulonephritis refers to a diffuse, inflammatory process in the glomeruli caused by an antigen–antibody reaction to an infection (usually streptococcus) elsewhere in the body or to changes in the glomeruli caused by disease, such as systemic lupus erythematosus. Most often seen in children or young adult males, 80% recover within about 2 weeks, but a few go into latent or chronic glomerulonephritis.

The disease is considered chronic when symptoms extend beyond a year, though this may develop without the patient having exhibited symptoms of the acute phase. *Chronic glomerulonephritis* is characterized by periods of exacerbations and remissions with progressive decline in renal function.

ACUTE GLOMERULONEPHRITIS
Common Diagnostic Tests

- Antibody titer against causal organism is usually elevated.
- Urinalysis: shows presence of protein, RBCs, and RBC casts. *(See LAB)*
- BUN and serum creatinine: elevated. *(See LAB)*
- Complete blood count and hemoglobin and hematocrit may show presence of anemia. *(See LAB)*
- Kidney function tests may show decreased renal ability to concentrate urine. *(See SS, Kidneys, common diagnostic tests)*

What to Look for

- Usually a history of sudden onset of symptoms occurring about 10 to 12 days following a streptococcal infection (*e.g.,* strep throat, scarlet fever, impetigo), exposure to hydrocarbons, or evidence of systemic lupus erythematosus (SLE).
- Urine scanty; may appear red, brown, or smokey.
- Hypertension (course of the disease may be followed by monitoring blood pressure).
- Edema: periorbital (around the eyes), but particularly peripheral. Retinal edema causes decreased visual acuity.
- Headaches, malaise, and nausea and vomiting.

Treatment

- Bed rest until urinary symptoms have subsided.
- Penicillin and other broad-spectrum antibiotics may be ordered. *(See PH, Antimicrobials)*

- Antihypertensive medications may be ordered. *(See PH, Cardiovascular system)*
- Diet: high in carbohydrates, low in sodium. Protein is usually restricted.
- Fluid restriction if edema is present.
- Treatment for renal failure, if indicated. *(See SS, Acute renal failure)*

Nursing Tips

- Monitor blood pressure carefully.
- Monitor intake and output carefully. Note color of urine.
- Daily weights should be taken in the same clothing, before breakfast each day.
- Assess for complications, such as congestive heart failure, convulsions, and renal failure.
- Try to prevent infections, especially upper respiratory ones.
- Elevate the head of the bed to minimize facial edema.
- Provide good skin care, especially important for the edematous patient.

CHRONIC GLOMERULONEPHRITIS

Common Diagnostic Tests

- Urinalysis: reveals proteinuria. Hematuria and RBC casts are also frequently seen. *(See LAB)*
- BUN and serum creatinine: elevated if renal function is markedly impaired. *(See LAB)*
- Renal biopsy for differential diagnosis. *(See NR, Renal biopsy)*
- Renal function tests. *(See SS, Kidneys, Common diagnostic tests)*

What to Look for

- Hypertension.
- Edema.
- Easy fatigue, weakness, and lassitude (signs of anemia).
- Visual disturbances caused by retinopathy.
- Nocturia: evidence of kidneys' decreased concentrating ability.
- Symptoms of complications or progression of renal impairment: cardiac failure, uremia, and convulsions. *(See SS, Acute renal failure; chronic renal failure)*

Treatment

(See treatment for acute glomerulonephritis)
- Patient is usually advised that pregnancy should be avoided.

Nursing Tips
- Provide the same general, supportive care as that for acute glomerulonephritis and renal failure, if indicated.
- Educate patient and family as to importance of following prescribed regimen. Emotional support is required for dealing with long-term illness.

POLYCYSTIC KIDNEY
Description

The development of a polycystic kidney is an inherited disorder that usually affects both kidneys, in which multiple, enlarging cysts gradually destroy functioning renal tissue by pressure.

What to Look for
- Usually the adult patient presents with hematuria, mild hypertension, flank pain, and recurring infection leading to uremia.

Common Diagnostic Tests
- X-ray, sonography, and scans.

Treatment
- Treatment is symptomatic and similar to that of any kidney insufficiency (*e.g.,* chronic glomerulonephritis or chronic renal failure).
- These patients are sometimes candidates for dialysis and renal transplant.

TRAUMA OF THE KIDNEYS AND BLADDER
Description

Trauma to the lower thorax or upper abdomen may cause injury to the kidneys. When the pelvis is fractured, damage to the bladder or urethra may occur. Hematuria, a common sign of injury to the kidney, frequently subsides spontaneously.

Common Diagnostic Tests
- Gross and microscopic examination of the urine for blood.
- Intravenous pyelogram (IVP).
- Renal arteriogram.
- Cystogram or cystourethrogram to rule out injury to bladder or urethra.
- Establishment of function in uninjured kidney is a vital part of evaluation.

What to Look for

- Blood in the urine.
- Signs of shock (*e.g.,* falling blood pressure; rapid, weak pulse; rapid breathing; cold, moist, pale skin). *(See SS, Postoperative care)*
- Signs of hemorrhage (*e.g.,* restlessness, thirst, rapid pulse, falling blood pressure, and cool, moist, pale skin). *(See SS, Postoperative care)*
- Inability to void may indicate renal shutdown, rupture, or obstruction of the urinary tract. Oliguria or anuria usually occurs when the bladder or urethra is damaged.

Treatment

- Bed rest.
- Treat shock and hemorrhage, if present.
- Surgical repair of the kidney may be attempted after shock is under control, and diagnostic studies are completed. (Whenever possible the injured kidney is preserved.)
- Surgical repair of a traumatized bladder or urethra is performed as promptly as possible. A cystostomy tube may be introduced.

Nursing Tips

- Provide bed rest.
- Monitor for signs of shock and hemorrhage, and provide treatment as indicated. *(See SS, Postoperative care)*
- Collect a specimen from each voiding (racking the urine) for gross inspection or microscopic examination for blood.
  (See SS, Postoperative care following renal surgery)
  (See NR, Urinary bladder catheterization and drainage)

TUMORS OF THE KIDNEY

Description

Most tumors of the kidneys are malignant. They are most often unilateral, encapsulated, solitary, and, frequently, silent. They tend to metastasize rapidly. Only a small percentage of patients with renal cancer have all three of the classic signs—hematuria, pain, and palpable mass.

Common Diagnostic Tests

- X-ray (intravenous pyelography, retrograde pyelography), ultrasound, nephrotomography, and renal angiography.
- Urinary cytology.
- Polycythemia (increased RBCs) may be seen in routine lab studies.

What to Look for

- Hematuria, usually painless and intermittent.
- Back pain, a palpable mass, low-grade fever, and mild hypertension.

Treatment

- Radical nephrectomy.
- Chemotherapy.
- Preoperative infarction. *(See SS, Preoperative infarction of renal tumors)*
- Postoperative irradiation.

Nursing Tips

(See SS, Postoperative care following renal surgery and SS, Oncology)

PREOPERATIVE INFARCTION OF RENAL TUMORS

Description

Preoperative infarction of renal tumors is achieved by renal artery catheterization and occlusion of the renal artery supplying the tumor area. This technique is believed to encourage the development of the patient's own immune response and to limit the spread of tumor cells at the time of nephrectomy, which is usually scheduled a few days later. It may also be done as a palliative treatment for the patient with advanced cancer.

What to Look for

- Following this procedure, patients usually feel very ill.
- Symptoms include severe pain and high temperature elevations, nausea and vomiting.

Nursing Tips

- Elevated white blood count is frequently seen.
- Nursing care is supportive.

OBSTRUCTION OF THE URINARY TRACT

Description

Obstruction to the flow of urine anywhere from the kidneys to the external urethral meatus, if uncorrected, will lead to increased intraluminal pressure, urinary stasis, infection, and eventual renal failure.
- The effects of obstruction depend upon its location in the urinary tract (the closer to the kidney, the more serious), the amount of occulsion, and the length of time it continues.

- *Hydroureter* (dilatation of the ureter), *hydronephrosis* (dilatation of the renal pelvis beyond its normal capacity with eventual damage to functioning part of the kidney), and *diverticula of the bladder* are the result of obstruction over a period of time.
- Common causes of obstruction include neoplasms, urethral strictures, ureteral strictures of spasms, enlargement of the prostate (benign or malignant), and urinary stones.
- The goal of treatment is to relieve the obstruction, usually surgically.

PROSTATIC ENLARGEMENT

Description

Prostatic enlargement, whether benign prostatic hyperplasia (BPH) or malignant, is the most common cause of bladder-neck obstruction in older males. The symptoms caused by this obstruction are called prostatism. Carcinoma of the prostate frequently accompanies BPH but is not believed to be responsible for it. A differential diagnosis is essential. Since symptoms of carcinoma usually appear late, yearly rectal examinations (done by the same examiner) of men over forty are the best method of early detection.

Common Diagnostic Tests

- Rectal examination.
  1. Enlarged prostate with rubbery consistency indicates BPH.
  2. Enlarged, hard, and nodular prostate usually indicates carcinoma.
- Intravenous pyelograms. *(See NR, x-ray preparations)*
- Excretory urogram.
- BUN and serum creatinine. *(See LAB)*
- Serum acid phosphatase is usually elevated in prostatic carcinoma. *(See LAB)*
- Serum alkaline phosphatase is elevated in bone metastasis. *(See LAB)*
- Bone scan and x-ray of bones for confirmation of metastasis. *(See NR, Scans)*
- Catheterization for residual urine, urinalysis, and culture.
- Cystoscopy.
- Biopsy, either by needle or by surgical incision.

What to Look For

- History of slowing of the urinary stream, hesitancy, intermittency, frequency, nocturia, and dribbling.
- Complete urinary retention may occur.

- Hematuria and signs of urinary tract infection may be present if condition is long standing. *(See SS, Urinary tract infections)*
- Low back pain or pains in hips or legs may signal metastasis to the bones in prostatic carcinoma.

Treatment

- Relief of urinary obstruction: a Coudé catheter is frequently used (it is a little stiffer, and the curved tip rides over obstruction).
- Transurethral resection of the prostate (TURP): used for smaller benign tumors. A resectoscope is used through the urethra to trim away the prostate. Prostatic fossa fills in with epithelial tissue to form a new urethra.
- Enucleation of the prostate gland. Bilateral vasectomy may be done at the same time to decrease incidence of epididymitis and orchitis postoperatively.
  1. Suprapubic prostatectomy: enucleation of the prostate through the bladder (lower abdominal incision—not done for carcinoma).
  2. Retropubic prostatectomy: enucleation of the prostate is achieved by making a lower abdominal incision with the bladder pulled forward, and than an incision into the anterior prostatic fossa.
  3. Perineal prostatectomy: approach is made through the perineum with care to avoid entering the rectum. (This procedure usually causes impotence; about 5% of perineal prostatectomies result in incontinence.)
- Radical resection of the prostate either by perineal or retropubic route is done for carcinoma. This includes removal of entire prostate gland, including capsule, seminal vesicles, and adjacent tissue. The urethra is resected and reanastomosed. It may be followed by bilateral orchiectomy. If done before metastasis, prognosis is excellent, but carcinoma of the prostate can metastasize rapidly with few local symptoms. Impotence is almost 100% in radical retropubic and perineal prostatectomy. Urinary incontinence is also fairly common in both.
- In addition to radical resection, the following methods of treatment are used for carcinoma of the prostate:
  1. Radiation preoperatively and postoperatively (external or interstitial). *(See SS, Oncology)*
  2. Chemotherapy, including hormonal therapy. *(See SS, Oncology)*
  3. Levodopa for relief of severe pain.
  4. Symptomatic treatment: may include transurethral resection to relieve obstructive symptoms.

Nursing Tips

- Decompression of a distended bladder must be done slowly.
  1. Remove 300 ml of urine; clamp catheter; after 15 minutes release another 300 ml; continue in this manner. Remove only 300 ml of urine at one time. Ordinarily one *never* clamps a catheter.
- If patient is to have vasectomy with prostatectomy be sure surgeon has explained reasons as well as consequences to him before informed consent is signed.
- Hemorrhage is a potential complication in all prostatic surgery. Check vital signs, urinary drainage, and dressings every 20 minutes immediately postoperatively. Following TURP, urine is usually reddish pink to light pink within twenty-four hours. Deepening color may indicate renewed bleeding. Patients who have undergone TURP may have delayed bleeding 7 to 14 days postoperatively.
- Catheters must be kept clear and should be large enough (#22, #24, #26) to allow for passage of blood clots.
  1. Check for patency every 20 minutes.
  2. Check the bladder for distention.
  3. If ordered, irrigate p.r.n. by introducing 30 ml of sterile normal saline at room temperature with a Toomey or bulb (Asepto) syringe and aspirating gently. Bladder must be kept clear of clots. Irrigation is a sterile procedure.
  4. Continuous irrigation through a "Y" tube or a three-way catheter, or sometimes with irrigant flowing into a suprapubic catheter and out a urethral one, requires checking for patency of the catheter, character of the drainage, and distention of the bladder. To calculate urinary output, subtract amount of irrigant that has gone in from amount in drainage bag.
  5. Clots may be too large to be dislodged by irrigant alone. If manual irrigation is required, first stop the three-way irrigation, irrigate manually using sterile technique, and then restart the three-way irrigation.
  6. Traction may be applied by the surgeon by the use of applied pressure to the Foley catheter. The catheter is pulled taut and taped to patients thigh. Its 30-ml. balloon fits into the prostatic fossa and may control hemorrhage following TURP. Traction is usually released on the surgeon's order after 4 or 5 hours because of potential danger to internal sphincter.
  7. Catheters are usually removed in about 4 to 7 days following TURP, in up to 2 weeks following perineal surgery.
- Bladder spasms are sudden, sharp, brief pains accompanied by the

feeling of the need to move the bowels and urinate at the same time. Traction on catheter may aggravate them. They are relieved when catheter is out. Anticholinergic drugs, *e.g.,* propantheline bromide (Pro-Banthine), and analgesics may be prescribed.

- Bloody drainage from the meatus (around catheter), usually caused by spasms, is commonly seen. Dressings in open prostatectomies are frequently saturated, so change them frequently. Keep wounds clean. Use Montgomery straps (see Fig. 5-3)
- A suprapubic cystostomy tube (frequently a Malecot catheter) may be in place for decompression of the bladder. There may be urinary drainage around tube. Excessive amounts may indicate clogged Foley. Skin must be protected.
- Tissue drains near incision must not be dislodged.
- A perineal wound must be kept clean. Heat lamp, Sitz baths, and irrigations with $\frac{1}{2}$ hydrogen peroxide and $\frac{1}{2}$ water may be ordered. Nothing should be introduced into the rectum (no enemas, rectal tubes, suppositories).
- Keep stools soft. Avoid straining, which could cause hemorrhage.
- Radical resection of prostate will in addition require
  1. Preoperative bowel prep: enemas and neomycin sulfate.
  2. Postoperative (after perineal prostatectomy): low-residue diet, medication to slow bowel motility, and a urethral catheter secured with tape or suture that also acts as a splint for urethral anastomosis.
- After removal of catheter, temporary voiding problems are common (especially after TURP). Observe voiding patterns and measure intake and output. Note frequency and character of urine. Fluids may be forced up to 2500 ml to 3000 ml per day. Diuretics may be ordered. *(See PH, Urinary system)*
- Watch for renewed bleeding, especially following TURP.
- Perineal exercises may correct incontinence.
  1. Patient contracts abdominal, gluteal, and perineal muscles as though trying not to void.
  2. Patient practices starting and stopping the urinary stream.
- Sexual activity may be resumed on advice of the surgeon.
- For the patient with carcinoma of the prostate who is receiving radiation or chemotherapy, see *SS, Oncology, Nursing care of patients receiving chemotherapy or radiation.*

URETHROTOMY
Description

Urethral strictures, one of the most common causes of urinary tract obstruction, have traditionally been treated by dilatation with sounds. Increasingly, though, internal urethrotomy (incision of the stricture) is becoming the treatment of choice.

Nursing Tips

- The patient will usually return to the floor from the operating room with a catheter in place and some sort of compression dressing (*e.g.*, vaginal packing for the female, an external penile compression dressing for the male patient).
- After the catheter is removed (usually after 24 hours), observe for bleeding and the reestablishment of normal voiding patterns.

URINARY CALCULUS
Description

Urinary calculi (stones) may be found in the kidney pelvis, the ureters, and the bladder. Stasis of urine, especially when infection is present, predisposes to stone formation.

- Metabolic disorders (*e.g.*, hyperparathyroidism and gout), immobility, extended presence of an indwelling catheter, excessive intake of milk and vitamin D, deficiency of vitamin A, and familial tendencies may all be factors.
- Abnormal pH of the urine is associated with different types of stones, and prophylaxis may center around altering it through diet and medication.
- Straining urine and retrieving the stones for chemical analysis is essential. About 90% of calculi contain calcium in combination with phosphate or oxalate and are radiopaque. Some stones cannot be visualized by x-ray.
- Ninety per cent of stones pass spontaneously in a period of days to weeks, but if a calculi lodges in a ureter, causing complete obstruction, it can lead to severe hydronephrosis and constitutes a surgical emergency. Calculi 1 cm or less usually pass spontaneously.

Common Diagnostic Tests

- X-ray; intravenous urography; retrograde pyelography. (*See NR, x-ray preparations*)
- Urinalysis: high specific gravity, abnormal pH, RBCs indicative of injury caused by passage of stones, WBCs indicative of infection. (*See LAB*)
  1. Twenty-four hour specimen may show high levels of calcium, uric acid, oxalate, phosphorous, or cystine.
  2. Urine for culture and sensitivity. (*See LAB*)

- Blood chemistry and electrolytes: variations from normal. *(See LAB)*
- Examination of the stone for chemical composition.
- Appropriate tests to try to find underlying cause of stone formation.

What to Look for

- Excruciating intermittent flank pain, which may radiate to groin, testes, or labia; may be accompanied by nausea, chills, and fever.
- Gross or microscopic hematuria.
- Evidence of chronic urinary tract infection. *(See SS, Urinary tract infections)*

Treatment
Medical

- Force fluids: up to 3 liters (3000 ml) daily.
- Ambulation is usually encouraged in an effort to move the stone.
- Analgesics for the relief of renal colic (pain). *(See PH, Central nervous system)*
- Hot baths may be helpful. Watch for feelings of faintness.
- Antibiotics, if there is evidence of infection. *(See PH, Antimicrobials)*
- Attempt to determine cause of stone formation.
- Recover and analyze composition of the stone.

Prophylactic

- High fluid intake.
- Diet should be modified to reduce intake of component of stone. Medication and diet are modified to acidify or alkalinize urine, as indicated.
- Ascorbic acid to acidify urine. Some studies have shown that the amounts of cranberry juice needed to acidify urine are too great to be practical.
- Sodium bicarbonate to alkalinize urine.
- Allopurinol (Zyloprim) to reduce uric acid excretion in the patient with uric acid stones. *(See PH, Analgesic antipyretics, anti-inflammatory agents, drugs for gout)*
- Orthophosphates *e.g.*, potassium acid phosphate (K-phos) to reduce calcium absorption from gastrointestinal tract and to lower pH of the urine, thus increasing calcium solubility.
- Aluminum hydroxide to bind with phosphorus, to increase fecal phosphate excretion in the patient who develops phosphorus stones. *(See PH, Gastrointestinal system)*

Surgical

- Surgical removal of an obstructive stone with as little trauma as possible.
  1. *Nephrolithotomy:* incision into kidney for removal of stone.
  2. *Pyelolithotomy:* removal of stones in kidney pelvis.
  3. *Ureterolithotomy:* removal of stone from ureter.
  4. *Nephrectomy:* removal of kidney, performed only if the kidney is functionless and the other kidney is functional.
  5. *Cystolithotomy:* removal of stone from bladder by incision through the abdomen.
  6. Crushing the stone by means of instrument introduced through the urethra into the bladder.

Nursing Tips

(See SS, Postoperative care)

- All urine should be strained through a strainer or fine gauze, and stones should be saved for chemical analysis. Stones vary in size (may be as small as a pin head), so rinse out the urinal or bedpan carefully, straining the water to be sure you have found stones that may have adhered to the sides. If patient is discharged before stone is passed, he will need to be taught how to do this.
- Analgesics for the relief of pain. *(See PH, Central nervous system)*
- Postoperative care specific to urinary tract surgery. *(See SS, Postoperative care following renal surgery)*
- Patient education is the key to preventing recurrence.
  1. Patient may be taught to test his urine *p*H with phenaphthazine (Nitrazine paper) daily, if ordered.
  2. Diet modification is essential—a visit from the dietician is a must.

POSTOPERATIVE CARE FOLLOWING RENAL SURGERY

Nursing Tips

In addition to considerations of postoperative care in general, *(See SS, Postoperative care)* the following are special considerations in the management of these patients.

- Hemorrhage is the greatest danger following renal surgery. Carefully monitor vital signs immediately postoperatively. Check dressings, catheters, and tubes for signs of bleeding.
- High abdominal incision in renal surgery (sometimes with entrance into the chest cavity) increases the danger of pulmonary complications. Prevent them by planning administration of an analgesic

15 minutes before encouraging patient to deep breathe and cough while splinting wound *(see NR, Deep breathing techniques)*. The patient may have chest tubes. *(See NR, Chest tube drainage)*.

- Paralytic ileus is another common complication. *(See SS, Paralytic ileus)*
- Relieve pain with analgesics and relieve discomfort caused by position during renal surgery with moist heat, massage, and analgesics.
- Accurate measurement of intake and output is essential. Always check and mark the level of drainage at the beginning of each shift.
- In cases of acute obstruction, the surgeon, in order to ensure adequate urinary drainage until corrective surgery can be done, may place temporary tubes above the obstruction, (*e.g.,* a nephrostomy tube—opening into the kidney—or a pyelostomy tube—opening into the renal pelvis. These tubes are always attached to closed gravity drainage.
- Management of catheters and tubes. *(See also NR, Urinary bladder catheterization and drainage)*

   1. They are connected to closed drainage systems.
   2. Check for patency of tube every hour by observing urine in the tube and the amount collecting in the drainage bag. Mark the time on the bag with tape or magic marker so that you can make an accurate comparison. Use a urometer for more accurate measurement. Notify surgeon if less than 50 ml collects in 1 hour.
   3. Observe and note color of urinary drainage. It is usually bloody the first days following renal surgery, except after nephrectomy, when there should be no blood.
   4. *Never* clamp *any* urinary drainage tube, unless there is a specific order.
   5. A *nephrostomy tube* (by percutaneous or surgical placement) must be kept patent and can usually be unclogged by periodically "milking" it by rolling it between the fingers. *Caution:* never clamp a nephrostomy tube.
      a. Must be handled with greatest care so that it is not dislodged.
      b. Sterile occlusive dressing around the tube: antiseptic ointment (*e.g.,* Betadine ointment).
      c. Never irrigate without a physician's order. If ordered, always aspirate before irrigating, and never introduce more than 5 ml to 8 ml of sterile saline (the capacity of the kidney pelvis).
      d. Position patient carefully so that tube is not kinked or obstructed.

6. *Ureteral catheters* usually exit from the urethra with a Foley. Catheters to either kidney should be appropriately marked "right" or "left" with tape. Separate drainage collection with urometer may be requested. Careful monitoring of amount of drainage is essential to confirm patency. The urologist will irrigate the ureteral catheter, if indicated.

- Management of drainage.
  1. Copious amounts of drainage from drains placed in the operative area (pink at first, then becoming serous) immediately postoperatively require frequent sterile dressing changes. Check under the patient for drainage. Montgomery straps are useful (see Fig. 5-3).
  2. Whenever there is surgical entry into the urinary tract, especially the ureters, the incision is never water tight, since tightening it too much could cause a stricture; therefore there is some urine drainage from the Penrose (which is irritating to the skin).
  3. If drainage is particularly heavy, a disposable colostomy pouch placed over the drain will collect it and protect the skin. Remember that karaya rings are not practical because urine dissolves them, though karaya powder may be used on irritated skin. *(See NR, Ostomies, fistulas, and draining wounds)*
  4. The drain will be gradually withdrawn by the surgeon. Drainage following ureterolithotomy or pyelolithotomy may last several days. Patient may be discharged with ostomy pouch.
  5. *(For care of urostomy or ileal conduit, see NR, Ostomies, fistulas, and draining wounds)*
- Fluid intake (usually intravenous) the first days after surgery is high enough to ensure adequate flushing of kidneys. In most cases, oral fluid intake is encouraged thereafter (except in the case of repair of the kidney pelvis, where it may be restricted).

URETHROPEXY (MARSHALL–MARCHETTI)

Description

Urethropexy provides for lengthening of the urethra, reestablishment of the normal urethral–vesical angle, and placement of periurethral sutures in the periosteum of the pubic bone. Though others have made modifications, this operation, which treats stress incontinence in women, was originally devised by Drs. Marshall and Marchetti and usually bears their names.

Nursing Tips

- When the patient returns from surgery, bed rest may be ordered.
- A catheter may be in place from 5 to 7 days.

- After the catheter is removed, observe for urinary frequency and the establishment of normal voiding patterns.

URINARY TRACT INFECTIONS

Description

Most urinary tract infections (UTI) ascend from the urethra. They are more common in females than in males. Some kidney infections are believed to be blood or lymphatic born.

Bacteria normally found in feces *(Escherichia coli, Klebsiella, Proteus,* and *Pseudomonas)* are the most common organisms found in UTIs *(E.coli* accounting for 85% of them). Bacteria inadvertently carried from the anus to the urethra, catheterization, cystoscopy, stasis of residual urine, and any type of obstruction to urinary flow are all potential causes of UTI.

Patients with diabetes mellitus, those on corticosteroids or other immunosuppressive agents, and those with neurological disorders that interfere with bladder emptying are also more prone to urinary tract infections. UTIs are rather common during pregnancy, when they require particular attention and, frequently, modifications of drug therapy.

Urine is normally sterile. Infection is implied when the colony count of a clean-catch or catheterized urine specimen is over 50,000.

CYSTITIS

Description

Cystitis, an inflammation of the bladder wall, is most often seen in women in their sexually active years. It is also seen in young girls and elderly women. The short female urethra is easily traumatized and easily contaminated from the vagina or anus. Male cystitis most often arises from urethritis or prostatitis.

Common Diagnostic Tests

- Urine culture and sensitivity (a clean-catch specimen). *(See LAB)*
- Cystoscopy: may be done to find underlying cause for the patient who has recurrent infections.
- Intravenous pyelograms (IVP) and voiding cystourethrograms. *(See NR, x-ray preparations)*
- Cystometric and other urodynamic studies. (No preoperative medications are given; no anesthesia.)
- Suprapubic needle aspiration of the bladder contents is sometimes done.
- Multiple glass test to locate area of infection *(e.g.,* urethra, bladder, or prostate).

- Introital (refers to the entrance to the vagina) culture (most frequent origin of infection).

What to Look for

- Colony count of over 50,000 in urine culture.
- Patterns of urination: urgency, frequency, nocturia, pain and burning (dysuria), and bladder cramps and spasms.
- Suprapubic pain and sometimes low back pain.
- Gross hematuria, especially at the end of the urinary stream, is sometimes seen.
- Fever is usually not present.
- Vaginitis: purulent vaginal discharge; irritation and itching of the vulva and perineum; urinary frequency; dysuria.
- Foul-smelling urine.

Treatment

- Antibacterial therapy: sulfonamides, ampicillin, or tetracyclines depending upon sensitivity of organism. *(See PH, Antimicrobials)*
- Urinary acidification with ascorbic acid to improve effectiveness of methenamine mandelate (Mandelamine) and tetracyclines. *(See PH, Antimicrobials)*
- Urinary tract germicides *(e.g.,* nitrofurantoin (Furadantin). *(See PH, Antimicrobials)*
- Topical urinary analgesics: phenazopyridine hydrochloride (Pyridium) and methylene blue.
- Antispasmodics and barbiturates may be ordered. *(See PH, Autonomic nervous system and central nervous system)*
- Force fluids.
- Sitz baths and heat may relieve discomfort.
- Prophylaxis for women who have several infections a year: low-dose antibacterial, *e.g.,* nitrofurantoin or trimethoprim with sulfamethoxazole (Bactrim or Septra), taken daily or after sexual intercourse.
- Introital antibiotic ointment.
- Surgical correction of the underlying cause may be required.

Nursing Tips

- To prevent recurrence, education of the female patient is essential.
  1. Wipe from front to back (urethra to anus) after each bowel movement.
  2. Void after sexual intercourse.
  3. Take prescribed medication following intercourse.
  4. Shower instead of tub bathing.
  5. Force fluids.

6. Empty the bladder completely by pressing it with the heel of the hand. This should be done every 2 or 3 hours to prevent stasis.
7. Take all of the medication prescribed, even if symptoms have subsided.
8. Wear cotton panties. Keep perineal area dry.

PYELONEPHRITIS

Description

Pyelonephritis is an acute or chronic pyogenic infection of one or both kidneys, usually acquired by the ascending route, though sometimes blood borne. It is usually associated with obstruction, stasis, and urinary tract infection. If uncontrolled, acute pyelonephritis may become chronic with irreversible kidney damage leading to hypertension and uremia.

Common Diagnostic Tests

- Culture and sensitivity of multiple clean-catch, midstream urine specimens. (See LAB)
- Urinalysis shows large quantities of bacteria, pus, and RBCs.
- Voiding cystourethrograms (VCUG).
- Intravenous pyelograms (IVP). *(See NR, x-ray preparations)*

What to Look for

- Sudden onset of chills, fever, vomiting, flank pain, suprapubic tenderness, frequency and burning on urination, nocturia, and foul-smelling urine all may be seen in acute pyelonephritis.
- Fatigue, sallow complexion, and low-grade fever, with insidiously appearing signs of azotemia and chronic renal failure may be seen in chronic pyelonephritis. *(See SS, Chronic renal failure)*

Treatment

- Bed rest in the acute stage.
- Specific antibiotics. *(See PH, Antimicrobials)*
- Force fluids, if renal status permits.
- Relief of obstruction.
- In chronic pyelonephritis
  1. Maintenance on low-dose antibiotics.
  2. Control of hypertension.
  3. Dialysis or nephrectomy, if indicated.

Nursing Tips

- Nursing care directed at relief of symptoms.
- See preceding sections dealing with patients with impaired renal function, especially acute glomerulonephritis, and chronic renal failure.

Specialties

BLOOD DISORDERS
PERNICIOUS ANEMIA
Description

Pernicious Anemia (PA) results from a vitamin B_{12} deficiency or its decreased absorption. This lack of B_{12} causes the red blood cells (RBCs) to fail to mature in the bone marrow, and they are destroyed before entry into the circulation. The body cannot produce new cells fast enough to maintain an adequate RBC level. The nerve cells also require B_{12} for normal function; therefore neurological changes are often an indirect indication of pernicious anemia.

Assuming that there is an adequate dietary intake of vitamin B_{12}, two internal processes are necessary for its use by the body. Vitamin B_{12} utilization requires the action of a protein (intrinsic factor) that is released by the gastric mucosal glands; thus, the stomach must be properly functioning. This B_{12} intrinsic factor complex must then be absorbed by the mucosa of the small intestine. Malabsorption problems or parasites in this area may prevent absorption. The symptoms do not appear immediately because long-term supplies of B_{12} are stored in the liver.

Common Diagnostic Tests

- Bone marrow biopsy to confirm maturation of megaloblasts (immature RBCs).
- Serum B_{12} and Folic acid levels. (Folic acid deficiency is distinguished from PA by normal B_{12} levels and normal Schilling tests).
- Schilling tests (see hospital lab manual).
- Gastric analysis to determine presence of hydrochloric acid. *(See NR, Gastrointestinal intubation)*

What to Look for

- Anemia.
- Sore, smooth tongue.
- Mild jaundice.
- Dyspnea.
- Numbness, tingling, peripheral neuritis, and gait changes due to spinal cord degeneration.
- Fatigue.
- Anorexia.
- History of gastric or small bowel surgery, chronic pancreatitis, chronic gastritis, or alcoholism.

Treatment

- Vitamin B_{12} injections (IM) every month for life. They may be started on a weekly schedule for 1 to 2 months. *(See PH, Cardiovascular system)*

Nursing Tips

- Elderly people are the most susceptible to PA.
- Vegetarians who eat no animal products may develop PA. Plant foods do not contain B_{12}.
- Folic acid is never given to patients with PA because it increases the rate of neurological involvement in PA.
- As in all anemias, there is a decrease in the oxygen-carrying capacity of the blood, and heart failure is a complication of long standing PA.
- These patients are especially sensitive to cold.
- A family member or the patient can be taught to give the monthly injections.
- It must be stressed that lifetime, monthly B_{12} injections are necessary.

SICKLE CELL ANEMIA

Description

Sickle cell anemia (SCA) is a chronic hemolytic anemia resulting from a genetic defect in the hemoglobin molecule. Sickle cells live only 6 to 12 days, as contrasted to 120 days for normal red blood cells (RBCs). The body cannot produce new cells at the greatly increased rate required to maintain the usual count of RBCs, so anemia occurs. Normal RBCs are disc-shaped with a cell flexibility that allows them to pass through the tiniest of capillaries. But red blood cells containing sickle hemoglobin assume rigid sickle shapes when they yield oxygen. These abnormal cells are easily trapped in capillaries, where the resulting obstruction of blood flow causes ischemia and infarction of tissue. Sickle cell crisis is the result of the painful infarcts, which most commonly occur in the lungs, bone marrow, and abdomen. The pain and fever associated with sickle cell crisis is the result of these infarcts.

Sickle cell anemia is almost exclusively found in blacks. It results when a sickle cell gene is inherited from each parent. Sickle cell trait occurs when a sickle cell gene is inherited from only one parent. It produces no symptoms.

Common Diagnostic Tests
- Complete blood count (CBC) and reticulocyte count will show severe hemolytic anemia. *(See LAB)*
- Blood smear will display sickled cells.
- Hemoglobin electrophoresis detects all major sickle cell variants, of which there are several.

What to Look for
- Anemia.
- Jaundice.
- Sickle cell crisis, due to acute infarction or ischemia of an organ or bone marrow. This produces mild to severe pain lasting hours to weeks, along with an elevated temperature.
- Frequent pulmonary infections and leg ulcers.
- A tendency toward dehydration because of an inability to concentrate urine, with resultant high volume output.

Treatment
- During sickle cell infarct crisis, pain relief is imperative. Increased hydration is necessary because this decreases the viscosity of the blood. Intravenous fluids are usually given in large amounts, anywhere from 2 to 5 liters a day.
- All effort is directed toward avoiding sickle cell crisis by preventing dehydration, infection, and fatigue. There is no cure.
- The daily fluid intake should be at least 2 liters.

Nursing Tips
- Mild sickle cell crisis may be treated at home with p.o. analgesics for pain and increased p.o. fluids.
- Pain in the extremities mimics arthritis.
- Leg ulcers are common because of vascular insufficiency in the legs.
- Infarcts in the jaw bones can result in tooth problems.

- Patients often assume grotesque positions in an effort to relieve the pain.
- Chronic anemias lead to cardiac problems and, ultimately, congestive heart failure.
- Sickle cell anemia most frequently produces its symptoms in early childhood, and the patients seldom live past 40 years of age.
- There are some milder varieties of sickle cell anemia that manifest later in life and may primarily produce retinopathy rather than painful bone crisis.
- Genetic counseling is extremely important. The possibility of an offspring having a sickle cell anemia can be determined and its significance explained to parents.

BURNS

Description

Burns are produced by harmful thermal, chemical, or electrical actions on the body that result in varying degrees of destruction at the points of contact. Electrical burns also cause internal damage due to the electrical current flow within the body. All chemical burns should be flooded with a hose or shower for 10 to 15 minutes to remove the chemical. If a chemical powder is present, brush it off before flooding with water. The severity of a burn is described as first, second, or third degree.

First degree burns are superficial but painful. A sunburn is a good example. There is no systemic reaction unless the burn is extensive, and then nausea, vomiting, and elevated temperature may be present.

Second degree burns resemble a severe, painful sunburn accompanied by blisters and swelling. There are often areas of broken skin, and the underlying surface is usually wet. The epidermis (first layer of skin) and part of the dermis (second layer) is affected, making it a partial-thickness burn. These burns will blanche with pressure.

Third degree burns appear as dry and leathery, white or charred, and painless areas involving the epidermis, dermis, and subcutaneous tissue. These full-thickness burns destroy the nerve endings and hair follicles and require skin grafts. These burns will not blanche with pressure.

What to Look for

- Hoarseness, inspiratory wheezing, and stridor indicating edema of the respiratory tract. Notify the physician *immediately*. This may occur anytime within 24 hours following smoke inhalation. Change in the level of consciousness is an indicator of hypoxia.
- Severe generalized edema, caused by plasma shifting from capil-

laries to interstitial space after second- and third-degree burns. This is called "burn shock" and is seen during the first 72 hours following burn injury.

- The amount and color of urine. Output must be maintained at no less than 30 ml to 60 ml per hour. Black urine indicates impending renal failure.
- Cardiac irregularities due to electrical burns with current passing through the heart or electrolyte imbalances *(e.g.,* of sodium and potassium). Digitalis toxicity may result if a patient is receiving digitalis.
- A tourniquet effect on the hands and feet—the result of circumferential burns of the arms and legs. Peripheral pulses should be checked every 2 hours. Call the physician *immediately* if a pulse cannot be detected.
- Difficulty in breathing may result from chest constrictions caused by circumferential burns of the chest. *Call physician immediately.*
- Extreme pain in partial-thickness burns but no pain in full-thickness burns because the nerve endings are destroyed.
- Paralytic ileus when second- or third-degree burns cover more than 20% of body surface. Check for bowel sounds every 2 hours.
- Gastrointestinal bleeding is s real possibility with burn patients because of Curling's ulcer, a duodenal ulcer specific to burn patients.
- Sepsis indicated by chills, change in level of consciousness, and a very high or abnormally low temperature. Report these to the physician *immediately.*
- Wound infections become apparent by increased redness around the burn area, change in color or odor or increase of drainage, and elevated temperature. Report these findings *immediately.*
- Electrical burns usually have two external sites, one entering and one leaving the body. The site of entry is usually smaller than the exit site. The area of superficial injury is usually smaller than the internal injury. Internal hemorrhage is possible following electrical burns. The severity of damage to internal organs or to muscles may require immediate surgery *(e.g.,* amputation or colostomy)
- An increased blood and urine sugar content without any history of diabetes. This is the body's response to stress, and the patient may require insulin for a short period of time.

Treatment

- Intravenous fluids started *immediately* to replace circulating volume and electrolyte loss *(see NR, Intravenous therapy).* Lactated Ringers or normal saline with additives is usually the solution. The amount, *p*H, and specific gravity of urine are major determinants for type, amount, and rate of IV fluids. An indwelling catheter connected to a drainage bag equipped for hourly urine measurement is essential *(see NR, Urinary bladder catheterization and drainage).* A CVP line *(see NR, Central venous pressure)* or pulmonary artery catheter may be inserted to determine cardiac status and to avoid hypovolemia or fluid overload while delivering the high volumes of IV solutions needed by patients with major burns.

- Oxygen is given by high-humidity face mask or tent to increase moisture in respiratory tract, particularly in the presence of singed nasal hairs or mouth, which indicate smoke inhalation. *(See NR, Oxygen administration)*
- All extremities with a burn injury are elevated above the level of the heart to prevent severe edema from developing.
- Blood, urine, sputum, and the burn wound (after washing) are cultured on admission and then usually every 2 to 3 days to identify and treat pathogens. Surgical incision in burned tissue may be performed to relieve constriction affecting circulation or respiration. Circumferential neck burns almost always require intubation. *(See LAB)*
- Nasogastric tube to prevent gastric distention because peristalsis often slows or stops after severe burns *(see NR, Gastrointestinal intubation).* Paralytic ileus is common. Antacids are commonly given every 2 hours to prevent Curling's ulcer.
- Reverse (protective) isolation, because loss of skin removes a natural barrier to infection.
- The burn area is aseptically scrubbed with warm sterile saline mixed with an antimicrobial agent, *e.g.,* povidone-iodine (Betadine), and then rinsed with warm sterile saline. Wearing sterile gloves, apply an antimicrobial ointment or cream, *e.g.,* silver sulfadiazine (Silvadene) to a one-eighth inch thickness. The ointment or cream may also be impregnated in gauze and then applied. *(See PH, Antimicrobials)*
- Gauze soaked in prescribed solution and moistened frequently is essential for burns that expose tendons, bones, or cartilage.
- Wet-to-dry dressings are used to aid in removing eschar (burned tissue). *(See MNS, Decubitus ulcer prevention and treatment*

Nursing Tips

- It is crucial to determine the patient's weight on admission and then daily thereafter (without dressings) because this is a factor in determining IV therapy.
- Burns of the face, neck, and head that have occurred in an enclosed area or have resulted in unconsciousness increase the prob-

ability of respiratory failure secondary to smoke inhalation. Look for singed nasal hairs, soot around the mouth or in the sputum, or respiratory distress. Pulmonary injury is a major cause of death after serious burns.

- Dressing changes should be done as quickly and efficiently as possible. Uncovered burn wounds increase the risk of infection, increase fluid loss, decrease body temperature, and increase pain to patients. These patients are very sensitive to low room temperature.
- Burn-wound care is directed toward maintaining a clean eschar (burned tissue), which gradually falls away or is surgically removed, allowing new skin to form or grafting to be done. *It is absolutely necessary that impeccable sterile technique be used.* Gloves, gown, mask, and hair cap are always worn during dressing changes.
- Medicate for pain (usually IV) before starting wound care. It is seldom possible to completely ease the pain.
- At least once each day, burn-wound care should be done when the physician is there to see the condition of the wound.
- Patients with circulatory problems and diabetes and those on steroids or chemotherapy have delayed healing ability.
- Burn patients over 60 years of age have an increased susceptibility to myocardial infarctions. *(See SS, Myocardial infarction)*
- There is a very high demand for protein in the healing process of burns. When they are able to eat, patients are often on 5000-calorie diets. Keep a daily calorie count. Hyperalimentation is often used.
- Partial-thickness burns that become infected can change to full-thickness burns.
- Burns in the perineal area require special attention to maintain cleanliness. A temporary colostomy is sometimes done.
- The position of the patient must be changed hourly to relieve pressure on burned areas. The limbs should be positioned to avoid contractures, and the hands and feet should be splinted in the position of function. Range of motion (ROM) exercises are extremely important and are usually done during dressing changes. *(See NR, Range of motion exercises)*
- Newly healed, burned skin is easily injured and sunburned.
- The nurse is with the patient for long periods and should be a careful observer of changes. Each time the wound is redressed, the color, extent of granulation, sensation, tenderness, and odor should be documented, and changes should be reported to the physician.
- Burns do not cause the patient to become unconscious. Look for other reasons if this happens (*e.g.,* head injury).

- The "rule of nines" is a method used in assessing the extent of burns in patients over the age of 14. It is necessary to know the percentage of the body that is burned to determine caloric and fluid requirements.

Head	9%
Each arm	9%
Each leg	18%
Front of torso	18%
Back of torso	18%
Perineum	1%

- Burns are considered major if more than 20% of total body surface area is involved because IV fluid replacement is then required.
- Burns of the face, neck, hands, feet, and perineum are always considered major, as are electrical burns and those involving smoke inhalation.
- Burn patients are frequently in the hospital for long periods of time and require care which is very painful. Their personalities may change drastically, with periods of depression and apathy.
- A nursing-care plan that lists step-by-step care must be prepared and updated every 24 hours.

EYE-PATIENT CARE

Nursing Tips

- Know the purpose of eye medications. They are very potent, and their specific action may be desired in one eye disease but contraindicated in another.
- If there is ever any question about which eye gets what medication, *check* before giving any. Remember that o.d. is right eye; o.s. is left eye; and o.u. means both eyes.
- Different medications are often ordered for each eye.
- Always triple check to be sure you have the proper patient, the proper eye, and the proper medication before instilling anything into the eye.
- Some eye drops are suspensions and must be shaken.
- Ophthalmic solutions must be sterile. Read package directions concerning proper storage of product.
- When eyelashes must be cut off, coat scissors with a sterile lubricant so the lashes will adhere and not fall into the eyes.
- Frequently, patients with eye diseases are hospitalized for other problems. They must *never* omit their daily schedule of eye medications. The physician treating their eyes should be contacted if any questions arise.

- Eye ointments are placed along the center rim of the lower lid. They will then be "blinked" into the eye.
- Eye drops are instilled by tilting the patient's head back and having him look up. Lightly press a sterile cotton ball or gauze sponge at the inner canthus of the eye. Pull cheek down with conjunctiva exposed. The drop goes into the conjunctival fold, not on the cornea or into the lacrimal duct. Immediate absorption through the lacrimal duct may cause toxic systemic effects with a drug such as atropine.
- If more than one drop is needed, have the patient blink one away before instilling the next one.
- Metal eye shields are often applied over an eye pad to prevent injury to the eye when the patient sleeps. To hold shield in place, use five strips of tape, each 5 inches long. Apply vertically over the shield, with the shield ends resting on the boney prominences of the face.
- Patients with patches over both eyes frequently become disoriented *(see MNS, Disoriented patients)*. Always speak before touching these patients. Try to avoid use of sleeping pills with elderly patients, especially when their eyes are covered, to avoid increased mental confusion.
- If only one eye is patched, determine the vision in the other eye. Also, inform patient that depth perception will be impaired.
- If bed rest is ordered, check daily for signs and symptoms of thrombophlebitis. *(See SS, Thrombophlebitis)*
- To enable patients with limited vision to feed themselves, place the food on the tray as though it were numbers on a clock and explain this system.
- Assist ambulating patient on the unpatched side.

CATARACT
Description

A cataract is an increasing opaqueness of the lens of the eye. Eighty percent of people over 70 years of age have them, and they are frequently seen at younger ages. Cataracts are most commonly associated with the natural aging process, but congenital cataracts and those resulting from eye trauma, medications (steroids), or a systemic disease such as diabetes are also not uncommon.

Common Diagnostic Tests
- Eye examination.

What to Look for

- Gray or white opacity over the pupil area.
- Gradual blurring of vision, with distant vision primarily affected.
- Sensitivity to light and difficulty driving at night because of the glare of headlights.

Treatment

- Surgical removal is the only cure.

Nursing Tips

- The time for surgery is when the lens opaqueness has reached the point where it interferes with necessary vision.
- Many of the patients are diabetics.
- Eye drops to dilate the eyes are given before surgery. Also, antibiotic ophthalmic ointments are used to prevent infection, a serious, potential complication of surgery.
- Postoperative orders are written on an individual basis. Eye shields are worn at night for 4 to 5 weeks to prevent eye injury. Hemmorhage and damage to the suture line are prevented by avoiding lifting, bending over, squeezing of the eye, or straining.
- Unless there are permanent intraocular implant lenses, soft contact lenses are placed in the eye about 6 weeks after surgery. These may be left in and need to be removed only every few weeks.
- It may be necessary to teach another family member to remove and clean the contact lenses or the patient may have to go to the physician's office periodically for this purpose.

CONTACT LENS IDENTIFICATION AND REMOVAL

Nursing Tips

- Always check the eyes of an unconscious or confused patient for contact lenses. Darken the room, gently separate the lids, and shine a penlight on the side of the eye. Look closely for an unnatural margin around the cornea. Occasionally the lens wanders onto the sclera.
- Check to see if there is a bracelet identifying the type or reason for contact lenses, or ask a family member.
- Hard contact lenses must not be left in the eyes of patients who are not totally conscious.
- To remove hard contact lenses, wash the hands before attempting to touch the lens. Place a thumb near the margin of each eyelid and gently separate the lids. If the lens is directly over the cornea, move the lid margins back toward the top and bottom of the lens,

pressing ever so slightly on the bottom eyelid while moving it up. The lens should flip out. If it does not, gently move it with a finger off the cornea and onto the sclera where it can be left more safely until it can be removed. If it is not possible to remove lenses, be sure the physician is notified. Tiny suction cups for contact lens removal are usually available in emergency rooms, if needed. Store lenses in vials of sterile saline labeled with the patient's name.

- Some types of soft contact lenses may be left in the eye indefinitely. Check with the physician. In the event they need to be removed, wash the hands before attempting to touch the lens. With the thumb and index finger of one hand, gently separate the eyelids. Use the other index finger to carefully slide the lens off the cornea and onto the sclera. "Pinch" the lens off the eye between the thumb and index finger. These lenses must also be stored in sterile saline. Soft lenses are not marked as to right or left eye, so be sure the vials are properly marked.

GLAUCOMA
Description

Glaucoma describes a condition of elevated intraocular pressure. It causes damage to the blood vessels supplying the optic nerve. Primary glaucoma—the most common form, also known as open-angle glaucoma—results from a structural defect of the eye. Secondary glaucoma refers to an interference in the drainage system resulting from injury or disease, such as uveitis. Acute, or closed-angle glaucoma, occurs when a sudden increase of intraocular pressure takes place due to an acute obstruction of the drainage system.

Common Diagnostic Tests

- Tonometer test: A tonometer placed directly on the anesthetized cornea measures intraocular pressure. Pressure above 21mm Hg is indicative of glaucoma. A pressure above 40mm Hg indicates acute glaucoma.

What to Look for

- In simple and secondary glaucoma there are no symptoms until vision is decreased. Decreased vision usually begins with peripheral fields.
- Acute glaucoma occurs suddenly with the complaint of seeing a halo around lights, pain in the eye, and often nausea and vomiting. This is a medical emergency and must be treated within hours.

Treatment

- Timolol maleate (Timoptic), pilocarpine, epinephrine: miotics given topically as eye drops, which reduce the size of the pupil and pull the iris away from the drainage channels. *(See PH, Autonomic nervous system)*
- Acetazolamide (Diamox): reduces the rate of fluid formation in the eye. *(See PH, Urinary system)*
- Iridectomy: a permanent surgical procedure done to allow drainage through artificial openings.
- Acute glaucoma is a medical emergency, and immediate treatment is necessary to reduce the high intraocular pressures. Acetazolamide (Diamox) may be given IV, or if this is not effective, mannitol IV is often used *(see PH Urinary system)*. Miotics are begun when the pressure return to normal. An iridectomy may be done immediately to prevent further attacks.

Nursing Tips

- The eye is anesthetized for tonometer examination. Instruct the patient *not* to rub the anesthetized eye for at least 15 minutes after the examination.
- Primary glaucoma is usually bilateral.
- Patients hospitalized for other reasons may also have glaucoma. They must *never* miss their daily routine of eye drops and other medication for glaucoma. Be sure other medications ordered for them, *e.g.,* atropine or propantheline bromide (Pro-Banthine) *(see PH, Autonomic nervous system),* are not contraindicated because of glaucoma.
- Acetazolamide (Diamox) is a diuretic and will increase urine output.
- Glaucoma cannot be cured by the use of drugs. The aim of the therapy is to control the intraocular pressure and keep it below 21mm Hg. Therefore, these patients must see the physician for regular eye examinations and regulation of medication.
- If surgery is done, individual orders for postoperative care will follow. Generally the patient is kept flat for 24 hours, but he may turn to his unoperated side. Anything that may increase pressure, such as bending down, straining, or lifting, should be avoided for several weeks.
- These patients must always wear bracelets that indicate that they have glaucoma. Encourage them to always ask a pharmacist for advice before buying over-the-counter medications because of possible contraindications with glaucoma.

RETINAL DETACHMENT

Description

Retinal detachment is the separation of the neural retinal layer from the inner surface of the eyeball. This is usually initiated by a small tear or hole in the retina. Fluid within the eye can then flow into the subretinal space. This tends to increase the detachment.

Common Diagnostic Tests

- Eye examination.

What to Look for

- Patients will note floating spots before the eyes, flashes of light, and blocked peripheral vision appearing as shadows in the visual fields. These symptoms gradually increase with time as the detachment progresses.

Treatment

- Immediate bed rest with the head turned toward area of detachment, in order to use gravity as a force to bring the retina back against the inner surface of the eyeball.
- Surgery, the earlier the better. The success of the surgery depends on the extent of the detachment and how long it has existed before it is treated.

Nursing Tips

- Sedation is often necessary to minimize head movements while patient is kept on bed rest awaiting surgery.
- Postoperative orders are written on an individual basis. The head is usually kept turned toward the detached area immediately following surgery.
- Hemorrhage is a potential major complication.
- The eye may be inflamed for several weeks after surgery. Eye drops are usually given to decrease the inflammation.
- Warm eye compresses are used to relieve crusting on the eyelids.
- These patients usually must remain at home for several weeks after leaving the hospital, and reading, as well as heavy lifting, bending over, or any physical strain, must be avoided during this postoperative period in order to decrease the possibility of a recurring detachment.

ONCOLOGY (CANCER)

Overview

Cancer is a disease of uncontrolled cell proliferation that results in the growth of malignant tumors capable of spreading (a process called metastasis) to adjacent or distant tissues. It is currently treated with surgery, radiation, chemotherapy, and hormonal therapy. Additionally, immunotherapy, including the use of interferon, may prove to be an effective treatment, but this is still in the research and test phase.

Surgery removes as much of the tumor mass as possible and is therefore most effective when the cancer is localized.

Radiation must be focused on the cancerous area so that it directly kills the abnormal cells without causing excessive damage to healthy tissue. Deep focal penetration is now obtained with higher energy beam intensities, thereby providing more safety in treatment. Localized radiation is also achievable by implanting radioactive material at the cancerous site.

Chemotherapy is the use of drugs that are more toxic to the rapidly growing abnormal cells than to healthy tissue. All cells, though, whether malignant or normal, are adversely affected, and a balance must be maintained in order to kill the cancerous, faster-growing cells without permanently harming the healthy cells. Even so, normal cells that proliferate at a fast rate, such as cells in the hair follicles, bone marrow, and the mucosa of the oral and gastrointestinal tracts, are severely affected. This explains the well-known side-effects of chemotherapy, such as hair loss, depressed bone marrow function, gastrointestinal dysfunction, and stomatitis. Combinations of drugs, called drug protocols, are selected for the differing antineoplastic effects of the individual agents. Some of the drugs are "cycle specific" and have the greatest impact during certain phases of the cell life cycle; others are "nonspecific" and are capable of cell kill regardless of the life cycle of the cell.

Hormonal therapy, including corticosteroids, sex steroids and surgery (oophorectomy, adrenalectomy), is used to treat tumors sensitive to an alteration of the body's endocrine balance.

Combined modality protocols employing the various modalities of surgery, radiation, chemotherapy, and hormonal therapy are called "combined modality treatment protocols" and are designed to obtain a cure, remission, or relief of symptoms of cancer.

The National Cancer Institute (NCI) offers a public cancer information service (CIS) that answers questions regarding the medical facilities in the area of the caller, home-care assistance programs, and financial aid sources. Local phone numbers may be obtained by contacting the Office of Cancer Communications, NCI, Bethesda, MD, 20014.

Patients with cancer of the lung, breast, and colon, as well as leukemia and lymphoma, are frequently treated in medical or surgical units of hospitals. Each of these disorders is separately described in the following pages.

BREAST CANCER

Description

Breast cancer is the most prevalent form of cancer in women. It is generally detected by manual examination of the breast, but it can only be confirmed by tissue biopsy. It metastasizes to the axillary lymph nodes, skin, and bones. Later it may progress to the liver, lung, and brain.

Common Diagnostic Tests

- Breast examination.
- Tissue biopsy.
- Mammograms and xerography: breast x-rays capable of detecting some breast cancers before they reach a palpable size of 1 centimeter.

What to Look for

- A solid, fixed, painless lump, found most often in the upper outer quadrant of the breast. The lump may be accompanied by a nipple discharge or by nipple retraction or elevation.
- Dimpling of the skin, so that it resembles the skin of an orange, often develops as the disease progresses.

Treatment

Surgical

- Radical mastectomy: removal of the breast, axillary nodes, lymphatic vessels that drain the arm on the affected side, and pectoralis muscles.
- Modified radical mastectomy: removal of the breast and all axillary nodes.
- Simple mastectomy: removal of the breast and palpable axillary nodes.
- Removal of only the tumor, commonly referred to as a "lumpectomy."

Chemotherapy

- Adjuvant chemotherapy is commonly used for women postoperatively when cancer involves the lymph nodes. It continues for a one-year period. It is usually not given in early, localized disease where there is no axillary node involvement.
- In premenopausal and postmenopausal women, chemotherapy is useful in treating metastatic disease.
- Tumors that are estrogen dependent may be treated with various hormonal therapies (surgery or medication).

Radiation

- In some breast cancer radiation is the treatment of first choice. If the disease is localized it may be used instead of surgery. In advanced cases it is followed with chemotherapy. Radiation in the breast area frequently causes inflammation of the mucosa of the trachea and bronchial tree, resulting in radiation pneumonitis, a complication that often occurs several weeks after the radiation treatment. Patients develop a productive cough and fever. These may progress to fibrosis of the lung, with a permanent decrease in effective lung volume.

Nursing Tips

- Radical mastectomies are not done as frequently as they once were. However, in any surgical procedure in which the lymph nodes and vessels on the affected side are removed, possible infection of the arm is a problem. *Never* allow injections or blood to be taken from that arm. To prevent trauma to the tissue, blood pressures should not be taken in the affected arm. The patient should wear a bracelet on that arm identifying this problem. Any redness, pain, or swelling in the affected arm should be immediately reported to the physician.
- Hemovacs are usually in place after mastectomies. Be sure they drain well, are emptied during each shift, and are irrigated by order if necessary. They are usually removed when drainage is under 100 ml each day.
- Check the hand for circulatory impairment.
- Keep the arm elevated on a pillow.
- A progressive plan of arm exercises (Fig. 5-11) should be ordered immediately postoperative. This usually begins with flexion and extension of fingers in the first few hours and progresses as ordered by the physician.
- Encourage "Reach to Recovery" program available through the local Cancer Society. A physician's referral is necessary and may be obtained while the patient is hospitalized.
- *(See Nursing care of the patient receiving chemotherapy or radiation)*

COLON CANCER
Description

Adenocarcinoma of the colon occurs most frequently in the sigmoid and rectal area. It is the most commonly occurring cancer in both sexes. Metastasis is by direct extension to adjacent organs or through the lymphatic or blood system to the liver and lung. An increased incidence has been found in populations with a high beef

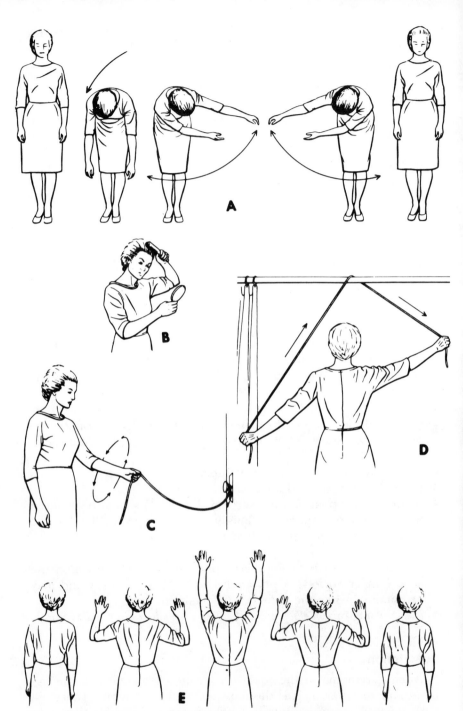

FIG. 5-11. *Exercises for the postmastectomy patient. A. Pendulum-swinging exercise. B. Hair-brushing exercise. C. Rope-turning exercise. D. Rope-sliding exercise. E. Wall-climbing exercise.*

and fat consumption and also in individuals with a history of chronic colitis, intestinal polyps, and a familial history of cancer of the colon. A decreased incidence occurs in those with rapid transit time of fecal material. This is the reason for the recent interest in the high-roughage diet.

Common Diagnostic Tests
- Rectal examination.
- Stools for occult blood. *(See LAB)*
- Barium x-rays of GI tract. *(See NR, x-ray preparations)*
- Colonoscopy with biopsy. *(See NR, Endoscopic procedures)*
- Liver scan. *(See NR, Scans)*
- Chest x-ray.
- CEA: blood test for carcinoembryonic antigen. An increase of CEA is frequently observed in patients with colorectal cancer. It is *not* definitive, however, because it may also be elevated in liver disease and pancreatitis and in other disorders.

What to Look for
- Rectal bleeding, often manifested by black stools.
- Cancer in the right side of the colon is frequently associated with an unexplained anemia; less often, a vague feeling of abdominal fullness or a palpable mass may occur.
- Cancer of the left side of the colon often is indicated by alternating constipation and diarrhea and small-caliber stools. These symptoms are caused by a gradually increasing intestinal obstruction.

Treatment
- Surgery. *(See SS, Intestinal surgery)*
- Radiation may be given before surgery to reduce the tumor size.
- Chemotherapy is sometimes used to treat metastatic disease.

Nursing Tips
- Radiation to the abdomen and pelvis frequently causes diarrhea and sometimes causes a bladder irritability leading to cystitis.
- *(See Nursing care of the patient receiving chemotherapy or radiation)*
- *(See Nursing Tips in SS, Intestinal surgery)*

LEUKEMIA
Description

Leukemia is a cancer involving the bone marrow, lymph nodes, and spleen that causes an overproduction of white blood cells (WBCs). It is classified by the type of immature WBCs that prevail (*e.g.*, myeloid, lymphoid, or monocytic) and also as "acute" or "chronic." The acute form may cause death within months; the patient with the chronic form has a life expectancy measured in years.

Common Diagnostic Tests
- Complete blood count (CBC) and platelet count. (*See LAB*)
- Bone marrow aspiration and biopsy. (*See LAB*)

What to Look for
- Abnormal bleeding, especially in skin and mucous membranes because of decreased platelet production (thrombocytopenia).
- Increased susceptibility to infection, resulting from increased numbers of immature WBCs that are unable to fight infectious organisms.
- Weakness and fatigue due to the abnormally rapid production of WBCs, and the resultant depletion of body reserves of amino acids and vitamins used in cell growth.
- Anemia, which develops because of displacement of red cell forms in the marrow by the increased white cell population.
- Shortness of breath, angina, and muscle pain occurs because of anemia and the lack of oxygen to the tissues.
- Enlargement of the spleen and liver, due to accumulations of large numbers of WBCs in these organs.

Treatment
- Chemotherapy. (*See PH, Antineoplastics*)
- Radiation.
- Blood and platelet transfusions. (*See NR, Intravenous therapy*)
- Bone marrow transplant is being investigated in some research centers.

Nursing Tips
- Be particularly aware of bleeding tendency and observe carefully for increase in petechiae, hematuria, or gastrointestinal bleeding.
- Infection is the leading cause of death in these patients.
- (*See Nursing care of the patient receiving chemotherapy or radiation*)

LUNG CANCER
Description
Lung cancer is classified according to the type of cancer cell identified by microscopic examination of biopsy material, (*e.g.*, squamous cell carcinoma, oat cell carcinoma). Frequently it metastasizes to the liver, bone, and brain. The lung is also a common site of metastases from other areas of the body.

Common Diagnostic Tests

- X-rays and tomograms of the chest.
- Bronchoscopy. *(See NR, Endoscopic procedures)*
- Sputum cytology.
- Alkaline phosphatase, an indicator of liver and bone metastasis. *(See LAB)*
- Bone, liver, brain, and CAT scans for signs of metastasis. *(See NR, Scans)*
- Mediastinoscopy, to evaluate mediastinal lymph nodes for metastasis. *(See NR, Endoscopic procedures)*

What to Look for

- A productive cough.
- Increasing fatigue.
- Anorexia (loss of appetite).
- Sudden weight loss.
- Dyspnea.

Treatment
Surgery

- Lobectomy, if cancer is confined to a segment or lobe.
- Pneumonectomy, if cancer involves more than one lobe.
- Over half the patients presenting with x-ray evidence of lung cancer are inoperable. A lung cancer has to be 2 cm distal to the origin of the bronchus (carina) in order to suture the bronchus following lobectomy (or pneumonectomy).
- See *SS, Pulmonary surgery* for additional information.

Radiation

- Radiation is useful for symptomatic relief of chest-wall metastasis or of pain resulting from bone metastasis.
- Radiation to the chest frequently causes inflammation of the mucosa of the trachea and bronchial tree, resulting in radiation pneumonitis, a complication that often occurs several weeks after the radiation treatment. Patients develop cough, sputum, and fever. This may progress to fibrosis of the lung, with a permanent decrease in effective lung volume.

Chemotherapy

(See PH, Antineoplastics)

Nursing Tips

(See SS, Pulmonary surgery)
(See Nursing care of the patient receiving chemotherapy or radiation)

LYMPHOMA
Description
Lymphomas are cancers of lymphatic tissue. They are broadly classified by microscopic determination of the type of malignant cell as Hodgkin's lymphoma (HL) or non-Hodgkin's lymphoma (NHL). Hodgkin's lymphoma primarily involves lymph nodes and is usually first seen in the cervical area. It spreads to adjacent nodes. Non-Hodgkin's lymphoma is more likely to involve other organs in addition to lymph nodes. Therefore, it is often widespread prior to detection.

Common Diagnostic Tests
- Biopsy of lymph nodes.
- Mediastinoscopy and laparoscopy enable viewing of mediastinal and peritoneal organs and so are done to determine the extent of the disease *(see NR, Endoscopic procedures)*. The disease may range from a single node or organ involvement on one side of the diaphragm to multiple nodes and organ involvement on both sides of the diaphragm. This is referred to as "staging" to determine the extent of the disease.
- Lymphangiogram is done to visualize nodes with a radiographic contrast material in order to evaluate nodal involvement in the abdomen and pelvis.
- Abdominal CAT scan. *(See NR, Scans)*
- Bone marrow and liver biopsy. *(See NR, Bone marrow aspiration and biopsy and NR, Liver Biopsy)*
- Sometimes a staging laparotomy and splenectomy are necessary for the examination of the lymph nodes and spleen.

What to Look for
- Increasing and painless enlargement of the lymph nodes.
- Weight loss of 10% or more in the past 6 months.
- Recurring temperature elevations to 100° F or higher.
- Night sweats.
- Pruritus (severe itching) is a common symptom of HL. Herpes zoster occurs in 25% of these patients.
- Symptoms of organ or major vessel compression because of enlargement of the lymph nodes and tissue. This may cause difficulty in breathing or swallowing and also edema of the lower extremities.

Treatment
- Surgery. Intestinal obstruction or other intra-abdominal complications may require surgery. Hypersplenism may require splenectomy. *(See SS, Gastrointestinal surgery)*
- Radiation may be curative for localized disease.

- Chemotherapy is the mainstay of treatment for most advanced lymphomas. *(See PH, Antineoplastics)*

Nursing Tips

- Lymphangiograms are done by insertion of contrast material into the lymphatic system. The site of insertion is between the first and second toe. The patients usually have sore feet and difficulty walking for several days. They should check their feet daily for signs of infection at the insertion site.
- Following a splenectomy, watch carefully for atelectasis (because splenectomy is high-abdominal surgery). Also, these patients are more susceptible to complications of bacterial infections (*e.g.,* pneumonococcal pneumonia).
- *(See Nursing care of the patient receiving chemotherapy or radiation)*

NURSING CARE OF THE PATIENT RECEIVING CHEMOTHERAPY OR RADIATION

Nursing Tips

- Anemia is a side-effect of chemotherapy and radiation. Rest periods from treatment may be necessary, and blood transfusions may be given.
- It is important to save good veins for therapy. Maintain IV sites for as long as possible. Some routine lab work can be accomplished by finger sticks for blood.
- Depressed WBC production predisposes the patient to infection. Anyone with a cold or other infection should not be in contact with the patient. This includes members of the hospital staff. Major sites of infection are the lung and urinary tract. Fungal infections are apt to occur in the mouth and perineal areas. There is an increased susceptibility to viral infections (*e.g.,* herpes zoster and measles).
- Reverse (protective) isolation is often ordered, and chemotherapy and radiation are deferred if the WBC falls below 3000.
- Hair loss depends upon the chemotherapeutic agent used in treatment.
- Nausea, vomiting, and diarrhea may accompany chemotherapy or abdominal and pelvic radiation. Antiemetics and antidiarrheal medications may be ordered, usually one hour before and after treatment. *(See PH, Gastrointestinal system)*
- Accurate I and O is necessary because excessive fluid loss requires IV replacement.
- Food should not be taken within an hour before or after chemotherapy or radiation. Frequent, small feedings are usually better tolerated. When diarrhea is a problem, eliminate as much fat as possible from the diet.

- There is often an alteration in the sense of taste while undergoing chemotherapy or radiation treatments. Foods may taste bitter or excessively sweet. Salty and very cold foods are often the most desired, while hot food and meat are frequently rejected.
- Fruit nectars, such as pear and apricot, are tolerated better than fruit juices when the mouth and throat are sore. Vitamin C needs to be supplemented with nectars.
- Physicians and nurses should know what dietary supplements (*e.g.,* Nutrament and Sustagen) taste like and that they come in different flavors and they should realize that the patient's taste and toleration must be considered.
- A decrease in platelets below 50,000 means an increased bleeding tendency. Many times all injections are prohibited.
- There are two main types of radiation: external radiation and internal implants. Patients receiving external radiation pose no threat to anyone caring for them or their families. Those with implants need to be cared for within the strict government guidelines required in every hospital licensed to use such therapy.
- Patients undergoing external radiation have the treatment area of the body outlined on the skin with a dye marker. This must not be scrubbed away. Friction, from such things as shoulder straps and shaving, as well as perfumes, lotions, and heating pads, should be avoided; additionally, sunbathing should not be done for a year following radiation treatment.
- Skin reactions may occur, and they are most likely to appear in friction areas, creases, and the groin. They appear as reddened, itchy, or weepy areas. Cornstarch may be applied to relieve the symptoms.
- Brain metastasis is often treated with radiation; this is always followed by hair loss in 2 to 3 weeks.
- Bone metastasis results in a tendency for pathological fractures. Move these patients very carefully, and never squeeze or pull on the body.

BIBLIOGRAPHY

POSTOPERATIVE CARE
BOOKS

LeMaitre GD, Finnegin JA: The Patient In Surgery: A Guide for Nurses, 4th ed. Philadelphia, WB Saunders, 1980

JOURNALS

Hall KV: Detecting septic shock before it's too late. RN Magazine 44(9):29–32, 1981
McConnell EA: After surgery. Nursing 77 7(3):32–39, 1977

McConnell EA: Toward complication-free recoveries for your surgical patients, Part I. RN Magazine 43(6):31–33, 82–90, 1980

McConnell EA: Toward complication-free recoveries for your surgical patients, Part II. RN Magazine 43(7):35–38, 70–76, 1980

Schumann D: How to help wound healing in your abdominal surgery patient. Nursing 80 10(4):34–40, 1980

CARDIOVASCULAR SYSTEM
BOOKS

Andreoli KG, Fowkes VH, Zipes DP et al: Comprehensive Cardiac Care, 3rd ed, pp 8–75. St. Louis, CV Mosby, 1975

Brunner LS, Emerson CP, Ferguson LK et al: Medical Surgical Nursing, 2nd ed, pp 789–798. Philadelphia, JB Lippincott, 1970

Burrell ZL, Burrell LO: Intensive Nursing Care, 1st ed, pp 9–81. St. Louis, CV Mosby, 1969

Chapman CM: Medical Nursing, 9th ed, pp 93–120. London, Cassell and Collier Macmillan, 1977

LeMaitre G, Finnegan J: The Patient in Surgery: A Guide for Nurses, 4th ed, pp 291–329, 341–343. Philadelphia, WB Saunders, 1980

Scherer JC: Introductory Medical Surgical Nursing, 2nd ed, pp 318–329 Philadelphia, JB Lippincott, 1977

Sexton DL, Fagan–Dubin L, Taggart E et al: The Nursing Clinics of North America, Vol 12, No 1, pp 87–168. Philadelphia, WB Saunders, 1977

Shafer KN, Sawyer JR, McCluskey AM et al: Medical Surgical Nursing, 6th ed, pp 352–363. St. Louis, CV Mosby, 1975

Smith DW, Germain CP: Care of the Adult Patient, 4th ed, pp 637–681. Philadelphia, JB Lippincott, 1975

JOURNALS

Atchison JS, Murray J: Post vascular surgery—when happiness can be a warm foot. Nursing 78 8:36, 1978

Benditt EP: The origin of atherosclerosis. Sci Am 236:74, 1977

Kousch D, Ward GW, Bandy P et al: Controlling high blood pressure, treating and counseling the hypertensive patient, promoting patient adherence. Am J Nurs 78: 824, 1978

Mastellar MJ Batterman B, Stegman M: Hypertension. Critical care update 6:3, 1979

Moore, MA:Hypertensive Emergencies. Am Fam Physician 21 (3):141, 1980

ENDOCRINE SYSTEM
BOOKS

Berkow R, Talbott JH, Abraham GN et al: The Merck Manual of Diagnosis and Therapy. Rahway NJ, Merck Sharp and Dohme Research Laboratories, Division of Merck & Co., 1977

Brunner L, Suddarth D: Textbook of Medical–Surgical Nursing, 4th ed. Philadelphia, JB Lippincott, 1980

Christman B, Nemchik R, O'Connor M et al: Managing Diabetics Properly. Horsham, PA, Intermed Communications, 1978

Economou S: The Surgical Clinics of North America: Symposium on Endocrine Surgery. Philadelphia, WB Saunders, 1979

Glenn J: Urological Clinics of North America: Symposium on Adrenal Diseases. Philadelphia, WB Saunders, 1977

Krueger J: Endocrine Problems in Nursing. St. Louis, CV Mosby, 1976

The Lab, Drugs, and Nursing Implications. Chestnut Hill, MA, Health-Care Education Programs of America, 1978 (taped lecture with workbook)

Luckmann J, Sorensen K: Medical–Surgical Nursing: A Psychophysiologic Approach. Philadelphia, WB Saunders, 1974

Phipps W, Long B, Woods N: Medical–Surgical Nursing: Concepts and Clinical Practice. St. Louis, CV Mosby, 1979

Porter A, Tribble N, Hollenberg E et al: The Nursing Clinics of North America: Symposium on Diabetic Patient Education and Care. Philadelphia, WB Saunders, 1977

Solomon B, Wake M, Bresinger J et al: The Nursing Clinics of North America: Symposium on Endocrine Disorders. Philadelphia, WB Saunders, 1980

Tilkian S, Conover M: Clinical Implications of Laboratory Tests. St. Louis, CV Mosby, 1979

JOURNALS

Camuñas C: Transphenoidal hypophysectomy. Am J Nurs 80(10):1820–1823, 1980

Emergency Medicine: Weathering thyroid storm. Emergency Medicine 11(9):75–78, 1979

Fredholm NZ: The insulin pump: New method of insulin delivery. Am J Nurs 81(11):2024–2026, 1981

Garofano C: Helping diabetics live with their neuropathies. Nursing 80 10(6):42–44, 1980

Gillies DA, Alyn IB: Caring for patients with thyroid disorders. Nursing 77 7(10):71–80, October, 1977

Guthrie D: DKA breaking the vicious cycle. Nursing 78 8(6):54–60, June, 1978

Guthrie D: Helping the diabetic manage his self-care. Nursing 80 10(2):57–64, February 1980

Jenkins E: Living with thyrotoxicosis. Am J Nurs 80(5):956–958, May, 1980

McCarthy JA: Diabetic nephropathy. Am J Nurs 81(11):2030–2034, 1981

Petrokas J: Commonsense guidelines for controlling diabetes during illness. Nursing 77 7(12):36–37, December, 1977

Plasse NJ: Monitoring blood glucose at home: A comparison of three products. Am J Nurs 8(11):2028–2029, 1981

Schumann D: Assessing the diabetic. Nursing 76 6(3):62–67, March, 1976

Stevens AD: Monitoring blood glucose at home: Who should do it. Am J Nurs 81(11)2026–2027, 1981

Walesky M, Slater N, Lundin D et al: Common problems in managing adult diabetes mellitus. Am J Nurs 78(5):871–890, May 1978

Wolf L: Insulin paving the way to a new life. Nursing 77 7(11):38–41, November, 1977

GASTROINTESTINAL SYSTEM

BOOKS

Brunner LS, Suddarth DS: Textbook of Medical–Surgical Nursing, 4th ed. Philadelphia, JB Lippincott, 1980

Jones D, Dunbar C, Jirovec M: Medical Surgical Nursing, A Conceptual Approach. New York, McGraw-Hill, 1978

Given BA, Simmons S: Gastroenterology in Clinical Nursing, 2nd ed. St. Louis, CV Mosby, 1975

Phipps W, Long B, Woods N: Medical–Surgical Nursing, Concepts and Clinical Practice, 7th ed. St. Louis, CV Mosby, 1980

JOURNALS

Auslander MO: Drug therapy of acute pancreatitis. Clinics in Gastroenterology 8(1):219–227, January, 1979

Austad WI: Pancreatitis: The use of pancreatic supplements. Drugs 17(6):480–487, June, 1979

Banks, PA: Answers to questions on pancreatitis. Hospital Medicine 14(5):8–9, 1978

Bath A: Total colectomy and ileostomy. Nursing Mirror 146(10):19–20, March, 1978

Bauer D: Preventing the spread of hepatitis B in dialysis units. Am J Nurs 80(2):260–261, February, 1980

Bell J: Just another patient with gallstones? Don't you believe it. Nursing 79 9(10):26–33, October, 1979

Broadwell DC, Sorrells SL: Loop transverse colostomy. Am J Nurs 78(6):1028–1031, June, 1978

Burkle W: What you should know about Tagamet. Nursing 80 10(4):86–87, April, 1980

Caprini JA et al: Nonoperative extraction of retained common duct stones. Archives of Surgery 111(4):445–455, 1976

Corman ML: Management of post op constipation in anorectal surgery. Diseases of the Colon and Rectum 22(3):149–151, April, 1979

de Tornay R, Stillman MJ: Nursing decisions, nursing intervention in acute pancreatitis. RN Magazine 41(12):67–73, December, 1978

Favero MS, Maynard J et al: Prevention and control of infections in specialized areas—viral hepatitis. Critical Care Quarterly 3(3):43–55, 1980

Fishbein RH, Handelsman JC: A method of primary reconstruction following radical excision of sacrococcygeal pilonidal disease. Ann Surg 190(2):231–235, August, 1979

For colitis, the corticosteroid watch. Emergency Medicine 11(9):141, September 15, 1979

Foulkes B: Inflammatory disease of the bowel. Nursing Mirror 146(4):19–21, January 26, 1978

Gaeke RF, Kirsner JB: When I say "colitis" I mean. . . J Nursing Care 11(3):14–15, March, 1978

Griffith D: Cholecystectomy and operative cholangiogram for gallstones. Nursing Times 74(26):1100–1104, June 29, 1978

Griffen WO: Management of diverticular disease. Hosp Med 14(11):108–126, November, 1978

Higson R: Types of hernia. Nursing Mirror 146(8):14–18, February 23, 1978

Jackson MM: Viral hepatitis. Nursing Clin North Am 15(4):729–746, December, 1980

Jones I: Colitis. Life Health 93(2):21–23. February, 1978

Keenan K, Parsons J, Philpotts EA et al: A trial of a new ostomy system. Nursing Times 75(30):1283–1285, July 26, 1979

Kodner IJ: Colostomy and ileostomy. Clin Symp 30(5):2–36, 1978

Long G: GI bleeding: What to do and when. Nursing 78 8(3):44–50, March, 1978

MacClelland DC: Kock pouch: a new type of ileostomy. AORN J 32(2):191–201, 1980

McConnell, EA: Curtailing a life-threatening crisis: GI bleeding. Nursing 81 11(4):70–73, 1981

Meyers R: Esophageal bleeding. Hospital Medicine 14(2):80–104, February, 1978

Nosis TM: Abdominal perineal resection. Point View 15(1):4–5, January, 1978

Prasad ML, Abcarian H: Urinary retention following operations for benign anorectal disease. Dis Colon Rectum 21(7):490–492, October, 1978

Schumann D: How to help wound healing in your abdominal surgery patient. Nursing 80 10(4):34–40, April, 1980

Stark, KJ. Nursing care of the Kock pouch patient. AORN J 32(2):202–206, 1980

Stevenson JD: A patient with carcinoma of the stomach. Nursing Times 75(23):960–964, June 7, 1979

Strauch B: Caring enough to give your patient control. Nursing 80 10(8):54–59, 1980

Swaffield L: Living with a stoma. Finding the problems. Nursing Times 75(10):66, March 8, 1979

Thompson JP: Anorectal bleeding. Nursing Times 75(4):142–146, January 25, 1979

Thorpe, CJ, Caprini JA: Gallbladder disease: Current trends and treatments. Am J Nurs 80(12):2181–2185, 1980

Wiley L: Realistic nursing goals in terminal cirrhosis. Nursing 78 8(6):43–46, June, 1978

Wilson RL: The use of ultrasound in suspected cholecystitis, Applied Radiology 7(1):119–121, January/February 1978

Zimmerman CE: Outpatient excision and primary closure of pilonidal cysts and sinuses. Am J Surg 136(5):640–642, November, 1978

NEUROLOGICAL SYSTEM
BOOKS

Brunner LS, Suddarth DS: The Lippincott Manual of Nursing Practice, 2nd ed, pp 750–751. Philadelphia, JB Lippincott, 1978

Burrell ZL, Burrell LO: Intensive Nursing Care, 4th ed, pp 134–147. St. Louis, CV Mosby, 1969

Carini E, Owens A: Neurological & Neurosurgical Nursing, 7th ed. St. Louis, CV Mosby, 1978

Flynn I, Schwetz K, Williams D: Muscular Dystrophy: Comprehensive Nursing Care in Nursing Clinics of North America, Vol 14, No 1. Philadelphia, WB Saunders, 1979

Gall GB: The Nervous System. In Handbook of Clinical Nursing. New York, McGraw-Hill, 1979

Hardy AG, Elson R: Practical Management of Spinal Cord Injuries for Nurses, 2nd ed. Edinburgh, London, New York, Churchill Livingston, 1976

Harrison's Principals of Internal Medicine, 9th ed, pp 1997–1999. New York, McGraw-Hill, 1980

Kinney M: Problems of the Nervous System. In Phipps WJ, Long B, Woods N: Medical Surgical Nursing—Concepts and Clinical Practice. St. Louis, CV Mosby, 1979

Mandell G, Douglas R, Bennett J: Principles and Practice of Infectious Diseases, pp 769–775. New York, John Wiley & Sons, 1979

Marshall J, Mau J: Neurological Nursing, 2nd ed. Oxford and Edinburgh, Blackwell Scientific Publications, 1967

Merritt HH: A Textbook of Neurology, 6th ed. Philadelphia, Lea & Febiger, 1979

O'Connor AB: Nursing in Neurological Diseases. New York, American Journal of Nursing, 1976

Phipp W, Long B, Wood N: Medical Surgical Nursing, pp 717–726, 1273–1278. St. Louis, CV Mosby, 1979

Pierce DS, Nickel VH: The Total Care of Spinal Cord Injuries, 1st ed. Boston, Little, Brown & Co., 1977

Swift N, Mabel RM: Manual of Neurological Nursing, 1st ed, pp 11–89. Boston, Little, Brown & Co., 1978

Winter C, Morela A: Nursing Care of Patients with Urologic Diseases, 4th ed, pp 319–331. St. Louis, CV Mosby, 1977

JOURNALS

Catanzaro M: Multiple sclerosis. RN Magazine 40(12):42, 1977

Dreyfus P: CNS disorders, a closer look at Alzheimer's disease. Consultant, 19:31, January, 1979

Fischbach F: Easing adjustment to Parkinson's disease. American Journal of Nursing 78(1):66, January, 1978

George W: Emergency care of a head-injury patient. RN Magazine 43:45, 1980

Gresh C: Helpful tips you can give your patients with Parkinson's disease. Nursing 80 10:26, 1980

Hansen A: Toward independence for paraplegics. Canadian Nurse 7:24, December, 1976

Jones IH: Senile dementia. Nursing Times 75:104, 1979

Kety S: Disorders of the human brain. Sci Am 241:202, 1979

Kinash R: Spinal cord injured patient. Journal Neurological Nursing, 10:29, March, 1978

Kunkel J, Wiley J: Acute head injury: What to do when and why. Nursing 79 9(3):22, 1979

Larrabee J, Pepper A, Macauley C: The person with spinal cord injury. Am J Nurs 77(8):1319, August, 1977

Meyd CJ: Acute brain trauma. Am J Nurs 78:40, 1978

Morell P, Norton WT: Myelin. Sci Am 242:88, 1980

Nicolson G: Cancer metastases. Sci Am 240:66, 1979

Porter S, Goldberg M, Buck D, et al: Family-centered conferences for better trauma care. Nursing 78 8(10):70, October, 1978

Ramirez B: When you're faced with a neuro patient. RN Magazine 42:67, 1979

Rudy E: Early omens of cerebral disaster. Nursing 77 7:59, 1977

Stauffer S: A master plan for teaching the patient with spinal cord injury, RN Magazine 42(7):55, July, 1979

Swift N: Why the MS patient needs your help. Nursing 79 9(9):57, 1979

Teasdale G, Jennett B: Assessment of coma and impaired consciousness. Lancet, 2:81, 1974

Underman A, Overturf G, Leedom J: Bacterial meningitis—1978. DM—Disease-a-month 24(5):8, February, 1978

ORTHOPEDICS
BOOKS

Brunner L, Suddarth D: Textbook of Medical–Surgical Nursing, 4th ed. Philadelphia, JB Lippincott, 1980

Donahoo CA Jr, Dimon JH: Orthopedic Nursing. Boston, Little, Brown and Co, 1977

Farrell J: Illustrated Guide to Orthopedic Nursing. Philadelphia, JB Lippincott, 1977

Farrell J: Casts, your patients and you. Part 1: A review of basic procedures. Part 2: A review of arm and leg cast procedures. Part 3: A review of hip spica procedures. Nursing 78 8(10):65, 8(11):57, 8(12):53, 1978

Larson CB, Gould M: Orthopedic Nursing, 9th ed. St. Louis, CV Mosby, 1978

Trainex Corporation: Care of the Patient in Traction. Warsaw, Indiana, Zimmer, 1978

JOURNALS

Bartholomew L, Rynes R, Hedberg S et al: Management of rheumatoid arthritis. Am Fam Physician 13:116–125, 1976

Brown–Skeers V: How the nurse practitioner manages the rheumatoid arthritis patient. Nursing 79 9(6):26–35, June, 1979

Cohen S, Viellion G: Programmed instruction: Nursing care of a patient in traction. Am J Nurs 79(10):1771–1798, 1979

Deyerle W, Crossland S: Broken legs are to be walked on. Am J Nurs, 77(12):27–30, 1977

Driscoll P: Rheumatoid arthritis: Understanding it more fully. Nursing 75 5(12):26–28, 1975

Driscoll P: Rheumatoid arthritis: Managing it more successfully. Nursing 75 5(12):29–32, 1975

Dunnery E: Fractured hip: How to position and mobilize patients without undoing their surgery. RN Magazine 42(6):45–57, 1979

Farrell J: Casts, your patients and you. Part 1: A review of basic procedures. Part 2: A review of arm and leg cast procedures. Part 3: A review of hip spica procedures. Nursing 78 8(10):65, 8 (11):57, 8(12):53, 1978

Gordon GW, Schumacher HR: Management of gout. Am Fam Physician 9:91–97, 1979

Jennings KR: The cheerful operation: total hip replacement. Nursing 76 6(7):32–37, 1976

Jones EM: Principles of traction. Nursing Mirror, 147(26):i–iv, 1978

Klinenberg JR: Hyperuricemia and gout. Med Clin North Am 61:299–312, 1977

Kryschyshen P, Fischer D: External fixation for complicated fractures. Am J Nurs, 80(2):256–259, 1980

Meredith S: Those formidable external fixation devices. RN Magazine 42(12):18–24, 1979

Meyers MH, McNelly D, Nelson K: Total hip replacement, a team effort. Am J Nurs, 78(9):1485–1488, 1978

Mooney U, Nickel V, Harvey JD et al: Cast-brace treatment for fractures of the distal part of the femur. J Bone Joint Surg (Am) 52-A(8):1563–1578, 1970

Nowatny M: If your patient's joints hurt, the reason may be osteoarthritis. Nursing 80 10(9):39–41, 1980

Patterson P: Awareness key to rheumatoid arthritis. AORN J 32(4):614–621, 1980

Pitorak E: Rheumatoid arthritis: Living with it more comfortably. Nursing 75 5(12):33–35, 1975

Ritchey JA: Traction review. O.N.A.J. 6:330, 1979

Spruck M: Gold therapy for rheumatoid arthritis. Am J Nurs 79(7):1246–48, 1979

Walters J: Coping with a leg amputation. Am J Nurs 81(7):1349–1352, 1981

RESPIRATORY SYSTEM
BOOKS

A Breath of Life, a Breath of Hope. New York, Breon Laboratories

Blodgett D: Manual of Respiratory Care Procedures. Philadelphia, JB Lippincott, 1980

Burrell ZL, Burrell LO: Intensive Nursing Care, 1st ed, pp 85–126. St. Louis, CV Mosby, 1969

Bushnell SS, Bushnell LS: Respiratory Intensive Care Nursing, 1st ed, pp 15–43, 193–216, 247–261. Boston, Little, Brown & Co, 1973

Chapman CM: Medical Nursing, 9th ed, pp 45–72. London, Cassell and Collier Macmillan, 1977

Wade JF: Respiratory Nursing Care, 2nd ed. St. Louis, CV Mosby, 1977

LECTURE

White HA: Acute respiratory failure (lectures), April 9th and April 16th, 1979. Georgetown University School of Nursing Continuing Education

JOURNALS

Cameron M: What patients need most before and after a thoracotomy. Nursing 78 8:28, 1978

Ciuca R: Cor Pulmonae. Nursing 78 8:46, 1978

Kaufman JS, Woody JW: For patients with COPD: Better living through teaching. Nursing 80 10:57, 1980

McConnell EA: How to truly help the patient with a radical neck dissection. Nursing 76 6:59, 1976

Sandham G, Reid B: Some Q's and A's about suctioning and a guide to better technique. Nursing 77 7(10):60, October, 1977

Stanley L: You really can teach COPD patients to breathe better. RN Magazine 41(4):43, 1978

Weber–Jones JE, Bryant MK: Over the counter bronchodilators. Nursing 80 10:34, 1980

URINARY SYSTEM AND THE PROSTATE
BOOKS

Berkow R, Talbott JH, Abraham GN et al: The Merck Manual of Diagnosis and Therapy, 13th ed. Parkway, NY, Merck Sharp and Dohme Research Laboratories, Division of Merck & Co., 1977

Brunner L, Suddath D: Textbook of Medical–Surgical Nursing, 4th ed. Philadelphia, JB Lippincott, 1980

Coe F, Simon N, Rosenberg M et al: The Medical Clinics of North America: Renal Therapeutics, Vol 62, No. 6. Philadelphia, WB Saunders, 1978

Conway BL: Carini and Owens' Neurological and Neurosurgical Nursing, 7th ed. St. Louis, CV Mosby, 1978

Hekelman FR, Ostendarp CA: Nephrology Nursing, Perspectives of Care. New York, McGraw-Hill, 1979

West PJ: The Urological Clinics of North America: Office Urology, Vol 7, No. 1. Philadelphia, WB Saunders, 1980

Winter C, Morel A: Nursing Care of Patients with Urologic Diseases, 4th ed. St. Louis, CV Mosby, 1977

JOURNALS

Anderson ER: Women and cystitis. Nursing 77 7(4):50, April, 1977

Baumrucker GO: A new male incontinence clamp. J Urol 121(2):201, February, 1979

Butts PA: Assessing urinary incontinence in women. Nursing 79 9(3):72, March, 1979

Castronovo F: Nursing decisions: Pulling a patient through acute renal failure. RN Magazine 41(11):61, 1978

Chodak GW: Systemic antibiotics for prophylaxis in urological surgery: A critical review. J Urol 121(6):695, 1979

deTornyay R, Stillman M: Nursing decisions. Pre and postoperative care of a kidney transplant patient: What you need to know. RN Magazine 42(4):55, 1979

deTornyay R, Stillman M: Pre and postoperative care of a kidney donor: What you need to know. RN Magazine 42(5):59, 1979

DiPalma JR: Drugs that induce change in urine color. RN Magazine 40(1):34, 1977

Gault P: How to break the kidney stone cycle. Nursing 78 8(12):24, December, 1978

Gault P: The prostate: Coping with dangerous and distressing complications. Nursing 77 (4):34, April, 1977

Gillies DA, Alyn IB: Test your knowledge of the patient in renal failure. Nursing 78 8(9):53, September, 1978

Gittes R: Retrograde renal and ureteral brush biopsy. Am J Nurs 78(3):410, 1978

A gland for no reason? (a basic guide to prostate troubles). Harvard Medical School Health Letter 5(5):1, March, 1980

Hodgson S: Anemia associated with chronic renal failure and chronic dialysis. Nephrology Nurse 2(3):43–46, 1980

Irwin BC: Hemodialysis means vascular access and the right kind of nursing care. Nursing 79 9(10):48, October, 1979

Juliani L: Assessing renal function. Nursing 78 8(1):34, January, 1978

Juliani L: When infection leads to acute glomerulonephritis, here's what to do. Nursing 79 9(9):40, September, 1979

Kinney A: Effect of cranberry juice on urinary pH. Nurs Res 28(5):287, 1979

Lazarus JM: Uremia: A clinical guide. Hospital Medicine 15(2):52, 1979

Marchart DJ: Urinary incontinence in the female. Hospital Medicine 13(3):60, 1977

Oestreich SJ: Rational nursing care in chronic renal disease. Am J Nurs 79(6):1096, 1979

Orme BM: Chronic renal failure: Guide to management. Hospital Medicine 14(11):92, 1978

Roberts HL: Renal assessment: A nursing point of view. Heart Lung 8(1):105, 1979

Soloway M: Role of nurse clinician in urologic oncology. Urology 12(6):685, 1978

Sorrels AJ: Continuous ambulatory peritoneal dialysis. Am J Nurs 79(8):1400, 1979

Stark JL: BUN/creatinine: Your key to kidney function. Nursing 80 10(5):33, May, 1980

Tobiason SJ: Benign prostatic hypertrophy. Am J Nurs 79(2):286, 1979

Ulrich B: The psychological adaptation of end stage renal disease: A review and a proposed new model. Nephrology Nurse 2(3):48–52, 1980

Underwood MA: Urinary tract infections. Critical Care Quarterly 3(3):63–70, 1980

Warwick R et al: Symposium on clinical urodynamics. Urol Clin North Am 6:1, 1979

Zeluff GW, Eknoyan G, Jackson D: Pericarditis in renal failure. Heart Lung 8(6):1139–1145, 1979

SPECIALTIES

BLOOD DISORDERS

Anionwu EN: Sickle cell, menace in the blood, Nursing Mirror 147:16, 1978

Castle W: Megablastic anemia. Postgrad Med 64(4):117, 1978

Doswell W: Sickle cell anemia. Nursing 78 8(4):65, April, 1978

Fosnot H: SCA—Tell the facts, quell the fables. Patient Care 12(11):164, 1978

Linehan MS: Sickle cell anemia—The painful crisis. Journal of Emergency Nursing 4:12, 1978

Marchand A, VanLente F, Galen R: Pernicious anemia. Diagnostic Medicine 2(2):7, 1979

McFarlane J: Sickle cell disorders. Am J Nurs 77(12): 1948, 1977

Robbins E: Pernicious anemia. Nursing Mirror 143:66, 1976

Schrier S: Anemia: Hemolysis. Scientific American Medicine. 5(IV):11, 1978

Wintrobe M: Anemia: The two things you should do first. Med Times 107(11):32, 1979

Wood C: Macrocytic megablastic anemia. Nurse Pract 2(6):33, 1977

BURNS

BOOKS

Barry J: Emergency Nursing, The Emergency Treatment of Burns, pp 347–354. New York, McGraw-Hill, 1978

Braen GR, Chandler A: Minor Burns, Evaluation and Treatment. Kansas City, Missouri, American College of Emergency Physicians, Marion Laboratories, 1979

Burrell ZL, Burrell LO: Critical Care, Burns, 3rd ed, pp 358–363. St. Louis, CV Mosby, 1977

CONFERENCE

Treatment of Burns. Sibley Hospital Inservice, June 11, 1980

JOURNALS

Bayley E, Costello K, Friel V et al: Burns: Breaking the anger despair cycle. Nursing 75 5(5):45, May, 1975

Christoferson B, Piercey M: The role of the nurse practitioner in the early management of thermal burns. The Nurse Pract 2(1): 20, 1976

Dyer C: Burn care in the emergent period. Journal of Emergency Nursing 6(1):9, 1980

Hayter J: Emergency nursing care of the burned patient. Nurs Clin North Am 13(2):223, 1978

Head J: Inhalation injury in burns. Am J Surg 139:508, 1980

Jones CA, Feller I: Burns. What to do in the first crucial hours. Nursing 77 7(3):23, March, 1977

Kinzie V, Lau C: What to do for the severely burned. RN Magazine 43(4):47, 1980

Rubenstein E: Smoke inhalation. Scientific American Medicine 8(VII):1, 1978

Schumann L, Gaston S: Commonsense guide to topical burn therapy. Nursing 79 9(3):34, March, 1979

Wagner M: Emergency care of the burned patient. Am J Nurs 77(11):1788, 1977

EYE-PATIENT CARE
BOOKS

Brunner L, Suddarth D: Medical Surgical Nursing, 4th ed, pp 1138–1145. Philadelphia, JB Lippincott, 1980

Saunders WH, Havener WH, Keith CP et al: Nursing Care in Eye, Ear, Nose and Throat Disorders, 4th ed, pp 1–194. St. Louis, CV Mosby, 1979

CONFERENCES

Eye Trauma. Georgetown University Emergency Medicine Update Series, Georgetown University, June 18, 1980

Glaucoma and Cataracts. Sibley Hospital, June 4, 1980

JOURNALS

Boyd–Monk H: Cataract surgery. Nursing 77 7(6):56, 1977

Boyd–Monk H: Screening for glaucoma. Nursing 79 9(8):42, 1979

Shiery S: Insight into the delicate art of eye care. RN Magazine 5(6):19, 1975

ONCOLOGY (CANCER)
BOOKS

Baldonado A, Stahl D: Cancer Nursing, Nursing Outline Series. Garden City, New York, Medical Examination Publishing, 1978

Bouchard R, Owens N: Nursing Care of the Cancer Patient, 2nd ed. St. Louis, CV Mosby, 1972

Burkhalter P, Donley D: Dynamics of Oncology Nursing. New York, McGraw-Hill, 1978

A Cancer Source Book for Nurses. American Cancer Society, 1975

Helping Cancer Patients Effectively, Nursing Skillbook Series. Horsham, PA, Intermed Communications, 1977

Heisel J: Food for Those Who Hesitate: Tips That They Might Tolerate. Durham, Duke University, 1976

Nutrition for Patients Receiving Chemotherapy and Radiation Treatment. American Cancer Society, 1974

Tiffany R: Oncology for Nurses and Health Care Professionals, Vol I and II. London, George Allen and Unwin, 1978

JOURNALS

Bodey G, Rodriguez V: Approaches to the treatment of acute leukemia and lymphoma in adults. Semin Hematol 15 (3):221, 1978

Buchanan–Davidson D: Where is that cancer. Journal of Practical Nursing 27:22, 1977

Cline M, DeVita V, Friedman M, et al: Cancer chemotherapy. Patient Care 13:52, 1979

Cox S, Wark E: Cancer, the delivery of nursing care. Nursing Mirror 147:7, 1978

Finney C: Leukemia. Journal of Nursing Care 11:12, 1978

Gormecan A: Influencing food acceptance in anorexic cancer patients. Postgrad Med 68(2):145, 1980

Hernandez B: Platelets, a short course. RN Magazine 43(6):36, 1980

Laatsch N: Nursing the woman receiving adjuvant chemotherapy for breast cancer. Nurs Clin North Am 13:337, 1978

LeBlanc D: People with Hodgkin's disease—The nursing challenge. Nurs Clin North Am 13:281, 1978

Levene M: A new role for radiation therapy. Am J Nurs 77(9):1443, 1977

Levine M: Cancer chemotherapy—A nursing model. Nurs Clin North Am 13:271, 1978

Levitt DS: Cancer chemotherapy: Those dreaded side effects and what to do about them 43(6):53, 1980

Rose K: The stress of chemotherapy. Canadian Nurse 74:18, 1978

Rosenberg S: The common cancers encountered in clinical practice. Oncology II(12):111-1, 1978

Souvik C: The nursing care of lung cancer patients emphasizing chemotherapy. Nurs Clin North Am 13:301, 1978

Welch D, Lewis K: Chemotherapy and alopecia. Am J Nurs 80(5):903, 1980

6

Appendix

Conversion tables
    Metric doses with approximate apothecary equivalents
    Equivalent weights in metric and in apothecary scales
    Conversion of avoirdupois body weight to metric equivalents
    Conversion of height to metric equivalents
    Equivalent Centigrade and Fahrenheit temperature readings
Medical abbreviations and symbols

CONVERSION TABLES

TABLE 6-1. **Metric Doses with Approximate Apothecary Equivalents**

Liquid Measure	
Metric	*Apothecary*
4000 ml	1 gallon
1000 ml	1 quart
500 ml	1 pint
30 ml	1 fluid ounce
4 ml	1 fluid dram
0.06 ml	1 minum

Note: a milliliter (ml) is the approximate equivalent of a cubic centimeter (cc).

TABLE 6-2. **Equivalent Weights in Metric and in Apothecary Scales**

Metric	Apothecary
30 g	1 ounce
15 g	4 drams
1 g	15 grains
60 mg	1 grain
30 mg	1/2 grain
15 mg	1/4 grain
1 mg	1/60 grain
0.4 mg	1/150 grain
0.25 mg	1/250 grain
0.2 mg	1/300 grain
0.12 mg	1/500 grain

TABLE 6-3. **Conversion of Avoirdupois Body Weight to Metric Equivalents**

lb	kg	kg	lb
10	4.5	10	22
20	9.1	20	44
30	13.6	30	66
40	18.2	40	88
50	22.7	50	110
60	27.3		
70	31.8		
80	36.4		
90	40.9		
100	45.4		

One pound = 0.454 kilograms

One kilogram = 2.2 pounds

TABLE 6-4. **Conversion of Height to Metric Equivalents**

Inches	Centimeters
18	46
24	61
30	76
36	91
42	107
48	122
54	137
60	152
66	

One inch = 2.54 cm

One cm = 0.3937 inch

TABLE 6-5. **Equivalent Centigrade and Fahrenheit Temperature Readings**

Centigrade	Fahrenheit
35	95.0
36	96.8
37	98.6
38	100.4
39	102.2
40	104.0
41	105.8

To convert Centigrade readings to Fahrenheit, multiply by 1.8 and add 32.

To convert Fahrenheit readings to Centigrade, subtract 32 and divide by 1.8.

MEDICAL ABBREVIATIONS AND SYMBOLS

a.c.   before meals
ad. lib.   freely as desired
b.i.d.   two times a day
$\bar{c}$ with
C   Celcius
c/o   complains of
cc   cubic centimeter (ml)
DC   discontinue
dr   dram (measurement) also written ʒ
elix   elixir
F   Fahrenheit
g   gram
gr   grain
gtt   drop
Hct   hematocrit
Hgb   (abbreviation); **Hb** (symbol) hemoglobin
h.s.   hour of sleep (bedtime)
I and O   intake and output
IM   intramuscular
IV   intravenous
kg   kilogram
lb   pound
LLQ   left lower quadrant (of abdomen)
LUQ   left upper quadrant
m   minum
mg   milligram
n.g. tube   nasogastric tube
noc.   night
n.p.o.   nothing by mouth
O$_2$ oxygen
o.d.   right eye
o.s.   left eye
o.u.   each eye
oz   ounce (also written ʒ)
p.c.   after meals
p.o.   by mouth
p.r.n.   when necessary
PT   prothrombin time
PTT   partial thromboplastin time
q.d.   every day
q.h.   every hour
q.i.d.   four times a day
q.s.   quantity sufficient

RLQ   right lower quadrant (abdomen)
RUQ   right upper quadrant
s   without
sp. gr.   specific gravity
$\overline{ss}$ one-half
stat.   at once
sub. q.   subcutaneously
t.i.d.   three times a day
>   greater than
<   less than

Pharmacology Index

Subject Index